Pocket Consultant

Gastroenterology

S.P.L. Travis DPhil, FRCP
Consultant Gastroenterologist
Derriford Hospital, Plymouth, UK

R.H. Taylor BSc, MD, MBA, FRCP
Medical Director and Consultant Gastroenterologist
Royal Hospital Haslar, Gosport, UK

J.J. Misiewicz BSc, FRCP
Honorary Joint Director, Department of Gastroenterology and Nutrition
Central Middlesex Hospital, London, UK

Second edition

Blackwell
Science

© 1991, 1998 by
Blackwell Science Ltd
Editorial Offices:
Osney Mead, Oxford OX2 0EL
25 John Street, London WC1N 2BL
23 Ainslie Place, Edinburgh EH3 6AJ
350 Main Street, Malden
    MA 02148 5018, USA
54 University Street, Carlton
    Victoria 3053, Australia
10, rue Casimir Delavigne
    75006 Paris, France

Other Editorial Offices:
Blackwell Wissenschafts-Verlag GmbH
Kurfürstendamm 57
10707 Berlin, Germany

Blackwell Science KK
MG Kodenmacho Building
7–10 Kodenmacho Nihombashi
Chuo-ku, Tokyo 104, Japan

The right of the Authors to be
identified as the Authors of this Work
has been asserted in accordance
with the Copyright, Designs and
Patents Act 1988.

First published 1991
Second edition 1998

Set by Semantic Graphics, Singapore
Printed and bound in Great Britain
at the University Press, Cambridge

The Blackwell Science logo is a
trade mark of Blackwell Science Ltd,
registered at the United Kingdom
Trade Marks Registry

DISTRIBUTORS

UK

    Marston Book Services Ltd
    PO Box 269
    Abingdon, Oxon OX14 4YN
    (*Orders*: Tel: 01235 465500
                Fax: 01235 465555)

USA
    Blackwell Science, Inc.
    Commerce Place
    350 Main Street
    Malden, MA 02148 5018
    (*Orders*: Tel: 800 759 6102
                781 388 8250
                Fax: 781 388 8255)

Canada
    Login Brothers Book Company
    324 Saulteaux Crescent
    Winnipeg, Manitoba R3J 3T2
    (*Orders*: Tel: 204 224-4068)

Australia
    Blackwell Science Pty Ltd
    54 University Street
    Carlton, Victoria 3053
    (*Orders*: Tel: 3 9347 0300
                Fax: 3 9347 5001)

A catalogue record for this title
is available from the British Library
and the Library of Congress

ISBN 0-632-04887-5

For further information on Blackwell
Science, visit our website:
w.w.w.blackwell-science.com

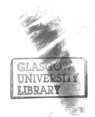

Contents

Preface and acknowledgements

Preface to the second edition

The Authors are delighted to present the second edition of the *Pocket Consultant in Gastroenterology*. Significant advances have taken place in our specialty during the 7 years that have elapsed since the first edition. We have therefore taken this opportunity to revise the text thoroughly and to bring it up to date with respect to advances in the knowledge of causes of various conditions, new techniques and new treatments. A new chapter dealing with systemic disorders and the gut has been added. We have adhered to the principle that the book should be of immediate practical value to doctors in training and to general practitioners, but we believe that nurses, and even consultants, will also find it helpful. The terse and somewhat didactic style has been retained, not only because it has apparently proved popular in a rapid-reference book, but also because it is the only way to keep the text within manageable limits and make the information readily accessible.

Preface to the first edition

This book is for House Officers on the wards, Senior House Officers or Registrars involved in outpatient clinics, and General Practitioners in their surgeries. The purpose is to provide a practical, concise text on gastroenterology. It will, we hope, be a useful guide and checklist when dealing with unfamiliar situations, and an *aide-mémoire* before follow-up consultations, ward rounds or discussion with senior colleagues. It should also help junior doctors in the management of emergency and elective admissions of patients with alimentary diseases. The style is terse and somewhat dogmatic by necessity, but we have attempted to address common clinical dilemmas.

We are most grateful to our colleagues, listed below, who have helped by reading drafts of the text or by making suggestions; we are, however, solely responsible for any errors. Above all, our thanks go to our families for their forbearance, patience and support.

....

Acknowledgements

Mrs E. Bardolph BSc SRN SCM, DR G.C. Cook DSc MD FRCP, Mr C.W. Imrie BSc FRCS, Miss R. James BSc, Dr D.P. Jewell DPhil FRCP, Dr D. Loft MD FRCP, Dr D.J. Nolan MD FRCR, Mrs H. Simpson BSc SRD, Dr R.P.H. Thompson DM FRCP, Dr C.B. Williams MD FRCP.

1 Alimentary Emergencies

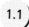 ## 1.1 Swallowed foreign body

Toddlers, the mentally disturbed and the elderly most commonly swallow foreign bodies. If no history is available, look for excessive salivation, regurgitation, choking, or distress. Objects impact in the pharynx, lower end of the oesophagus or pylorus. Pain or fever suggest perforation. Once through the pylorus, spontaneous passage is the rule, but perforation can occur in the ileocaecal region.

All cases

- Look in the mouth
- If the object is impacted in the fauces, call the ENT surgeons
- X-ray the chest and abdomen, but failure to visualize an object does not exclude its presence
- Look for surgical emphysema, mediastinal and sub-diaphragmatic gas on X-ray
- Barium or Gastrografin examination is *not* indicated and may hinder endoscopy
- Address the underlying issues to avoid repeated ingestion, especially in prisoners or the mentally disturbed who may have ingested foreign bodies for individual gain

Bones, pins, glass and batteries

- Chest pain suggests perforation and a small haematemesis may herald perforation of a major vessel. In either case, contact the thoracic surgeons urgently
- Sharp objects should otherwise be removed by an experienced endoscopist, unless they have passed the duodenum. A plastic sleeve over the endoscope helps prevent trauma during withdrawal
- After endoscopic removal, further chest pain may indicate delayed perforation
- Batteries, especially small alkaline batteries ingested by toddlers, should be retrieved immediately if in the oesophagus. Corrosive perforation or heavy metal intoxication has been reported. Once in the small intestine, safe passage is the rule

Coins, beads and blunt objects

- Almost always pass spontaneously unless more than 5 cm long or 3 cm in diameter

- Reassure the patient or parents and advise them to check stools for 3 days
- Repeat abdominal X-ray after 36 h if there is doubt about progress. Documented arrest by X-rays for 72 h is an indication for surgical exploration

Body-packing (ingested packets of drugs)

- Smuggled packets of drugs may be swallowed, or secreted per rectum
- Intact packets can cause intestinal obstruction and if packets do not pass within 72 h, surgical removal is advisable
- Endoscopic removal is contraindicated because of the risk of rupturing the bags
- Packets may burst spontaneously and cause life-threatening overdose
- Heroin overdose causes constricted pupils, bradypnoea, or coma. Hypoglycaemia or non-cardiogenic pulmonary oedema may occur later. Give intravenous naloxone 0.8 mg rapidly, to a maximum 2.4 mg if necessary
- Cocaine causes dilated pupils, tachycardia and agitation. Convulsions, metabolic acidosis or coma may occur. Sedate with intravenous diazepam 5–10 mg and give oral propranolol 40 mg three times daily for a few days
- Severe overdose of any narcotic is an indication for ventilation and surgical removal of the packets, to stop drug absorption
- The doctor's immediate duty is the treatment of the patient if body-packing is discovered. Once treatment has been initiated, the local police and hospital administrator should be informed. The police will inform other authorities (such as Customs and Excise, Drug Squad)
- Questioning of the patient must wait until the patient is fit, and be sanctioned by a senior doctor. Doctors have a moral duty to ensure that the patient understands their legal right to consult a Crown-appointed solicitor, through an interpreter if necessary

1.2 Complete oesophageal obstruction

Bolus obstruction causes sudden, complete dysphagia for solids and liquids, with inability to swallow saliva. Food impacted against a benign or malignant stricture is the usual cause. Occasionally the presentation is delayed for a few days in the mentally handicapped or severely debilitated. The obstruction must be relieved urgently.

Clinical features

Ask about and look for:
- Duration of symptoms preceding obstruction
- Predisposing disease (stricture, carcinoma, Schatzki ring)
- Triggering factors (steak, toast, fibrous foods, tablets)
- Dehydration
- Weight loss (suggest malignant obstruction)
- Supraclavicular nodes (from a carcinoma of the cardia)
- Complications (aspiration pneumonia, perforation)

Investigations

The endoscopist should be contacted as a priority.
- Full blood count—anaemia suggests carcinoma
- Serum electrolytes—high urea indicates dehydration
- Chest X-ray—look for a mediastinal fluid level (obstruction), absent gastric air bubble (obstruction) or right lower lobe consolidation (aspiration)
- Urgent endoscopy—must be performed by an experienced endoscopist
- A barium swallow risks aspiration and is not necessary, unless the diagnosis is in doubt. This is not the same as in dysphagia without obstruction (Section 2.1, p. 59)

Management

- Intravenous fluids
- Endoscopic removal of the obstructing bolus
- Endoscopic dilatation can be done immediately after disimpaction
- Fizzy drinks occasionally disimpact fibrous debris, but endoscopy is needed when a food bolus has been stuck for a few hours
- Fine-bore nasogastric feeding, or nutritional supplements are needed (Section 12.2, p. 408) if dilatation is delayed. Endoscopic placement of the tube is awkward, but indicated if it cannot be inserted in the normal way (p. 445)
- Intravenous metronidazole 500 mg and cefotaxime 1 g three times daily for 5 days, if aspiration pneumonia is present

Prevention

Simple measures decrease the risk of acute obstruction in patients with

oesophageal strictures or prosthetic oesophageal tubes (pp. 68 and 73):
- Avoid fibrous food (apples, oranges), steak and toast
- Wear dentures if edentulous
- Chew all solids well
- Fizzy drinks with meals
- Avoid oral potassium supplements, salicylates and large tablets
- Omeprazole 20–40 mg or lansoprazole 30 mg daily delays or prevents restricturing in most patients and heals associated oesophagitis. Proton-pump inhibitors should be continued indefinitely

Oesophageal rupture

Sudden chest pain after forceful vomiting is the cardinal symptom when the distal posterior oesophageal wall tears longitudinally in spontaneous perforation (Boerhaave's syndrome). Traumatic perforation after instrumentation or chest injury is more common than spontaneous rupture.

Differential diagnosis

Perforation presents with chest pain, respiratory distress, painful swallowing, or subcutaneous emphysema. Early diagnosis is crucial to survival. Failure to consider the possibility is the commonest reason for misdiagnosis.
- Myocardial infarction (ECG, cardiac enzymes)
- Dissecting aneurysm (pulses, chest X-ray, urgent echocardiogram)
- Perforated peptic ulcer (rigid, silent abdomen, erect chest X-ray)
- Acute pancreatitis (amylase more than fourfold elevated)
- Spontaneous pneumothorax (chest X-ray in expiration)

Investigations

Confirm the diagnosis and site of perforation.
- Chest X-ray—look for mediastinal or sub-diaphragmatic gas, or a hydro/pneumothorax (Fig. 1.1)
- Gastrografin swallow—in spontaneous rupture, tears are usually large and leak contrast; after instrumental rupture, tears are often small and do not leak contrast. Upper oesophageal perforations tend to leak into the mediastinum; mid-oesophageal perforations into the mediastinum and right pleura; and distal oesophageal perforations into the mediastinum, left pleural cavity or abdomen

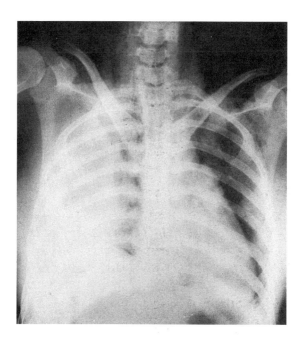

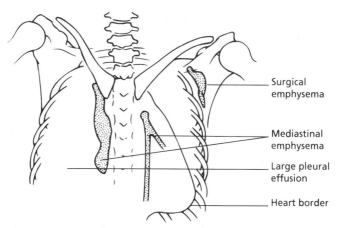

Fig. 1.1 Chest X-ray in oesophageal rupture showing consequences of oesophageal perforation. There is a large right pleural effusion, mediastinal emphysema and gross surgical emphysema in the neck and upper chest wall.

Management

Oesophageal perforation is a lethal condition. Conservative management is confined to highly specific situations. If the perforation has involved the pleural cavity, or has been contaminated by saliva, gastric contents or food, then surgery is mandatory.

Resuscitation
- Intravenous fluids
- Analgesia—intravenous diamorphine 2.5 mg every hour until pain relieved, then every 4 h
- Involve thoracic surgical colleagues at an early stage

Spontaneous rupture
- Nil by mouth
- Surgical repair and drainage is almost always needed and should occur within 24 h
- Antibiotics (intravenous metronidazole 500 mg and cefotaxime 1 g three times daily for 5 days)
- Enteral nutrition through a fine-bore nasojejunal tube, if feeding has not restarted within 72 h
- Parenteral nutrition is indicated if complications (such as mediastinitis) develop

Instrumental rupture
- Small tears (with minor symptoms and no leakage of contrast) may be managed conservatively in conjunction with the surgeons. Large tears that leak contrast are managed as for spontaneous rupture
- Nil by mouth
- Nasogastric aspiration for 3 days
- Intravenous fluids
- Antibiotics as above
- Indications for surgery are a persistent pyrexia, or pneumothorax after 48 h
- When perforation complicates palliative treatment of a malignant stricture, patients who are unfit for surgery may be managed by endoscopic insertion of a cuffed oesophageal tube

1.4 Caustic oesophageal injury

Ingestion of caustic cleaning fluids can cause progressive and devastating injury to the oesophagus and stomach. Most occur as accidents in children under 5 years old. Symptoms and the appearance of the pharynx do not correlate with the extent of oesophageal or gastric injury.

Clinical features

- There may be no symptoms initially, but diagnosis is not difficult if an accurate history is obtained
- Identify the specific fluid ingested
- Hoarseness and stridor indicate pharyngeal or laryngeal injury
- Painful dysphagia or haematemesis indicate oesophageal oedema and ulceration. This may occur rapidly or be delayed for several hours
- Respiratory distress and shock occur when mediastinitis develops due to oesophageal necrosis
- Acute symptoms may resolve, to be followed by dysphagia after several weeks or months as scar tissue causes an oesophageal stricture

Investigations

- Chest X-ray—look for mediastinal air or oedema
- Direct laryngoscopy and endoscopy—to record the extent of injury. This should be performed under general anaesthetic, since sedation is unsatisfactory in children and does not allow adequate views of the larynx or hypopharynx. Circumferential burns lead to strictures

Management

Resuscitation
- Nil by mouth
- Establish the airway by intubation or tracheostomy if respiratory symptoms or stridor are present
- Intravenous fluids
- Do *not* give neutralizing agents

Minor, non-circumferential burns
- Allow liquids and then a light diet if tolerated
- Arrange psychiatric assessment if ingestion was a suicide attempt

Deep ulcers or circumferential burns
- Remain nil by mouth for 48 h
- Monitor for chest pain or fever, indicating delayed perforation or

mediastinitis. If these occur, give intravenous antibiotics, liaise with thoracic surgical colleagues and start nasojejunal feeding
- Allow liquids and a light diet if asymptomatic after 48 h
- Omeprazole 20 mg twice daily for 4 weeks may reduce the rate of late stricturing, but steroids have no effect

Late complications

- Oesophagogastric strictures occur in about 25%, but almost invariably in those with deep ulcers or circumferential burns
- Review patient after 4 weeks and at 3, 6 and 12 months
- Arrange a barium swallow if dysphagia occurs, before oesophageal dilatation
- Repeated dilatation is frequently necessary. Shortening of the oesophagus may promote gastro-oesophageal reflux, so omeprazole 20 mg daily is reasonable to reduce restricturing
- Attention to nutrition is vital
- Surgery is indicated if patients cannot tolerate repeated dilatation
- The risk of carcinoma of the oesophagus is substantially increased

1.5 Acute bleeding: upper gastrointestinal tract

The aims of management in upper gastrointestinal bleeding are to stabilize the patient, stop active bleeding and prevent recurrent bleeding. There are about 90 admissions per 100 000 adults annually in the UK, with an overall mortality of 11% unless patients are admitted to a specialized bleeding unit, where a mortality of about 5% can be expected. Most bleeds from peptic ulcers stop spontaneously and about 25% can be identified who have no risk of rebleeding and can be rapidly discharged. The task is to distinguish the 20% who rebleed in hospital and need surgical intervention. A standard clinical approach is recommended for every patient, so that patients at highest risk of rebleeding and death are identified early.

Clinical approach

- Assess severity
- Resuscitate
- Establish the site of bleeding
- Liaise with the surgical and intensive care teams on call
- Medical intervention
- Early surgery when appropriate

Assessment

The aim is to identify patients at high risk of rebleeding and death, by clinical and endoscopic examination. All patients with haematemesis or melaena must be treated actively until a stable baseline has been established. There is no room for complacency.

High-risk patients

These are patients with three or more of the following criteria:

- Age > 60 years
- Fresh haematemesis with melaena—twice the mortality of either alone
- Non-steroidal anti-inflammatory drug (NSAID) intake
- Continued bleeding, or a rebleed in hospital
- Cardiac failure
- Chronic airflow limitation
- Chronic liver disease
- Onset of bleeding in a patient already in hospital for another reason
- Pulse > 100 b.p.m.—suggests the need for transfusion
- Systolic BP < 100 mmHg—but it may be preserved until very late in young patients
- Postural drop in systolic BP > 15 mmHg on sitting up
- Endoscopic stigmata present. These are: active arterial bleeding (80% risk of rebleed); visible vessel in the ulcer base (50% risk of rebleed); fresh adherent clot or oozing (30% risk of rebleed); or black dots on the ulcer base (5% risk of rebleed)
- Endoscopic evidence of oesophageal varices or portal hypertensive gastropathy (p. 174)

Lower risk patients

- Age < 60 years
- Coffee-ground vomitus without melaena
- No endoscopic stigmata of recent bleeding, varices or portal hypertensive gastropathy
- Haemodynamically normal (pulse < 100 b.p.m., systolic BP > 100 mmHg, warm peripheries)
- No serious concomitant disease
- No anticoagulation therapy or coagulopathy
- Haemoglobin > 10 g/dL

Document the following

In addition to a record of the assessment of the patient:

- Preceding symptoms (dyspepsia, vomiting, weight loss)

Table 1.1 Differential diagnosis of haematemesis or melaena.

Common	Less common (< 5%)	Rare (1%)
Duodenal ulcer (35%)	Duodenitis	Hereditary telangiectasia
Gastric ulcer (20%)	Oesophageal varices	Aortoenteric fistula
Gastric erosion (6%)	Oesophagitis	Haemostatic defect
Mallory–Weiss tear (6%)	Tumours	Pseudoxanthoma elasticum
No lesion found (20%)		Haemobilia
		Pancreatitis
		Angiodysplasia
		Portal hypertensive gastropathy

- Drug and alcohol ingestion
- Presence or absence of melaena on rectal examination
- Signs of chronic liver disease (Table 5.2, p. 156)

Causes

See Table 1.1.

Investigations and management

Resuscitation on arrival

- Ensure a patent airway
- Insert a 14- or 16-gauge intravenous cannula (grey or yellow Venflon)
- If pulse > 100 b.p.m., give 500 mL colloid (such as Haemaccel) over 30–60 min and repeat if necessary whilst waiting for blood
- Transfuse blood until haemodynamically stable in the first few hours, because initial haemoglobin is a poor indicator of the severity of the bleed. Subsequently transfuse up to haemoglobin of 10 g/dL
- Synthetic colloid or crystalloid will cause haemodilution: 1000 mL decreases the pretransfusion haemoglobin by about 10%
- Reserve group O rhesus negative blood for dire emergencies (such as continuing massive bleeding and systolic BP < 80 mmHg despite 1000 mL intravenous colloid), when the risk from hypotension exceeds that from uncrossmatched blood
- Insert a urinary catheter in patients who need a central venous line (p. 13), to monitor urine output for haemodynamic information
- Ensure that the patient remains nil by mouth until endoscopy
- Do not insert a nasogastric tube, because this increases the risk of haemorrhage from gastric and oesophageal lesions

- Admission to designated high-dependency unit for gastrointestinal bleeding reduces mortality to 5% or less. If this is not available, consider admission of high-risk patients to intensive care and contact surgical colleagues as soon as the patient is resuscitated

Initial investigations

- Full blood count, crossmatch, coagulation studies (when liver disease is present, or suspected) and electrolytes
- Crossmatch 4 units of blood for high-risk patients, but group and save alone for lower risk patients
- Haemodynamic status is a better guide to transfusion requirements than measured haemoglobin
- Arterial gases in those with cardiorespiratory disease
- ECG in high-risk patients
- Chest X-ray in high-risk patients (abdominal films rarely help)

Indications for a central venous line

- Signs of major haemorrhage (pulse > 100 b.p.m., systolic BP < 100 mmHg). Reasons for *not* inserting a central line in high-risk patients (p. 11) must be carefully considered
- Rebleed during the same admission
- Inadequate peripheral venous access
- If a central venous line is needed, monitoring in a high-dependency area is advisable because these patients have a very high risk of further bleeding

Establish site of bleeding

- Arrange endoscopy after resuscitation, ideally on the next endoscopy list, within 12–24 h. Mucosal lesions and stigmata for rebleeding are otherwise missed. Ensure that the presence or absence of stigmata (p. 11) is recorded
- Indications for emergency endoscopy are continued bleeding, a rebleed in hospital or if the patient is being considered for surgery
- Profuse haemorrhage may obscure the bleeding site. Gastric lavage to remove clots rarely alters management and can be hazardous. Repeat endoscopy after a further 12 h resuscitation is recommended. Immediate surgery should be a joint decision between surgeons and physicians
- Table 1.1 (p. 12) shows the differential diagnosis

Monitoring and discharge

- Pulse, BP, central venous pressure and urine output hourly, until stable
- Re-examine after 4 h
- Coagulation studies if > 4 units transfused

- Daily full blood count, urea and electrolytes in high-risk patients
- Keep 2 units in the blood bank for 48 h after bleeding has stopped
- Lower risk patients (p. 11) can safely start eating and drinking immediately after endoscopy and be discharged at any time thereafter, as long as there is adequate support at home
- High-risk patients (p. 11) should be keep in hospital for 48 h after bleeding has stopped

Medical intervention

These measures are not an alternative to surgery if an operation is indicated (p. 15), but may help stop bleeding or reduce the risk of rebleeding. Endoscopic haemostasis is indicated for patients with a peptic ulcer and active bleeding or non-bleeding visible vessel.

- Endoscopic haemostasis: all techniques halve the risk of rebleeding, but depend on local expertise and may not be available. Injection of adrenaline (up to 10 mL 1:10 000) around peptic ulcers, thermocoagulation and laser photocoagulation all have similar efficacy. Sclerosant (ethanolamine) is best avoided as necrosis and perforation has been reported. A combination of adrenaline (1:10 000) and thrombin (1000 U/mL) may be the most efficacious at preventing rebleeding
- Tranexamic acid (1 g intravenously, three times daily for 72 h) is the only pharmacological agent that has been shown on meta-analysis to reduce rebleeding and mortality. Individual trials have conflicted, but in the absence of a previous thromboembolic event, it is a reasonable adjunct in the treatment of high-risk patients until further trials are available
- Ranitidine, omeprazole or other acid-suppressing drugs have **no** place in the initial treatment of bleeding. Proton-pump inhibitors and H_2-receptor antagonists should be reserved for treatment once a peptic ulcer has been diagnosed
- Determination of *Helicobacter pylori* status should be done at the time of emergency endoscopy, using a biopsy urease (CLO) test (p. 99). Eradication therapy for *H. pylori*-positive patients (Table 3.2, p. 91) is indicated as soon as oral feeding is restarted
- Other drugs (octreotide, vasopressin or glypressin for varices; omeprazole or tranexamic acid for haemorrhagic gastritis) are occasionally indicated (p. 20). A combination of ethinyloestradiol (50 µg) and norethisterone (1 mg/day) decreases episodes of recurrent acute bleeding from angiodysplasia (such as hereditary telangiectasia)

Rebleeding

Rebleeding greatly increases mortality. Patients at high risk of rebleeding (p. 11) need to be identified and the surgeons told of their admission. Patients (especially those with more than two risk factors) are best admitted to a high-dependency area, where signs of rebleeding should be detected early. Signs of rebleeding are:

- Rise in pulse rate (a sensitive and early sign)
- Fall in central venous pressure
- Decrease in hourly urine output
- Haematemesis or melaena
- Looking at the patient (pallor, pulse, postural pressure drop and peripheral circulation) is as important as looking at the charts

Indications for surgery

Contact surgical colleagues at the outset, before an operation is necessary rather than when it is inevitable. Delay increases mortality. When the following criteria are met, surgery is appropriate forthwith. Any decision *not* to operate should only be taken after discussion with the consultant surgeon.

- Age > 60 years and
  - > 4 units transfused in 24 h, or
  - one rebleed in hospital, or
  - continued bleeding, or
  - spurting vessel at endoscopy
- Age < 60 years and
  - > 8 units transfused in 24 h, or
  - one rebleed in hospital, or
  - continued bleeding, or
  - spurting vessel at endoscopy
- A visible vessel in the ulcer base, or adherent clot, are indications for endoscopic therapy and close observation rather than surgery, unless bleeding continues

The differential diagnosis of upper gastrointestinal bleeding is shown in Table 1.1 (p. 12). Individual topics are discussed below.

Oesophageal varices

Cirrhosis is the commonest cause of portal hypertension (p. 174) and oesophageal varices in the UK. Whilst oesophageal varices can be found at endoscopy in almost 50% of patients with cirrhosis, less than a third of these will bleed from their varices. Mortality during an acute bleed depends on the severity of liver disease on admission. Mortality according to Child's grade A is 10%, grade B is 25% and grade C is 50% (Table 5.5, p. 166), but 60–80% of all patients who bleed from varices will be dead within 4 years.

Assessment

• Bleeding from oesophageal varices is a complex clinical emergency for which control of bleeding is only one aspect
• Attention to infection, control of ascites (p. 169), encephalopathy (p. 166), alcohol withdrawal (p. 202) and nutrition (p. 401) are vital for a successful outcome

Acute bleeding

• Resuscitate and monitor (p. 13), but do not use intravenous saline. Dextrose, or colloid (synthetic, albumin or blood) are indicated
• 30% with known varices have another source of haemorrhage
• During active bleeding, correct disordered coagulation to international normalized ratio (INR) < 1.5 or prothrombin time < 22 s with fresh frozen plasma (FFP). However, FFP is contraindicated in the absence of bleeding, because this increases intravascular volume and variceal pressure, which may precipitate haemorrhage. Platelet transfusion may be necessary for thrombocytopenia (platelet count < 60 × 10^9/L). Discuss with the haematologists
• Arrange urgent endoscopy for sclerotherapy or banding by an experienced endoscopist
• Give oral lactulose, starting at 90 mL/day, for hepatic encephalopathy (p. 166), intravenous vitamins (p. 423) and chlormethiazole for detoxification (p. 202)
    If sclerotherapy is not available, or bleeding continues:
• Insert a Sengstaken tube until sclerotherapy can be performed or repeated after 12 h
• After a second attempt at sclerotherapy, if bleeding persists the tube should be repositioned and an octreotide infusion commenced (50 µg bolus, then infused at 50 µg/h for up to 96 h)
• Vasopressin (10–20 U/h), or glypressin (2 mg bolus, then 2 mg every 4 h, for up to 96 h) are alternatives to octreotide, but have a higher complication rate. Either are contraindicated in patients with angina and transdermal or buccal nitrate 5–10 mg every 12 h is advisable in all patients
• For recurrent bleeding after two or three attempts at sclerotherapy, the alternatives are oesophageal transection with splenectomy and proximal gastric devascularization, or transjugular intrahepatic portosystemic shunt (TIPSS) (see below)

- Oesophageal transection has a mortality of 50% and should only be considered for patients without other organ failure, who were admitted in Child's group A or B (Table 5.5, p. 166). Splenectomy and proximal gastric devascularization are needed to prevent subsequent bleeding from gastric varices
- TIPSS, where a stent is inserted between the hepatic and portal vein under radiological control, can only be performed at specialist centres, but is the procedure of choice if hepatic transplant is being considered. Control of bleeding is excellent (approaching 100%), but 1 month mortality is still high (30–40%) owing to liver failure. Late complications (blocked stent) are still common
- Bleeding gastric varices are one cause of failed endoscopic haemostasis. Surgery or TIPSS have been the only option, but preliminary reports suggest that endoscopic injection of bovine thrombin (2–10 mL of 1000 U/mL) controls active bleeding, although varices are not eradicated. Endoscopic band ligation may lead to further haemorrhage or perforation

Balloon tamponade
- Indicated for uncontrolled variceal bleeding, or recurrent haemorrhage despite sclerotherapy or banding
- To be inserted by experienced operators only
- Sedation, or a general anaesthetic to insert an endotracheal tube and secure the airway, is necessary
- Insert a cooled, lubricated Sengstaken or Minnesota tube beyond 45 cm. The tube can usually be stiffened by inserting a well-lubricated pair of paediatric endoscopic biopsy forceps down the central lumen
- Inflate the gastric balloon with 300 mL tap water containing 50 mL of any intravenous X-ray contrast medium
- Tie a 250 mL bag of saline to the tube to provide traction, but carefully protect the mouth to prevent pressure necrosis
- Aspirate gastric and oesophageal ports hourly, as well as connecting to a bag for continuous drainage
- Do not inflate the oesophageal balloon unless oesophageal bleeding continues for 15 min after the gastric balloon has been inflated. Then inflate the oesophageal balloon to 30 mmHg with air, measured by manometer
- X-ray to check position (Fig. 1.2)
- Active bleeding is arrested in 90%. Continued bleeding usually means that the tube is misplaced or that there are gastric varices
- Deflate the oesophageal balloon after 6 h and the gastric balloon after 12–24 h to allow further endoscopic sclerotherapy or banding
- Complications include tracheal intubation, oesophageal rupture from

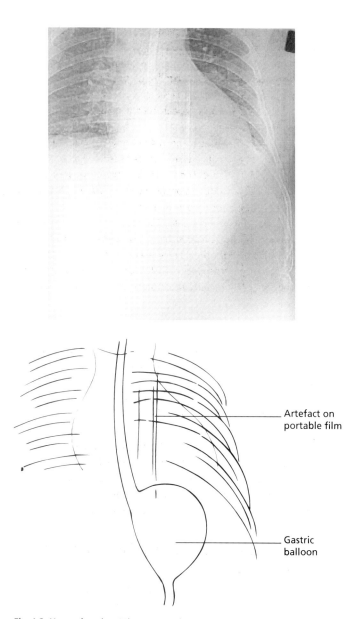

Artefact on
portable film

Gastric
balloon

Fig. 1.2 X-ray showing Minnesota tube in correct position. Gastric balloon has been inflated with 300 mL water mixed with 50 mL contrast medium.

inflating the gastric balloon in the oesophagus, or mucosal necrosis from leaving the balloon inflated for too long

Prevention of rebleeding from varices

- The highest risk of rebleeding is in the first 6 weeks
- Most gastroenterologists repeat sclerotherapy at 1–2 week intervals until varices are obliterated
- Varices recur after obliteration in 40%, usually within 1 year
- Propranolol 40 mg three times daily decreases the risk of bleeding and may reduce mortality. It is worth trying in patients who have bled, but may not be tolerated. Isosorbide mononitrate 10–40 mg daily may also be given to further reduce portal venous pressure
- Portal hypertensive gastropathy may cause bleeding after variceal obliteration. The gastric mucosa has a characteristic 'snake skin' appearance at endoscopy. Propranolol is the treatment of choice (p. 174)
- Surgical or percutaneous portosystemic shunts are indicated for recurrent bleeding, especially in non-cirrhotic portal hypertension (p. 174)

Mallory–Weiss tears

A mucosal tear at the oesophagogastric junction due to forceful vomiting results in haematemesis. The typical features are:
- Initial vomitus does not contain blood
- Vomiting has often been provoked by alcohol
- 90% settle with conservative treatment
- Acid-suppressing drugs are unnecessary
- Continued bleeding can be controlled by endoscopic injection or thermocoagulation. Surgery is very rarely needed
- Bleeding after forceful vomiting may also be caused by prolapse of the gastric mucosa resulting in a focal area of haemorrhagic gastropathy ('hernia gastropathy') distal to the gastro-oesophageal junction

Acute gastric erosions and haemorrhagic gastropathy

Erosions are diagnosed endoscopically, but may be obscured by oozing from haemorrhagic gastropathy (gastritis is a misleading term that should be reserved for a histological diagnosis). Major haemorrhage from superficial gastric injury is unusual and the cause is often readily apparent.

Causes
- NSAIDs
- Alcohol
- Stress (trauma, major surgery or patients in intensive care)

Specific treatment
- A proton-pump inhibitor (lansoprazole 30 mg/day, omeprazole, or pantoprazole 40 mg/day) is usually given for 1–4 weeks, depending on the cause
- Persistent bleeding is treated with intravenous tranexamic acid 400 mg three times daily, or vasopressin 20 U/h, in addition to omeprazole which can be given intravenously for named patients
- Total gastrectomy is the last resort for continued bleeding after all medical treatment has been vigorously applied for 24–48 h, and should only be performed by an experienced surgeon
- It should be noted that whilst antacids, rantidine, or sucralfate prevent stress erosions in intensive care patients, there is very little evidence that they reduce clinically significant bleeding or mortality

Gastric ulcer (Section 3.4, p. 104)

- Consider provoking causes (such as NSAIDs)
- Appropriate endoscopic haemostasis (p. 14) reduces rebleeding and mortality
- Give a proton-pump inhibitor (lansoprazole 30 mg or omeprazole 20 mg daily) for 4 weeks once bleeding has stopped, together with *H. pylori* eradication therapy if endoscopic biopsies confirm infection
- Misoprostol 200 µg twice daily may be appropriate after this for patients with NSAID-associated ulcers who cannot stop NSAIDs (p. 126)
- Arrange a repeat endoscopy after 8–12 weeks, to biopsy and take brushings for cytology from the ulcer site
- If surgery is needed for continued bleeding, a Billroth 1 gastrectomy is usually performed. Undersewing with a vagotomy and pyloroplasty is a simpler operation, but the ulcer cannot be examined histologically to exclude cancer. Wedge resection removes the ulcer and has the lowest morbidity in high-risk elderly patients, but long-term acid suppression is then necessary because it does not prevent recurrent ulceration

Duodenal ulcer (Section 3.8, p. 116)

- Combine ulcer healing with eradication of *H. pylori*

- The optimum treatment is triple, or quadruple eradication therapy (Table 3.2, p. 91)
- Repeat endoscopy is unnecessary, except after endoscopic haemostasis in high-risk patients
- Always confirm that eradication of *H. pylori* has been successful after an ulcer has bled, preferably by an isotope breath test (p. 99)
- Successful eradication of *H. pylori* significantly reduces the risk of rebleeding and also the risk of bleeding from another ulcer to an extent similar to maintenance H_2-antagonists, although there have been no comparative trials. *H. pylori* treatment is cheaper in the long term and also provides a cure
- Risk of repeat haemorrhage without eradication or maintenance therapy is 20% over 5–10 years, but still higher if associated with NSAIDs
- NSAID-associated ulcers heal with proton-pump inhibitors or H_2-antagonists even if NSAIDs have to be continued, but are not directly associated with *H. pylori* (p. 126). Misoprostol 200 µg twice daily prevents NSAID-associated duodenal ulcers, but is less effective for duodenal than gastric injury
- Maintenance therapy (cimetidine 400 mg at night, or a proton-pump inhibitor) is indicated for patients at high risk of dying from the complications of recurrent ulceration (p. 126) when eradication therapy has been unsuccessful, or when NSAIDs have to be continued

'No source of bleeding found'

Unfortunately this is quite common and can produce difficult management problems. Possible causes are:
- Lesion missed on endoscopy
- Mucosal lesion healed before patient endoscoped:
    - erosions
    - Mallory–Weiss tear
    - Dieulafoy lesion (bleeding vessel with no surrounding ulceration, usually high on the greater curve)
- Bleeding from third part of the duodenum, or beyond:
    - jejunum (ulcerative jejunitis)
    - Meckel's diverticulum
    - colon
- Other:
    - nose bleed
    - rare causes of bleeding (Table 1.1, p. 12)

Management

The management of gastrointestinal bleeding from obscure and occult sources is discussed in more detail on p. 23 and Section 9.7 (p. 361; Fig. 9.8, p. 362).

- Reassess the patient—no further action is necessary for low-risk patients (p. 11)
- Repeat endoscopy in high-risk patients (p. 11)
- Investigate rare causes of bleeding (recheck coagulation, discuss small bowel radiology, endoscopic retrograde cholangiopancreatography (ERCP), ^{99}Tc sulphur colloid red cell scan (p. 24) or ^{99}Tc pertechnate scan with radiologists)
- Selective angiography during active bleeding (which must be at a rate of 1 unit/4 h) is indicated after two negative endoscopies, preferably in a specialist unit
- Small bowel enteroscopy may be available in specialist units, but in most hospitals laparotomy and peroperative endoscopy is the ultimate procedure for recurrent episodes of active bleeding from obscure origin

Aortoenteric fistula

Consider this rare diagnosis in any patient with an aortic graft and gastrointestinal bleeding. Exsanguination at the first bleed is uncommon. Small 'herald' bleeds occur for up to 2 weeks. Aortography is usually unhelpful and endoscopy to the fourth part of the duodenum, if possible, is the best investigation. An abdominal CT scan may show haematoma around the graft, but surgery should not be delayed if hypotension has occurred. Aggressive surgery is needed as soon as the diagnosis is made, preferably in a specialist unit.

1.6 Acute bleeding: lower gastrointestinal tract

Bleeding from the colon is recognized by the passage of fresh red or reddish-brown altered blood per rectum. It is usually readily differentiated from upper gastrointestinal bleeding, because it has neither the smell, nor the tarry-black appearance of melaena. Upper tract bleeding rapid enough to cause red rectal bleeding is rare, and is invariably associated with haemodynamic disturbance.

Clinical approach

- Assess severity—as for upper tract bleeding
- Resuscitate

Table 1.2 Causes of rectal bleeding.

Common	Less common	Rare

Perianal conditions
  haemorrhoids
  fissures, prolapse
Colorectal polyps
Colorectal carcinoma
Ulcerative colitis
	Ischaemic colitis
	Crohn's disease
	Diverticular disease
		Angiodysplasia
		Anorectal varices
		Small intestinal
		  diverticula
		  lymphoma
		  Kaposi's sarcoma
		Solitary caecal ulcer
		Vasculitis

- First episode, or recurrent (obscure) bleeding?
- Establish the site of bleeding
- Specific treatment

Causes

See Table 1.2.

Investigations—first episode

Severe bleeding
- Full blood count, coagulation studies, crossmatch and check electrolytes
- Rigid sigmoidoscopy—blood is likely to prevent colonoscopy
- Gastroscopy—only to exclude brisk gastric or duodenal haemorrhage, although bright red rectal bleeding would be very unusual
- Angiography—if bleeding continues in excess of 1 unit/4 h (Fig. 1.3; Fig. 9.6, p. 362)

Slight/moderate bleeding
- Blood tests as above
- Rigid sigmoidoscopy and proctoscopy
- Colonoscopy once the bleeding has stopped

Investigations—obscure (recurrent) bleeding

Bleeding of obscure origin is defined as recurrent bouts of acute or chronic bleeding for which no source has been found after initial upper and lower gastrointestinal endoscopy. The topic is complex and further addressed in Section 9.7 (p. 361) and Fig. 9.6 (p. 362).

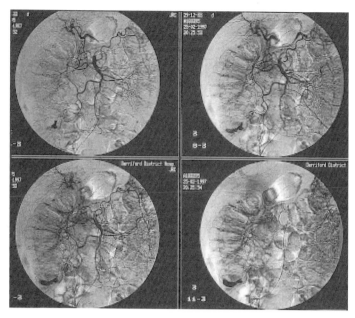

Fig. 1.3 Serial films from mesenteric angiography in a 63-year-old man with continuous bleeding (8 unit transfusion in 24 h) and a normal upper gastro-intestinal endoscopy. The bleeding vessel in the caecum could not be embolized and laparotomy was necessary.

Consider:
- Repeat colonoscopy—angiodysplasia can be missed
- Small bowel enema—better than a follow-through for identifying mucosal lesions (p. 458)
- ^{99}Tc sulphur colloid red scan—when active bleeding is too slow to be detected by angiography. Care must be taken not to overinterpret the scans which may indicate the wrong area in up to 40% of bleeding colonic lesions
- ^{99}Tc pertechnate Meckel's scan—at an early stage in young patients, but sensitivity is < 80%
- Angiography—during a subsequent episode of brisk bleeding (1 unit/4 h). Colonoscopy by an experienced operator using an instrument with a wide suction channel may identify the site more successfully
- Self-induced rectal trauma is a rare cause of recurrent bleeding

Management

Severe bleeding stops spontaneously in 80% of cases after adequate blood replacement. Treatment of the cause (Table 1.2, p. 23) is then needed. In the remainder, bleeding is continuous or recurs, sometimes frequently, over many months. Identifying the site of persistent or recurrent bleeding is one of the most difficult problems in acute gastroenterology. Once the site is identified, surgical resection is indicated. If the site cannot be found, treatment depends on the pattern of bleeding.

Continuous bleeding

Surgery is advisable if bleeding persists after replacement of 6 units of blood. The options are:

- Laparotomy with peroperative colonoscopy after lavage through an appendicostomy. The physician is well advised to attend the laparotomy
- Segmental resection if the site can be identified
- 'Blind' hemicolectomy can rarely be justified. If the site cannot be found and surgery is essential to stop bleeding, a sub-total colectomy should be performed

Intermittent bleeding

Referral to a specialist gastroenterology unit is advisable if the site of bleeding cannot be identified after three episodes of bleeding.

Rectal bleeding in children

The differential diagnosis is:

- Intussusception—commonest at 6–12 months
- Meckel's diverticulum
- Ulcerative colitis
- Foreign body
- Juvenile polyps—usually in the descending colon
- Intestinal haemangiomas
- Child (sexual) abuse

Acute abdominal pain

Clinical diagnostic accuracy is about 50%. Metabolic and extraintestinal causes (Table 1.3) should be considered if the diagnosis is in doubt.

Causes

The type of pain, relieving factors and progress are so variable that they rarely discriminate between diseases causing acute pain (Table 1.3; Table 1.4).

Table 1.3 Causes of acute abdominal pain.

Common	Less common	Rare
Appendicitis	Cholangitis	Necrosis
Biliary colic	Mesenteric infarction	hepatoma
Cholecystitis	Pyelonephritis	fibroid
Diverticulitis	Torsion	Splenic infarction
Intestinal obstruction	ovarian cyst	Pneumonia
Perforated viscus	testicle	Myocardial infarction
Pancreatitis	omentum	Diabetic ketoacidosis
Peritonitis	Rupture	Porphyria
Salpingitis	ovarian cyst	Addisonian crisis
Mesenteric adenitis	ectopic pregnancy	Lead poisoning
Renal colic	aortic aneurysm	Tabes dorsalis
'Non-specific'	Prolapsed disc	Inflammatory aneurysm
	Abscesses	Volvulus
	Exacerbation of peptic ulcer	sigmoid
	Ileitis	caecum
	Crohn's	gastric
	Yersinia spp.	Herpes zoster

Discriminating questions

- Site
- Duration
- Severity
- Radiation
- Aggravating factors

Also ask about

- Vomiting (if it precedes pain, a surgical cause is less likely)
- Time last ate or drank
- Bowel disturbance
- Urinary frequency
- Date of last menstrual period
- Previous abdominal surgery

Specifically examine for

- Distension
- Visible peristalsis
- Rebound tenderness, guarding or rigidity
- Pulsatile mass and peripheral pulses
- Hernial orifices
- Rectal *and pelvic* tenderness or masses

Table 1.4 Patterns of acute abdominal pain.

	Appendicitis	Cholecystitis	Perforated viscus	Renal colic	Pancreatitis	Diverticulitis	Salpingitis	Intestinal obstruction
Site	C/RLQ	RUQ	UQs	R/L loins	UQs	LQs	LQs	Symmetrical
Duration	12–48 h	Days	<12 h	<12 h	<48 h	Days	>24 h	<48 h
Severity	Moderate	Severe	Severe	Severe	Severe	Moderate	Moderate	Severe
Radiation	Nil	Shoulder, back	Nil	Groin	Nil	Nil	Groin, thigh	Nil
Aggravating factors	Movement cough	Inspiration	Movement cough	Nil	Movement	Movement cough	Nil	Eating

C/RLQ, central or right lower quadrant; RUQ, right upper quadrant; UQs, upper quadrants; R/L, right or left; LQs, lower quadrants.

- Bowel sounds
- Epigastric bruit (normally audible in about 10% of thin patients)
- Fever (> 39°C with rigors suggests pyelonephritis, cholangitis or pneumonia)

Investigations

Every patient with acute abdominal pain should have on admission:
- Full blood count—leucocytosis may be absent in the elderly
- Electrolytes and creatinine
- Amylase—but many causes of slight elevation other than acute pancreatitis (p. 34)
- Group and save serum
- Urine examination—including *pregnancy test* if doubtful
- Erect chest X-ray—look for basal atelectasis and gas under diaphragm
- Supine abdominal X-ray—look for biliary and renal calculi, dilated bowel (> 2.5 cm small intestine, > 6.0 cm colon), air in the biliary tree (p. 456)
- ECG
- Blood cultures—if febrile

Management—general principles

- Analgesia—do not withhold opiates for severe pain 'pending a surgical opinion', if the diagnosis is clear
- Perforation, peritonitis, or obstruction need emergency surgery
- Observation overnight often clarifies a difficult diagnosis
- Nil by mouth until a decision about surgery has been made
- Specific management of common causes of abdominal pain are discussed below

Appendicitis

See Section 7.4 (p. 267).

Biliary colic

Distinguishing features
- Biliary colic typically causes a few minutes of right upper quadrant pain, with intervals of an hour, and subsides after several hours. The pain may rarely be exclusively high epigastric in location. Recurrent colic is a feature of chronic cholecystitis

....

- Fever, leucocytosis or pain lasting more than 12 h, are likely to be due to acute cholecystitis
- Murphy's sign (tenderness in the right upper quadrant on inspiration) is positive during pain
- Flatulence, distension, fat intolerance and nausea are frequent but non-specific, and occur in other common conditions, especially irritable bowel syndrome or non-ulcer dyspepsia
- Daily pain is unlikely to be due to biliary colic, even if gall stones are present

Management
- Ultrasonography will detect gall stones, although difficult in the obese and those with a fibrosed gall bladder. Repeat ultrasound after a fatty meal is a test of gall bladder function, and is abnormal (no contraction) in acute or chronic cholecystitis
- An isotope (HIDA) scan (p. 461) or an oral cholecystogram will identify a non-functioning gall bladder, which is likely to be due to chronic cholecystitis
- Other laboratory investigations are usually unhelpful
- Cholecystectomy is appropriate if symptoms are typical (p. 27). Non-surgical options are discussed on p. 219

Acute cholecystitis

Distinguishing features
- Fever and persistent pain distinguish acute from chronic cholecystitis
- Impaction of a gall stone in the cystic duct causes > 90%
- Typical pain (Table 1.4, p. 27) occurs in < 50%
- Pain may be provoked by a fatty meal and builds up to a peak over 60 min, unlike the short spasms of biliary colic
- Fever develops after 12 h due to bacterial invasion and pain then becomes continuous
- Murphy's sign is sensitive, but not specific
- Calcified calculi (15%) and very rarely gas within biliary tree due to *Clostridium welchii* infection may be visible on plain abdominal X-ray

Complications
See Chapter 6 (p. 216).
- Recurrence (50%)
- Cholangitis due to associated common duct stones (10%)
- Mucocoele, empyema or gangrene of the gall bladder (1%)

- Biliary peritonitis (0.5%, with a mortality of 50%)
- Mirizzi's syndrome (obstructive jaundice due to external pressure on the common bile duct from inflammation around a stone impacted in the cystic duct)

Conservative management
- Confirm the diagnosis by ultrasound. Tenderness under the ultrasound probe in the presence of gall stones and a thickened gall bladder wall is effectively diagnostic. Isotope (HIDA) scans are also accurate, but not universally available
- Analgesia (intramuscular pethidine 100 mg and hyoscine 20 mg, but not morphine which can increase the pain)
- Intravenous fluids
- Nasogastric suction may be helpful, to alleviate vomiting if present
- Antibiotics (intravenous amoxycillin 500 mg three times daily and gentamicin 5 mg/kg once daily)
- Cholecystectomy at the earliest opportunity (see below)

Surgical management
- Optimum treatment is surgery on the same admission, on the next available list. Morbidity, total hospital stay, costs and mortality from complications of acute cholecystitis are lower compared to delayed cholecystectomy. Elderly patients and diabetics are especially appropriate for early surgery, because septic complications are more common
- Laparoscopic cholecystectomy is safe during acute cholecystitis in experienced hands. Cholecystostomy or percutaneous drainage of an empyema may be more appropriate in very sick elderly patients, but is rarely necessary
- The longer the interval between cholecystitis and surgery, the greater the risk of a recurrent attack: concern about an increased surgical complication rate 7–14 days after an acute attack is probably unfounded
- Other indications for surgery include signs of peritonitis and uncertainty about the diagnosis (when perforation or retrocaecal appendicitis cannot be excluded)

Cholangitis

See Section 6.4 (p. 228).

Diverticulitis

See Section 9.3 (p. 348).

Perforated viscus

The commonest cause is a perforated duodenal ulcer, followed by appendicitis, sigmoid diverticula or carcinoma, Crohn's disease and gastric ulcers. Beware a perforated peptic ulcer in patients already or recently in hospital for another reason.

Distinguishing features
- Sudden onset of severe, unremitting pain
- Temporary improvement 3–6 h later can trap the unwary
- Pain and peritonism may be absent in the elderly or those on steroids
- Abdomen fails to move with respiration
- Bowel sounds are usually absent
- Gas under the diaphragm on an erect chest X-ray is usual (70%), but not universal
- Lateral decubitus films for the very sick will also show free gas, but can be difficult to interpret
- Spontaneous sealing of the perforation occurs rarely

Surgical management
- Emergency surgery after vigorous intravenous resuscitation is almost invariably indicated
- Oversewing, omental patch and peritoneal lavage are customary for gastroduodenal perforation
- Hemicolectomy is indicated for right-sided colonic perforation, but distal perforation is probably best managed by resection, colostomy and rectal closure (Hartmann's procedure)
- The late complication of sub-phrenic abscess is best detected by ultrasound, but an abscess may cause an immobile diaphragm which can be readily detected by X-ray screening

Conservative management
- Indicated for the few patients in whom the risks are too high, or who refuse surgery
- Give intravenous fluids, antibiotics and nasogastric suction
  Some surgeons advocate starting intravenous fluids, antibiotics and suction for 4–6 h and operating on those who do not improve, since this may have a lower mortality than emergency surgery for all patients. Whilst preoperative resuscitation is always advisable, this conservative surgical approach is not widespread.

Peritonitis

Fever, guarding, rebound tenderness and rigidity may be minimal in the elderly, the very young, patients on steroids and the immunocompromised. Bowel sounds are absent.

Causes

- Perforated viscus
- Local:
  - appendicitis
  - cholecystitis
  - diverticulitis
  - pancreatitis
  - salpingitis
- Primary infective peritonitis
- Continuous ambulatory peritoneal dialysis (CAPD)
- Rare:
  - tuberculous
  - sclerosing
  - granulomatous
  - periodic (familial Mediterranean fever)

Management

- Intravenous resuscitation
- Intravenous antibiotics (cefotaxime 1 g and metronidazole 500 mg three times daily), after blood cultures
- Laparotomy
- Spontaneous bacterial peritonitis is usually due to *Escherichia coli* or *Streptococcus pneumoniae* in cirrhotic patients with ascites (p. 168). Ascitic fluid should be sent for immediate Gram stain and absolute neutrophil count. Intravenous antibiotics (cefotaxime 1 g three times daily) should be started if the neutrophil count is > 250/mL, pending the result of culture
- CAPD peritonitis is usually caused by Gram-positive skin flora. Cloudy effluent, abdominal pain and tenderness are usual. Patients are often afebrile. Send fluid for Gram stain and absolute neutrophil count: a neutrophil count > 100/mL or the presence of organisms is diagnostic. Renal unit antibiotic policies differ, but intraperitoneal vancomycin 15 mg/L dialysate and gentamicin 4 mg/L are appropriate. Always consider silent intestinal perforation if bacteria other than skin flora are isolated. Laparotomy without further delay by an experienced surgeon is then indicated

• Tuberculous peritonitis is usually diagnosed at laparotomy, but can be suspected by a high ascitic adenosine deaminase level, although this is not widely available. Standard antituberculous chemotherapy for 9 months is advised (p. 387)

Acute pancreatitis

Acute pancreatitis presents as isolated or recurrent attacks. Initial symptoms are a poor indicator of prognosis. Complications (p. 131) should be sought because early recognition improves prognosis and recovery is potentially complete. Isolated and recurrent attacks are distinguished from chronic pancreatitis by the absence of permanent impairment of exocrine or endocrine function.

Distinguishing features
Abdominal pain with a serum amylase > four times the upper limit of normal is usually diagnostic, but late presentation (> 12 h) of a perforated duodenal ulcer, or ectopic pregnancy, may cause a similar rise in amylase
• The severity, rather than the nature, of the symptoms (pain and vomiting) characterizes pancreatitis
• Diabetic coma is occasionally caused by acute pancreatitis

Predisposing factors
• Small gall stones—30–50%, more common in women, causing transient impaction at the ampulla
• No predisposing cause is found in about 15%
• Alcohol—10–40%, more common in men and in recurrent or chronic pancreatitis
• Trauma—about 5%, postoperative, post-ERCP or after blunt trauma
• Other causes of acute pancreatitis are rare:
• drugs (azathioprine, sulphonamides, sodium valproate, frusemide, tetracyclines)
• pancreatic duct obstruction by benign stenosis, dyskinesia, pancreatic or ampullary carcinoma
• pancreas divisum (congenital absence of pancreatic fusion)
• end-stage renal failure
• organ transplantation (drug, viral or lipid related)
• hypercalcaemia (acute or chronic pancreatitis)
• hypertriglyceridaemia (> 10 mmol/L)
• viral (mumps, coxsackie B4), pregnancy, hypothermia and arteritis cause isolated cases

Other abdominal causes of a moderately (< fourfold) raised serum amylase are:
- Acute on chronic pancreatitis in an alcoholic
- Perforated peptic ulcer (posterior perforation provokes pancreatitis)
- Ectopic pregnancy (amylase-secreting cells in the fallopian tube)
- Intestinal ischaemia, or infarction
- Aortic dissection
- Renal failure
- After any ERCP
- Consistent clinical features, a predisposing cause and an associated abnormality (such as hypocalcaemia or hypoxia) help discriminate acute pancreatitis from other causes of a moderately raised serum amylase

Complications
- Local:
  - inflammatory mass (phlegmon)
  - pseudocyst (fluid collection; persistently raised amylase, p. 131)
  - abscess (swinging pyrexia 1 week after attack)
  - jaundice (pancreatic oedema, or stones, can occlude the common bile duct)
- Paralytic ileus—exacerbates fluid and electrolyte imbalance
- Hypovolaemic shock—due to vomiting, hypoalbuminaemia, ascites or retroperitoneal haemorrhage
- Grey Turner's (flank) and Cullen's (periumbilical) signs are caused by tracking of blood-stained fluid
- Hypoxia—(PaO_2 < 8 kPa, or 60 mmHg) a prognostic factor and clinically underdiagnosed
- Hypocalcaemia—(< 2.0 mmol/L, corrected by adding 0.02 mmol/L for every g/L that the serum albumin < 40 g/L). Tetany is rare
- Acute renal failure—due to hypovolaemia, or disseminated intravascular coagulation (rare)
- Effusions—ascitic and pleural exudates with a high amylase
- Death—6–28%, depending on severity
- Recurrent attacks occur in a third, especially in alcoholics, or if cholecystectomy for associated gall stones is delayed

Management

Establish the diagnosis
- Serum amylase elevated > fourfold. Urinary amylase (spot sample) remains elevated for longer than serum amylase, but is not widely used

• Ultrasound may reveal pancreatic oedema and will also demonstrate gall stones if present. A well-visualized normal pancreas makes pancreatitis most unlikely

• CT scan is indicated if the pancreas cannot be visualized by ultrasound or the attack is severe

Assess the severity (Table 1.5)

• Three or more factors present out of eight possible characteristics indicates severe disease (Glasgow prognostic score). Unfortunately none may be abnormal in the early stages, and there is a move towards using the APACHE II scoring system for evaluating multisystem failure. This is widely used in intensive care units and whilst not specific for acute pancreatitis, it does identify sick patients at an early stage

• C-reactive protein concentration > 150 mg/L also discriminates between mild and severe pancreatitis, and is easier to apply than a multiple scoring system

• Peritoneal aspiration of more than 20 mL clear fluid, or any volume of dark fluid, also indicate severe acute pancreatitis, if Gram stain is negative and there is no odour

• Patients with severe disease have 30–40% major morbidity or mortality and greater need of intensive care management. Age (> 55 years), multiple organ failure and aetiology (post-ERCP, unknown) are associated with a higher mortality. Most patients (about 75%) have mild acute pancreatitis (mortality < 3%), but initial clinical appearances can be deceptive

Resuscitation

• Insert a central venous line if there is any doubt about cardiovascular stability or fluid replacement

Table 1.5 Markers of severe pancreatitis.*

White cell count > 15 × 10^9/L
Urea >16 mmol/L (no improvement with intravenous fluids)
Calcium < 2.0 mmol/L
Albumin < 32 g/L
Glucose >10 mmol/L (no history of diabetes)
Po_2 < 8 kPa (60 mmHg)
AST > 200 iu/L
LDH > 600 iu/L
C-reactive protein > 150 mg/L

*Most reliable when used 48 h after onset of attack, which limits clinical applicability.

• Intravenous crystalloid (0.9% saline) is usually sufficient for mild attacks, but some colloid (4.5% human albumin solution, or FFP) should be given for severe attacks
• Amount depends on urine output or central venous pressure, but 1500 mL colloid with 2000–3000 mL crystalloid daily are commonly needed in severe attacks
• Blood transfusion is indicated if the haematocrit is less than 0.30 (Hb < 10 g/dL)

Specific treatment (Fig. 1.4)
• Nil by mouth and nasogastric aspiration are designed to reduce pancreatic secretions
• Stop all drugs if possible
• Arrange urgent ERCP and sphincterotomy if there is jaundice or any gall stones are identified
• Lexipafant, a platelet-activating factor antagonist reduced multiorgan failure scores and some local complications in one controlled trial of severe pancreatitis, but is not yet licensed. No other drugs have been of proven value (including aprotinin, somatostatin, calcitonin), nor is peritoneal lavage helpful, even in severe attacks with haemorrhagic ascites. Surgery in the acute phase is only indicated for complications (p. 133)
• CT scan is better than ultrasound for determining prognosis: look for pancreatic necrosis, visible on a contrast-enhanced image, which is a poor sign (Fig. 4.1, p. 132). If necrosis is identified and there has been no clinical improvement within 48 h, repeat the scan to assist surgical decision-making
• Abdominal ultrasound or CT scan should be repeated if there is persistent pain or pyrexia, or if the amylase has not returned to normal after 5 days, to detect a pseudocyst or abscess. Management of complications is discussed on p. 131

Indications for surgery
See Section 4.1 (p. 133).

Treat predisposing causes
• Urgent ERCP and sphincterotomy if jaundice or gall stones are present
• Cholecystectomy immediately after recovery from gall stone associated pancreatitis, even if sphincterotomy has been performed (p. 133)
• Complete abstinence from alcohol
• Stop any implicated drugs
• Early elective ERCP for recurrent pancreatitis and sphincterotomy for ampullary dyskinesia or tumour

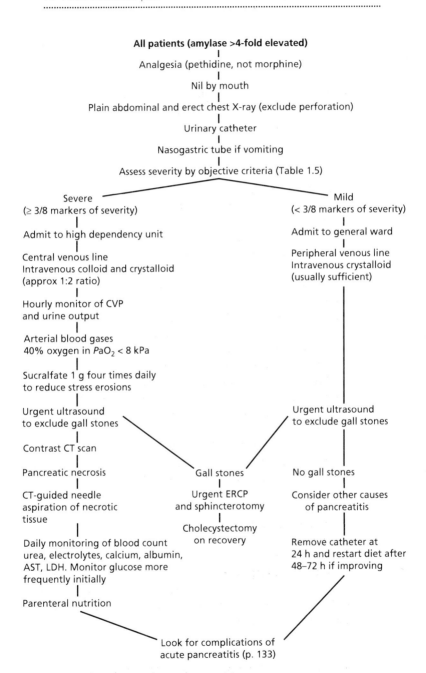

All patients (amylase >4-fold elevated)

Analgesia (pethidine, not morphine)

Nil by mouth

Plain abdominal and erect chest X-ray (exclude perforation)

Urinary catheter

Nasogastric tube if vomiting

Assess severity by objective criteria (Table 1.5)

Severe
(≥ 3/8 markers of severity)

Mild
(< 3/8 markers of severity)

Admit to high dependency unit

Admit to general ward

Central venous line
Intravenous colloid and crystalloid
(approx 1:2 ratio)

Peripheral venous line
Intravenous crystalloid
(usually sufficient)

Hourly monitor of CVP
and urine output

Arterial blood gases
40% oxygen in PaO_2 < 8 kPa

Sucralfate 1 g four times daily
to reduce stress erosions

Urgent ultrasound
to exclude gall stones

Urgent ultrasound
to exclude gall stones

Contrast CT scan

Pancreatic necrosis

Gall stones

No gall stones

CT-guided needle
aspiration of necrotic
tissue

Urgent ERCP
and sphincterotomy

Consider other causes
of pancreatitis

Cholecystectomy
on recovery

Daily monitoring of blood count
urea, electrolytes, calcium, albumin,
AST, LDH. Monitor glucose more
frequently initially

Remove catheter at
24 h and restart diet after
48–72 h if improving

Parenteral nutrition

Look for complications of
acute pancreatitis (p. 133)

Fig. 1.4 Management of acute pancreatitis.

• Consider distal pancreatic diversion by an experienced surgeon for recurrent pancreatitis associated with ductal stenosis or pancreas divisum

Acute intestinal ischaemia

The superior mesenteric artery supplies the jejunum and intestine to mid-transverse colon (Fig. 9.5, p. 351). Acute intestinal ischaemia usually refers to mesenteric infarction and is uncommon. It is difficult to diagnose early, when surgery is most likely to be effective. The other patterns of intestinal ischaemia (mesenteric angina, focal ischaemia and ischaemic colitis) are covered in Section 9.5 (p. 350). Causes of intestinal ischaemia are shown in Table 9.5 (p. 352).

Distinguishing features
• Severe abdominal pain in an elderly patient with arterial disease
• Paucity of abdominal signs, compared with the severity of pain
• Atrial fibrillation, or vasculitis with abdominal pain
• An epigastric bruit suggests the diagnosis if present, but is frequently absent
• Rectal bleeding after the onset of pain is a late sign
• Peritonism is a late sign, when the patient is usually beyond recovery
• Marked leucocytosis (20–30 × 10^9/L) is common, but not invariable
• Haematocrit > 0.50 indicates dehydration

Management
• Mesenteric infarction without resection is invariably fatal. Early liaison with an experienced surgeon is essential, because the situation is usually irretrievable by the time there is no clinical doubt about the diagnosis
• Suspect the diagnosis in a sick, elderly patient with severe abdominal pain and few signs
• Plain abdominal X-ray—often unremarkable. Paucity of gas, fluid levels or mucosal oedema (thickened small intestinal wall, or 'thumb printing' in the colon, p. 353; Fig. 9.6, p. 354) are usually late features
• Angiography does not help management in acute ischaemia, because non-obstructive infarction can occur and laparotomy is merely delayed
• Give analgesia—intravenous morphine 10 mg, then 2.5 mg aliquots every 3–4 h to control pain
• Vigorous intravenous rehydration—monitor haematocrit, central venous pressure and urine output
• Check arterial gases—metabolic acidosis responds to rehydration
• Antibiotics—intravenous cefotaxime 1 g and metronidazole 500 mg three

times daily, after blood cultures, if hypotensive
• Early exploratory laparotomy—especially for elderly patients, for diagnosis and to remove infarcted gut. A 'second look' to remove further non-viable tissue after 24 h is often advisable
• Mortality is above 80% and morbidity after extensive resection is substantial (short bowel syndrome, p. 262)

Abdominal pain in pregnancy (see also Section 13.1, p. 428)

Pregnancy displaces abdominal organs, alters the pattern and signs of pathology and interferes with the mechanisms that localize abdominal sepsis. Miscarriage after surgery occurs in a quarter of patients, but this is related to the stage of disease rather than laparotomy. The risks of overlooking peritonitis are substantial and negative laparotomy is well tolerated by mother and fetus.
• Appendicitis is the most common indication for laparotomy
• Ovarian cyst torsion, haemorrhage or rupture are the next most common causes
• Biliary colic during the first or second trimester is best treated surgically to avoid the risk of acute cholecystitis
• Pancreatitis is more common and usually gall stone related
• For all conditions, joint assessment by an experienced surgeon and obstetrician is appropriate, with ultrasound by an experienced radiologist rather than an obstetric ultrasonographer

Abdominal pain in the elderly (see also Section 13.2, p. 430)

Elderly patients often present late and tolerate delayed diagnosis or management poorly. The intensity of pain, fever, tachycardia and leucocytosis from intra-abdominal sepsis may be minimal.
• Biliary tract disease including cholangitis accounts for 25%. Early ultrasound and, if necessary, ERCP are indicated
• Intestinal obstruction and incarcerated hernias are the next most common conditions
• Appendicitis is the cause of an acute abdomen in about 10%
• Intestinal ischaemia should be considered if the severity of the pain is disproportionate to the signs

Abdominal pain in the immunocompromised

Abdominal pain in patients receiving chemotherapy for malignancy, organ transplant or renal replacement therapy, or immunosuppression for other diseases, is more common than in AIDS for most areas in the UK. The elderly and diabetics are relatively immunocompromised.

• Signs of perforation or abdominal sepsis may be minimal

• Neutropenic patients are prone to overwhelming sepsis. Laparotomy should not be delayed if appendicitis, diverticulitis or cholecystitis is suspected

• Neutropenic enterocolitis ('typhlitis') causes fever, diarrhoea and abdominal tenderness. The pathogenesis is unknown, but *Clostridium difficile* accounts for some and poor nutrition may contribute. Intravenous fluids, antibiotics and early surgery if perforation is suspected are appropriate

Metabolic causes

Metabolic derangements can masquerade as acute abdominal emergencies.

• Diabetic ketoacidosis—severe pain occurs in 10%, but acute pancreatitis must be excluded

• Hypercalcaemia—constipation and vomiting can occur without acute pancreatitis (Ca > 3.5 mmol/L)

• Acute adrenal insufficiency—with hyponatraemia, hyperkalaemia, elevated urea and hypotension

• Acute intermittent porphyria—neurological signs and abdominal pain, but no rash. Urine turns red on standing; porphobilinogen is detected by adding 2 mL Ehrlich's aldehyde to 2 mL urine. The pink colour is insoluble in chloroform

• Lead poisoning—ask about constipation, water supply and look at the gums for a fine blue line. Basophilic stippling and red cell lead are diagnostic

• Tabetic crisis—'lightning' pain; look for Argyll Robertson pupils and at posterior column function. It is extremely rare

Extraintestinal causes

Referred pain is more common in children and young adults.

• Lobar pneumonia—especially basal. Pneumothorax or pulmonary embolism may also cause abdominal pain

• Testicular torsion—do not forget to look, especially in teenagers

• Inferior myocardial infarction. Cardiac failure may cause severe epigastric pain due to hepatic venous congestion

• Herpes zoster—before the rash appears

• Spinal arthritis

• Root compression—classically with a thoracic meningioma; pain radiates from back to front

Munchausen's syndrome

Psychiatrically disturbed patients who manipulate recurrent admission to hospital by simulating an acute medical condition, often describe acute abdominal pain in a convincing manner. Features that should raise suspicion are:

• 'Textbook' story of an acute abdominal condition (renal colic, peptic ulcer, biliary colic), with normal investigations

• History of surgery, or admission to hospitals in other parts of the country. Recent admissions are frequently concealed (look for signs of venesection)

• Psychiatric history, or inappropriate affect

• Neuropsychiatric disorders and acute abdominal pain can occur in acute porphyria, lead poisoning or syphilis (tabetic crisis, see above)

• Previous hospital admissions should be pursued. The patient is often well known to hospitals in one area. Once the diagnosis is documented, a description should be circulated to local hospitals, but self-discharge is usual before a photograph can be taken

Undiagnosed abdominal pain

No specific diagnosis is made in a third of patients with acute abdominal pain. Take a careful history to identify any pattern of recurrent or acute on chronic abdominal pain. Complete resolution between episodes of recurrent pain makes organic disease more likely. If the pain is localized to a specific site, consider non-visceral pain in the abdominal wall. Pain from a rectus sheath haematoma or Spigelian hernia (lateral to the rectus sheath) may be very severe, but neuromuscular abdominal wall pain is more common. Otherwise the term 'non-specific abdominal pain' is best used, or 'irritable bowel' if the pain is acute on chronic (p. 367).

Distinguishing features

• Type, site and relief of pain fail to fit a common pattern

• Abdominal bloating is common

• Vomiting occurs in 50%, often preceding pain

• Constipation should not be overlooked and can be diagnosed on plain abdominal X-ray

• Non-visceral abdominal pain is exacerbated by a finger placed on the site of pain whilst tensing the muscles of the abdominal wall, but makes little difference to pain from an irritable bowel (Carnet's sign)

Management

• Observation with oral fluids and analgesics for 24 h will usually discriminate the non-specific from the pathological cases

• Confirm that the temperature, blood count, C-reactive protein and urine examination are all normal

• Any abnormalities should be pursued, by ultrasound, small bowel radiology or a gastroenterological opinion as appropriate

• A confident diagnosis of irritable bowel syndrome helps management (p. 367)

• Non-visceral abdominal pain can often be relieved by injection of local anaesthetic after consultation with anaesthetists or the pain team

1.8 Intestinal obstruction

Mechanical intestinal obstruction or failure of peristalsis (ileus) is life threatening. Figure 1.5 outlines the approach to management.

Clinical features

The cardinal features are:
• Pain
• Distension
• Vomiting
• Constipation

The pain is colicky, but once strangulation occurs the pain becomes continuous and rebound tenderness is present. Vomiting can be the only feature of high jejunal obstruction.

Subacute obstruction means incomplete occlusion of the lumen and an explosive episode of diarrhoea can follow the pain.

A succussion splash is often audible if the abdomen is shaken. Visible peristalsis may be seen. Hernial orifices must be examined carefully and previous abdominal surgery noted. Bowel sounds are increased in mechanical obstruction, but decreased in ileus.

Causes

Mechanical
• External herniae
• Adhesions
• Malignant colonic strictures

These three causes account for 75%.

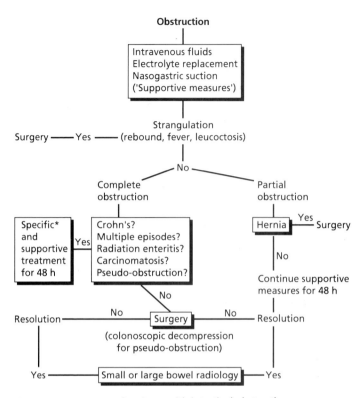

Fig. 1.5 Management of patients with intestinal obstruction.
*Specific treatment: intravenous steroids.

Less common mechanical causes

- Luminal:
  - ingested foreign bodies
  - fibrous food bolus
  - gall stone ileus
  - intussusception
- Mural:
  - sigmoid diverticular disease
  - Crohn's disease
  - NSAID-induced small intestinal strictures
  - radiation enteritis
  - ileocaecal tuberculosis
  - malignant small bowel strictures (carcinoid, lymphoma, carcinoma)

- Extrinsic:
    - volvulus (sigmoid, caecal, gastric)
    - internal herniation (through mesenteric foramina)

Ileus

- Following laparotomy
- Retroperitoneal lesions:
    - pancreatitis
    - haemorrhage
    - ureteric obstruction
- Drugs—anticholinergics and opiates, among others
- Metabolic:
    - diabetic ketoacidosis
    - acute renal failure
    - hypokalaemia
- Intestinal infarction
- Pseudo-obstruction

Investigations

- Plain abdominal X-ray—the upper limit of normal diameter of the small intestine is 2.5 cm and of the colon is 6.0 cm. Supine films alone are sufficient for diagnosis. Look for mucosal oedema, the site that luminal gas disappears, displacement of bowel loops by a mass, and air in the bowel wall or biliary tree. An occasional fluid level on an erect film is normal. On an erect chest X-ray, look for air under the diaphragm
- Blood tests—look for hypokalaemia or high urea. Leucocytosis suggests strangulation. Crossmatch 2 units prior to surgery
- Arterial gases—metabolic alkalosis occurs with severe vomiting

Management (Fig. 1.5, p. 43)

- Nasogastric suction
- Replace fluid and electrolytes—5 L 0.9% saline and 200 mmol KCl are commonly needed in the first 24 h. Sequestered fluid in obstructed bowel is not measured, so adjust infusion rate according to the urine output and central venous pressure in very sick patients
- Assess concomitant medical problems—drugs may not have been absorbed
- Relieve the obstruction—the site governs the type of operation. Suspicion of strangulation demands urgent surgery. Non-operative manoeuvres are

initially indicated for ileus, pseudo-obstruction, volvulus or intussusception

- Monitor:
  - urine output
  - nasogastric aspirate
  - central venous pressure in the shocked or elderly
  - daily electrolytes

Ileus

- Nasogastric suction, maintaining serum potassium at 4.0–4.5 mmol/L, intravenous fluids and patience are usually sufficient
- Check that anticholinergic drugs are not prescribed and decrease opiate analgesia to a minimum
- Try metoclopramide 10 mg intravenously three times daily, or cisapride 30 mg per rectum three times daily if ineffective, as prokinetic agents
- Consider parenteral nutrition if resolution is delayed for longer than 72 h
- Exclude mechanical obstruction by contrast radiology, if obstruction persists after a few days

Volvulus

- Sigmoid volvulus—common in developing countries, elderly males and the mentally handicapped. Plain X-ray shows massive sigmoid distension. Colonoscopy is more effective than a deflating rectal tube and should be attempted before surgery
- Caecal volvulus—obstruction is often incomplete initially but recurs without surgery, so laparotomy is advisable
- Gastric volvulus—associated with diaphragmatic eventration, visible on plain chest and abdominal X-rays. Distinguish from 'acute gastric dilatation' which is a misnomer for gastric ileus, caused by poor attention to nasogastric suction and electrolyte balance. Surgery is needed for gastric volvulus, with repair of the diaphragm

Intussusception

- Usually idiopathic in infants; due to a Meckel's diverticulum in adolescence; or a polyp or carcinoma in adults
- Intermittent pain, rectal bleeding, small intestinal fluid levels and an absent caecal gas shadow suggest the diagnosis. Facial pallor during pain occurs in infants
- Barium enema is diagnostic and may be therapeutic in the early stages

Pseudo-obstruction

- Clinical features of intestinal obstruction without a mechanical cause. The motility disorder commonly affects the whole gastrointestinal tract, although it is colonic distension that is often most prominent
- Consider the diagnosis in the elderly and mentally handicapped, or when obstruction is associated with other disorders (myocardial infarction, pneumonia, Parkinson's disease)
- An urgent single contrast barium enema is often necessary to distinguish pseudo-obstruction from mechanical obstruction, and may have a therapeutic effect
- Stop causative drugs (opiates, phenothiazines, tricyclics, clonidine) and treat associated disease
- Do not allow the patient to remain supine, but ensure mobility or turning regularly, including into the prone or head-down position as this may help deflation
- Rectal cisapride 30 mg three times daily may be helpful. Erythromycin 2 g daily is also prokinetic due to motilin-like activity. Stimulant laxatives (senna, codanthrusate) rarely help and lactulose may increase intraluminal gas. Enemas should be used with care as perforation can occur
- Repeat plain abdominal X-ray after 48 h to monitor caecal diameter
- 90% resolve spontaneously, but colonoscopic decompression is warranted if pain is severe, or the caecum > 10 cm. Surgery should be avoided if at all possible, but caecostomy is appropriate if two attempts at colonoscopic decompression fail and symptoms persist
- Chronic intestinal pseudo-obstruction is a feature of systemic sclerosis, neuromuscular diseases and amyloidosis amongst others

1.9 Toxic dilatation of the colon

Dilatation of the colon with signs of systemic upset ('toxic') is becoming less common as acute attacks of ulcerative colitis are recognized and appropriately treated (p. 308). The danger if surgery is inappropriately delayed is colonic perforation, which still carries a high mortality.

Clinical features

- Colitis—usually caused by severe ulcerative colitis, but can occur in Crohn's colitis, and rarely in ischaemic, or infective colitis (*Yersinia enterocolitica*, *Campylobacter* spp., *Clostridium difficile*, p. 321)

- Fever > 37.8°C
- Neutrophils > 10×10^9/L
- Tachycardia > 90 b.p.m.
- Radiological colonic dilatation (widest diameter > 6.0 cm; Fig. 1.6)
- Clinical appearance can be deceptive due to steroids

Management

Patients presenting with dilatation should start intensive medical treatment (see below) and the response carefully assessed after 24 h. About half respond, but a decision to continue for a further 24 h or proceed to emergency colectomy must be made by a senior physician in consultation with a colorectal surgeon. Patients who recover continue treatment as for severe colitis (p. 309). When dilatation develops during intensive medical treatment for colitis, colectomy is indicated without further delay.

Diagnosis
- Always take a daily plain abdominal X-ray in patients with severe colitis (p. 309). Mucosal islands (polypoid mucosal swellings projecting into the colonic lumen; Fig. 1.6, p. 48), in addition to dilatation indicate very severe ulceration and predict the need for colectomy. The presence of three or more distended loops of small bowel is also associated with the need for colectomy
- Stool culture and faecal *Cl. difficile* toxin assay
- Blood cultures
- Rigid sigmoidoscopy and rectal mucosal biopsy to confirm colitis, but colonoscopy or barium enema are dangerous

Supportive therapy
- Vigorously correct fluid and electrolyte imbalance with intravenous fluids and KCl supplements (serum K 4.0–4.5 mmol/L)
- Nil by mouth
- Involve the surgeons as soon as the diagnosis is made
- 2 hourly observation of pulse and temperature, 4 hourly BP, as well as fluid balance and meticulous stool chart, since nursing observations are essential prognostic factors when deciding the timing of colectomy (p. 311)
- Examine the patient at least twice daily (check pulse, BP and tenderness)
- Monitor daily full blood count, C-reactive protein, electrolytes and maximum colonic diameter on plain abdominal X-ray

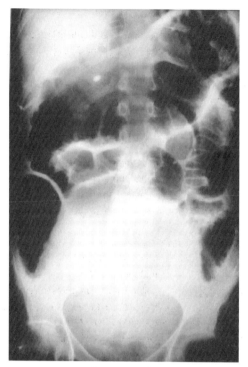

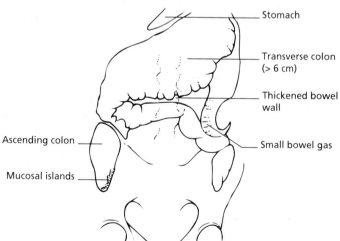

Fig. 1.6 Toxic dilatation of the colon in ulcerative colitis. Plain abdominal radiograph in toxic megacolon showing a grossly dilated transverse colon with mucosal islands in the ascending colon.

Specific therapy
- Stop antidiarrhoeal agents, opiates and anticholinergic drugs
- Intravenous hydrocortisone 100 mg four times daily, for ulcerative colitis or Crohn's disease
- Rectal hydrocortisone 100 mg in 100 mL twice daily (p. 309)
- There is no evidence that antibiotics alter outcome

Indications for emergency colectomy

The decision can be difficult, but prolonged medical treatment increases mortality, even in young patients. If the situation is stable after 24 h, a further 24 h trial of medical treatment may be justified. This decision should be taken by a senior physician, jointly with the surgeons. Indications for colectomy are:
- Persistent tachycardia, or fever
- Failure to improve clinically (no change in stool frequency, tachycardia or abdominal pain) or radiologically within 24 h
- Signs of perforation (may be minimal, due to steroids)
- Mucosal islands as well as dilatation (because such severe ulceration and oedema is very unlikely to respond to steroids)
- A prospective study in ulcerative colitis without colonic dilatation has shown that if after 3 days intravenous treatment the stool frequency is > 8/day, or the frequency is 3–8/day together with a C-reactive protein > 45 mg/L, then there is an 85% chance that colectomy will be needed on that admission (p. 311)

1.10 Acute hepatic failure

Acute hepatic failure occurs in a previously normal liver and is either fulminant or late onset (subacute). The time of onset and mortality distinguish the two types, although other features and management are similar.

The main differential diagnosis is between acute and acute on chronic liver failure (Table 1.7, p. 50). The potential for complete recovery distinguishes acute failure, although it has a worse prognosis.

Clinical features

Hyperacute hepatic failure
- Encephalopathy within 7 days of the onset of jaundice
- Encephalopathy includes all stages from personality change to coma. The grade may change rapidly (Table 1.6)

Table 1.6 Grade of hepatic encephalopathy.

Grade	Features
1	Altered mood or behaviour
2	Drowsy
3	Stupor
4	Coma
5	Coma with no response to painful stimuli

• Paradoxically, this group has the highest likelihood of recovery with medical management.

Acute liver failure

• Encephalopathy develops 8–28 days after the onset of jaundice
• This group has a high mortality and marked prolongation of prothrombin time

Subacute liver failure

• Encephalopathy after an interval of 4–12 weeks after the onset of jaundice
• Less marked prolongation of prothrombin time, but mortality remains high

Associated features

• Fetor—the smell of pear drops
• Jaundice—may be minimal in the early stages
• Liver size—usually small, due to hepatic necrosis. If enlarged, acute on chronic liver failure (Table 1.7) is more likely
• Spleen—usually impalpable
• No single feature entirely discriminates between acute and acute on chronic hepatic failure, although the history is the best guide

Table 1.7 Acute versus acute on chronic hepatic failure.

	Acute	Acute on chronic
History	Short	Long
Nutrition	Good	Poor
Liver	Small	Usually enlarged
Spleen	Impalpable	Enlarged
Spiders	Absent	Many
Encephalopathy	Early	Late
Jaundice	Late	Early
Ascites	Late	Early

Causes

Paracetamol overdose and viral hepatitis are the commonest causes in the UK. Presentation a few days after apparent recovery from paracetamol poisoning is typical.

• Viral—hepatitis B or D (δ agent). Rare after hepatitis A, C or E (community-acquired non-A, non-B), yellow fever or leptospirosis
• Drugs—paracetamol (especially associated with alcohol), halothane, isoniazid
• Alcohol—occasionally without underlying liver disease, but usually acute on chronic
• Wilson's disease
• Budd–Chiari syndrome—ascites is often prominent
• Fatty liver of pregnancy—third trimester (p. 428)
• HELLP syndrome (haemolysis, elevated liver enzymes and low platelet count)—a severe complication of pre-eclampsia in pregnancy (p. 428)

Investigations

Blood tests

• Coagulation studies, glucose and potassium immediately and creatinine as soon as possible
• Full blood count, group and save, bilirubin, albumin, aspartate transaminase, amylase
• Hepatitis serology, paracetamol levels, serum copper and caeruloplasmin, and 24-h urinary copper where appropriate

Other

• Chest X-ray
• Ultrasound of liver and pancreas. Hepatic vein Doppler studies if Budd–Chiari syndrome is suspected
• Blood cultures—even if afebrile
• EEG—may be diagnostic when there is doubt and may be prognostic, but is seldom necessary

Management

General

• Intensive care nursing
• Insert a central venous line early to ensure good hydration. Aggressive early rehydration appears to improve outcome. Patients drink little because

of nausea or encephalopathy. Hypovolaemia impairs hepatic and renal perfusion

- Monitor urine output, blood glucose and vital signs, every hour
- Check serum potassium and coagulation studies twice daily for the first 48 h, then daily with full blood count, creatinine and albumin
- Do not give intravenous saline
- Reassess the grade of encephalopathy (Table 1.6; although a number-connection or trail chart offers more objective assessment for subtle changes), ascites and fluid balance once or twice daily

Specific therapy

- Commence N-acetyl cysteine infusion for significant paracetamol poisoning and continue infusion until coagulation returns to normal
- Inotropic support if hypotensive

Encephalopathy

- No oral protein
- Lactulose, starting at 30 mL three times daily until diarrhoea develops. Then reduce to 10 mL three times daily. Neomycin is of little additional benefit
- Avoid sedation if possible, but chlormethiazole is appropriate for alcohol withdrawal (p. 202)
- Protect the airway as encephalopathy progresses beyond grade 2 (Table 1.6, p. 50)
- Intracranial pressure monitoring is appropriate in grade 4 encephalopathy (usually when the patient has been transferred to a liver unit). Mannitol 0.3–1.0 g/kg is given when intracranial pressure is increased. Oxygen and inotropic support are also necessary. Phenytoin decreases subclinical seizure activity and cerebral oedema

Hypoglycaemia and hypokalaemia

- 10% dextrose 100 mL/h with KCl 40 mmol/L, but 20–50% dextrose may be needed if hypoglycaemia is severe
- Empirical antibiotics (see below)

Bleeding

- Avoid arterial punctures
- FFP if clinically significant bleeding occurs, but coagulation studies seldom fully correct. A single dose of 10 mg vitamin K intravenously will ensure adequate stores, but will not correct the coagulopathy

• Acid suppression (omeprazole 20 mg orally, or sucralfate 2 g three times daily) is often given to reduce stress-induced gastric erosions, but the evidence of benefit is debated

• Disseminated intravascular coagulation can cause bleeding as well as clotting factor deficiency due to liver failure. If thrombocytopenia is present, check fibrin degradation products and haptoglobins (for haemolysis)

Renal failure

• 55% develop renal impairment. Good hydration is the key to preventing renal failure, but hepatotoxic drugs may be directly nephrotoxic

• Serum urea is falsely low in severe liver disease, so creatinine should be measured, but a bilirubin > 200 µmol/L interferes with creatinine assay

• Haemofiltration or dialysis is indicated if serum K > 6.0 mmol/L, HCO_3 < 15 mmol/L or creatinine > 400 µmol/L

Infection

• Meticulous care of intravenous and urinary catheters

• Blood, urine and catheter cultures are essential and must be performed before starting antibiotics

• Antibiotics are recommended, because patients are critically ill and signs of sepsis are commonly absent. Intravenous cefotaxime 1 g three times daily is appropriate, until culture results are available

Indications for transplant

Deciding when the chance of spontaneous recovery is less than the risks of a liver transplant is difficult. Discuss the situation with the nearest transplant centre (Appendix 1, p. 477) at an early stage.

Transfer is generally recommended in the following circumstances (Tables 1.8, 1.9)

• The prothrombin time (measured in seconds) at the time of referral is greater than the interval (hours) between poisoning and referral

• Prothrombin time exceeds 50 s

• Metabolic acidosis at presentation

• All patients with established encephalopathy. Table 1.10 shows the criteria used for transplantation in fulminant hepatic failure at King's College Hospital, but it is too late to transfer a patient at this stage. Hepatitis B and alcohol abuse are relative, but not absolute contraindications to transplantation. In one study 17/92 patients admitted to a liver unit with paracetamol

Table 1.8 Guidelines for referral of patients to a liver unit following paracetamol overdose.

Day 2	Day 3	Day 4
Arterial pH < 7.30	Arterial pH < 7.30	INR > 6.0 or PT > 75 s
INR > 3.0 or PT > 50 s	INR > 4.5 or PT > 60 s	Progressive rise in PT
Oliguria	Oliguria	Oliguria
Creatinine > 200 µmol/L	Creatinine > 200 µmol/L	Creatinine > 300 µmol/L
Hypoglycaemia	Encephalopathy	Encephalopathy

PT, prothrombin time.

poisoning were listed for transplantation. 70% of those transplanted survived compared to 14% who were listed but not transplanted. The overall mortality was 32%

Take into account
- Age (< 60 years)
- Previous liver function (should have been normal)
- Ability to cope with post-transplant regimen (p. 209)

Before and during transfer
- Insert a central venous line if the prothrombin time exceeds 30 s (INR 2.0) or if there is renal dysfunction. Good hydration and circulation improve outcome
- Give 10% glucose 100 mL/h with 40 mmol/L KCl to prevent hypoglycaemia or hypokalaemia
- Give 20% mannitol 20 mL/h if encephalopathic before transfer
- Intubate and ventilate patients with advanced encephalopathy before transfer, because cerebral oedema is exacerbated by movement

Table 1.9 Guidelines for referral of patients to a liver unit for non-paracetamol induced liver failure.

Hyperacute	Acute	Subacute
Encephalopathy	Encephalopathy	Encephalopathy
PT > 30 s	PT > 30 s	PT > 20 s
Renal failure	Renal failure	Renal failure
		Serum sodium < 130 mmol/L
		Shrinking liver volume

PT, prothrombin time.

Table 1.10 Criteria for liver transplant in fulminant failure.

Paracetamol cases	Non-paracetamol cases
Arterial pH < 7.30	INR > 6.7 or PT >100 s
or all of the following	*or any three of the following*
PT > 100 s	Aetiology non-A, non-B or drug reaction
Creatinine > 300 μmol/L	Age < 10 or > 40 years
Grade 3–4 encephalopathy	Jaundice > 7 days before encephalopathy
	INR > 4.0 or PT > 50 s
	Bilirubin > 300 μmol/L

PT, prothrombin time.

Prognosis

Factors
- Grade of encephalopathy—15% survival without transplant, when grade 3–4
- Age:
  - > 40 years 15% survival
  - < 30 years 40% survival
- Albumin:
  - > 35 g/L 80% survival
  - < 30 g/L 20% survival
- Cause—drug reactions and non-A, non-B (hepatitis C) induced failure have a worse prognosis than other causes
- Onset—late onset has a worse prognosis than fulminant failure

Transplant in acute liver failure
- 65% survive, but this is improving
- Auxiliary liver transplantation until the original liver has recovered has proved disappointing

2 Oesophagus

2.1 Dysphagia

Causes

Acute or progressive dysphagia demands urgent investigation. Oropharyngeal and oesophageal causes are recognized (Table 2.1). Bolus obstruction is covered in Section 1.2, p. 4.

Clinical features

A careful history usually distinguishes between oropharyngeal and oesophageal causes (Fig. 2.1). Four questions about the dysphagia are essential: interval, type of food, pattern and associated features.

Interval
• Difficulty in initiating swallowing, repeated attempts at swallowing

Table 2.1 Causes of dysphagia.

	Oropharyngeal	Oesophageal

Common	Aphthous ulcers
	Candidiasis
	Stroke
		Oesophagitis
		Oesophageal dysmotility
		Peptic stricture
		Carcinoma
		  oesophagus
		  cardia

Unusual	Parkinson's disease
	Globus hystericus
	Pseudobulbar palsy
	Motor neurone disease
	Pharyngeal pouch
	Xerostomia
		Motor disorders
		  achalasia
		  diffuse spasm
		  systemic sclerosis
		  polymyositis
		Oesophageal infection
		External pressure
		  bronchial carcinoma
		  mediastinal nodes
		  aortic aneurysm
		Postcricoid web
		Schatzki ring
		Radiation stricture

Rare	Oral tumours Syringobulbia Bulbar poliomyelitis Muscular dystrophy Botulism	Corrosive/pill stricture Aberrant vessels Left atrial enlargement Retrosternal goitre Chagas' disease

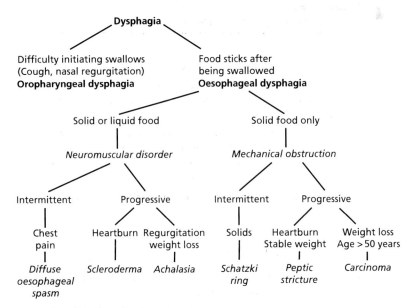

Fig. 2.1 Diagnosis of dysphagia. Adapted from Richter JE In: Sleisenger ME, Fordtran JS eds. *Gastrointestinal Disease.* Philadelphia: WB Saunders, 1993.

or dysphagia within a second of starting to swallow characterize oropharyngeal dysphagia
• Dysphagia a few seconds after starting to swallow indicates an oesophageal cause
• Where the patient points to is no help in locating the site of the lesion

Type of food
• Ask if dysphagia is for liquids (usually pharyngeal), solids (mechanical oesophageal cause likely) or both (oesophageal dysmotility more likely)
• Exacerbation by hot or cold liquids is common in oesophagitis

Pattern
• Progressive dysphagia indicates an organic cause, such as carcinoma, benign stricture or achalasia
• Intermittent symptoms are common in oesophageal dysmotility, diverticula, web or ring
• Short (< 3 months), progressive history indicates malignancy
• A 'lump in the throat' as the only symptom is unlikely to have a mechanical cause

Associated features
• Weight loss confirms that an organic cause is probable, but lack of weight loss is of no diagnostic value

- Heartburn suggests a peptic stricture
- Cough indicates spillover into the bronchial tree, commonly due to oropharyngeal dysphagia, or achalasia when at night. Very rarely it is due to an oesophagobronchial fistula
- Odynophagia (pain during swallowing) often accompanies dysphagia in oesophagitis, achalasia or diffuse oesophageal spasm
- Examine the mouth and teeth or dentures, and feel for supraclavicular nodes (from carcinoma of the cardia)
- Look for signs of systemic disease (anaemia, systemic sclerosis or neurological disorders)

Urgent investigations

- Indicated when dysphagia is for solids alone, when symptoms are progressive or when there is associated weight loss
- Telephone the radiologist or gastroenterologist to arrange urgent investigation. Confirmation by request form or letter can follow later
- Chest X-ray—look for a hilar tumour, mediastinal fluid level, absent gastric bubble or right lower lobe consolidation (aspiration)
- Barium swallow—within 48 h. A smooth, tapering stricture is often benign. Irregularity or asymmetry suggests malignancy (Fig. 2.3, p. 69)
- Endoscopy—after a barium swallow. Allow 12 h for barium to clear: it can block the endoscope
- Blood tests—anaemia may be due to malignancy, poor nutrition, bleeding, or Plummer–Vinson syndrome (p. 70). A high urea usually reflects dehydration

Elective investigations

- Barium swallow, chest X-ray and endoscopy can be performed electively in patients with intermittent dysphagia without weight loss, or when symptoms suggest oesophageal motility disorders
- Cine or bread barium swallow, or oesophageal manometry is usually appropriate if the barium swallow is normal (p. 82)
- ENT assessment is indicated for most pharyngeal causes of dysphagia
- Lung function tests (spirometry and transfer factor) establish a baseline in patients with systemic sclerosis

2.2 Gastro-oesophageal reflux disease

Gastro-oesophageal reflux does not always cause symptoms. Abnormal reflux is predominantly caused by dysfunction of the lower oesphageal sphincter and not necessarily by a hiatus hernia. Delayed clearance of refluxate prolongs mucosal exposure to the low pH (< 4), which damages the oesophageal mucosal barrier and initiates oesophagitis. In addition to acid, bile acids and pepsin also disrupt mucosal integrity or provoke oesophageal dysmotility. Peptic stricture of the oesophagus is an unusual complication, in view of the high prevalence of gastro-oesophageal reflux.

Clinical features

- Heartburn—retrosternal pain related to meals, lying down, stooping, straining and occasionally to exercise
- Regurgitation of acid or bile (waterbrash). Patients often have difficulty in describing the taste, usually bitter or sour
- Dysphagia may be due to peristaltic dysfunction. Pain during swallowing (odynophagia) is unusual unless there is severe oesophagitis or a stricture (when dysphagia for solids is also present)
- Excess salivation during pain
- Relief by antacids
- Chest pain, related to posture or exercise (both of which increase intra-abdominal pressure), can be difficult to distinguish from angina (p. 81)
- Nocturnal asthma (cough or wheeze) may be the only symptom, and can be relieved by treatment of reflux
- Oesophagitis can be asymptomatic. There is no clear relation between the symptom severity and endoscopic severity of oesophagitis

The sliding hiatus hernia myth

The common sliding hiatus hernia is compatible with normal lower oesophageal sphincter function. It is not necessarily pathological and no symptoms can be attributed to the hernia itself. Symptoms are due to oesophagitis or oesophageal dysmotility provoked by reflux.
- More than 30% of patients over 50 years have a hiatus hernia
- Less than 50% have symptomatic gastro-oesophageal reflux
- A report of a sliding hiatus hernia on barium radiology is not a diagnosis. If a patient's symptoms warrant investigation, endoscopy to identify oesophagitis is appropriate, with further investigation if this is normal
- Never accept a hiatus hernia as a cause of iron-deficiency anaemia—there is usually another cause, such as a silent caecal carcinoma
- Rolling (paraoesophageal) or incarcerated hiatal herniae are diagnosed radiologically. A chest X-ray may show a fluid level behind the heart. Episodic pain or vomiting are indications for a barium meal, as partial or complete gastric volvulus may occur, for which surgery is needed

Investigations

- Isolated symptoms of gastro-oesophageal reflux do not require investigation
- Endoscopy is indicated if symptoms are not relieved by general measures (see below) in preference to a barium meal because oesophagitis or Barrett's oesophagus are more reliably detected
- It is common to get symptomatic reflux with no signs of oesophagitis at endoscopy
- Macroscopic oesophagitis indicates reflux, but the severity frequently does not correlate with symptoms. Endoscopic oesophagitis is graded 1–4 for the purposes of clinical trials: (1) erythema, (2) linear erosions, (3) circumferential erosions, or (4) chronic mucosal lesions such as ulcers or Barrett's oesophagus
- If Barrett's oesophagus (see below) is found, multiple biopsies should be taken
- Microscopic oesophagitis within 5 cm of the gastro-oesophageal junction occurs in some normal subjects. More proximal changes occur in symptomatic reflux, even when the mucosa looks normal
- Iron-deficiency anaemia should not be attributed to oesophagitis
- *Helicobacter pylori* is unrelated to reflux oesophagitis
- The Bernstein (oesophageal acid perfusion) test reliably reproduces symptoms if these are due to reflux. It is not widely used in the UK, probably because a trial of a proton-pump inhibitor is simpler
- 24-h oesophageal pH monitoring is indicated when it is difficult to distinguish symptomatic reflux from other causes of chest pain (p. 82), but is not part of routine management

General measures

General measures to reduce reflux are more important than drugs in most patients.
- Reduce fat intake (fat promotes reflux by delaying gastric emptying)
- Weight reduction (height/weight charts: Appendix 3, p. 486; reducing diet: p. 414)
- Stop smoking
- Raise the head of the bed by about 10 cm, using blocks or bricks (especially if symptoms are nocturnal)
- Small, regular meals
- Allow 3 h between last meal and retiring at night
- Avoid hot drinks or alcohol before bed
- Avoid drugs that adversely affect oesophageal motility (nitrates,

anticholinergic agents, antidepressants, theophylline compounds), or that damage the oesophageal mucosa (NSAIDs, slow-release potassium)

• Use antacids or alginates (Gaviscon, Gastrocote) for occasional symptomatic relief. There is no evidence that one is better than the other and neither will heal oesophagitis

Management

If general measures alone are insufficient, drug treatment is indicated. Controversy persists about the best approach, but proton-pump inhibitors are unequivocally the most effective treatment and are best given in the morning. At first presentation, liquid alginates appear to be more cost-effective than acid suppression with H_2-receptor antagonists, since 50% respond equally well to either. After alginates, an incremental approach is recommended, using the minimum effective treatment to relieve symptoms. Only a minority of patients with reflux have severe oesophagitis (Fig. 2.2).

• Prokinetic drugs (such as cisapride 10–20 mg twice daily or metoclopramide 10 mg three times daily) or H_2-receptor antagonists (best given after supper, not at night) are effective for mild degrees of oesophagitis. Response is inversely proportional to the severity of oesophagitis. Both are better than either alone, but are more expensive and less effective than proton-pump inhibitors

• There is probably little difference between the proton-pump inhibitors (lansoprazole, omeprazole or pantoprazole) in terms of efficacy or side-effect profile, although costs may vary. Pantoprazole has fewer potential drug interactions, but is currently not licensed in the UK for more than 12 weeks continuous use. In one single-dose study the bioavailability of lansoprazole was reduced by 27% when given with food, whilst omeprazole was not affected. This may not be clinically relevant, since a comparative trial on 120 patients with moderate to severe oesophagitis found that lansoprazole 30 mg was equivalent to omeprazole 40 mg daily (96% healing at 4 weeks)

• Intermittent treatment of recurrent symptoms is often necessary

• Symptomatic erosive oesophagitis relapses within 6 months in 80% on no maintenance treatment, 40% on ranitidine 300 mg or omeprazole 10 mg daily and 15% on omeprazole 20 mg daily, but these represent a small proportion of all patients with reflux

• Maintenance treatment with cisapride 10 mg twice daily or cimetidine 800 mg after supper may be considered for patients with mild oesophagitis and frequent, recurrent symptoms

• Maintenance treatment with lansoprazole 15–30 mg daily or omeprazole 20–40 mg daily is indicated for patients with refractory

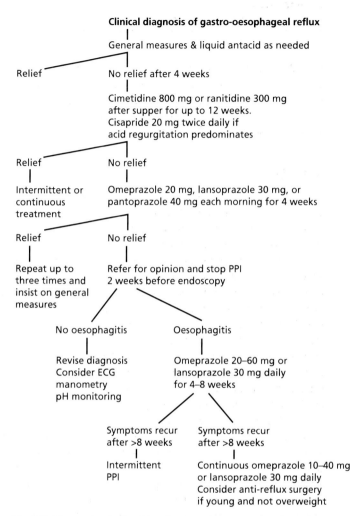

Fig. 2.2 Management plan for symptomatic gastro-oesophageal reflux.

symptoms or confluent oesophagitis, Barrett's oesophagus or a peptic stricture may need higher doses of omeprazole

• Concerns about long-term sequelae of PPIs appear unfounded, but postmarketing surveillance continues. Interference with vitamin B_{12} absorption, intestinal bacterial overgrowth, pronounced hypergastrinaemia with G-cell hyperplasia and accelerated atrophic gastritis in those with *H. pylori* are areas of interest in long-term treatment

• The current consensus is to eradicate *H. pylori* in patients who need PPIs long term

• Overweight, smoking drinkers characteristically continue to have symptoms

Refractory symptoms

Symptoms that persist despite treatment with a proton-pump inhibitor (omeprazole up to 60 mg or lansoprazole 30 mg daily) are usually due to coexistent oesophageal dysmotility, or a non-oesophageal cause.

• Retake the history. Abdominal bloating is common in oesophageal dysmotility. Exercise-related pain may be angina

• Repeat the endoscopy. Stop proton-pump inhibitors prior to endoscopy if oesophagitis has not previously been identified. Otherwise continue treatment, since up to 15% fail to respond

• If the endoscopy is normal, arrange oesophageal manometry or a bread–barium swallow to exclude achalasia or diffuse oesophageal spasm. 24-h manometry may be needed to identify oesphageal spasm

• Arrange 24-h pH monitoring (p. 466) if radiology or manometry is normal, or investigate for non-oesophageal causes by abdominal ultra-sound or exercise test as appropriate

• If the endoscopy shows persistent oesophagitis despite treatment, consider surgery

Indications for antireflux surgery

Surgery is rarely indicated. Laparoscopic antireflux surgery currently has similar risks (lack of efficacy, postoperative stricture, vagal denervation, inability to belch, splenic or oesophageal damage) to open procedures. Mortality is 1%, but results can be good in well-selected patients in experienced hands.

Consider surgery by an experienced surgeon if all the following criteria are met:

• Severe symptoms persist despite all medical treatments vigorously applied. Symptoms of volume reflux (waterbrash or fluid regurgitation into the mouth) have traditionally favoured surgery, but the concept of volume reflux is now questioned

• Objective evidence of gross reflux (by pH monitoring)

• Age < 60 years

• Oesophageal dysmotility has been excluded by manometry

Barrett's oesophagus

Features

• Endoscopic biopsy evidence of intestinal metaplasia proximal to the gastro-oesophageal junction

- Oesophageal carcinoma develops in 2–5% and dysplasia in 10% over 5 years
- The risk of carcinoma appears to be related to the length of Barrett's oesophagus

Management

- Multiple biopsies every 2 cm are needed to exclude dysplasia at diagnosis
- Prescribe omeprazole 40 mg daily. Lower doses do not induce regression
- Long-term treatment is usually indicated, because Barrett's oesophagus is assumed to be a consequence of severe gastro-oesophageal reflux
- Repeat endoscopy to rebiopsy after 6–12 months treatment in patients aged < 60 years
- If multiple foci of high-grade dysplasia are detected in young patients, oesophagectomy should be considered
- Annual surveillance endoscopy has not yet been shown to reduce mortality, but it is reasonable to continue vigorous antisecretory therapy and repeat endoscopy every 12 months in patients with low-grade dysplasia or long (> 5 cm) Barrett's oesophagus, for as long as patients remain surgical candidates
- Photodynamic therapy and ablation of Barrett's epithelium by endoscopic laser therapy remain experimental techniques

Oesophageal ulcers

Features

- Associated with severe oesophagitis or Barrett's oesophagus
- Endoscopy, biopsy and brush cytology are needed to exclude malignancy

Management

- Check that biopsies and brushings for cytology have been taken at endoscopy
- Prescribe lansoprazole 30 mg or omeprazole 20 mg daily for 4 weeks
- Repeat the endoscopy, biopsy and brushings at 6-week intervals until healing occurs
- Long-term treatment with a proton-pump inhibitor is appropriate for peptic oesophageal ulcers, because these indicate severe reflux with a high recurrence rate
- Refer for surgery if high-grade dysplasia is detected in ulcers that persist despite treatment

Alkaline reflux

Bile, pancreatic enzymes and bicarbonate due to duodenogastric reflux, as well as acid and pepsin, can cause oesophagitis. This occurs particularly after partial gastrectomy. Biliary reflux at endoscopy is normal if the patient is retching.

• Oesophagitis with a pH > 4 at all times during ambulatory monitoring is necessary for diagnosis

• General measures and antacids should be tried. Sucralfate binds bile and may help, but needs to be give four times daily to heal oesophagitis. Dilute hydrochloric acid BP (0.1 mL in 10 mL water) would be logical and is said to be better than placebo for heartburn in pregnancy, but is not in general use

• Surgical (Roux-en-Y) revision is reserved for severe, intolerable symptoms

2.3 **Benign strictures**

Causes

• Peptic—95%

• Anastomotic—following a surgical procedure

• Radiotherapy—for carcinoma of the breast or bronchus. Stenosis after radiotherapy for oesophageal carcinoma is almost always malignant

• Corrosives—bleach (p. 8) or drugs such as slow-release potassium tablets. Patients taking NSAIDs have a higher incidence of strictures. Pills (tetracycline tablets, slow-release potassium) may cause strictures. Advise elderly patients with poor oesophageal motility to take such drugs when standing, with plenty of fluid

• Mucocutaneous disorders—Behçet's syndrome, epidermolysis bullosa

Clinical features

Dysphagia is the main symptom (p. 59; Fig. 2.1, p. 60) and reflux is usually present. The main differential diagnosis is carcinoma. Dysphagia for < 3 months or rapid weight loss favour carcinoma.

Investigations and management

Initial investigations

• As for dysphagia (p. 69, Fig. 2.3)

• Check the results of biopsies and brushings

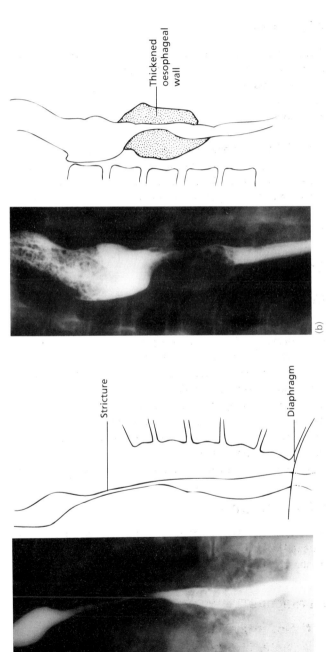

Fig. 2.3 Radiological appearances of benign and malignant oesophageal strictures. (a) Barium swallow showing a smooth stricture in the mid-oesophagus. Negative biopsies and cytology from the stricture confirmed its benign nature. (b) Barium swallow showing irregular stricturing in the lower oesophagus due to a carcinoma. The oesophageal wall is thickened by the tumour.

Dilatation

• Endoscopic dilatation as an outpatient procedure is safe in experienced hands. The technique is beyond the scope of this book (Appendix 2, p. 480)

• A subsequent chest X-ray is not necessary unless pain occurs or perforation is suspected

• Repeat dilatations may be needed

• Encourage the patient to make appointments direct with the endoscopy unit if dysphagia recurs, to save time

• Recurrent symptoms < 4 weeks after dilatation suggests a carcinoma

Other advice

• Omeprazole 20–40 mg daily has been shown to delay or prevent recurrent peptic strictures

• Prevention of oesophageal obstruction (p. 5)

2.4 Oesophageal carcinoma

Oesophageal carcinoma accounts for 2% of all cancers. The incidence is increasing rapidly for unknown reasons. Whilst only 30% are resectable and 5-year survival is 10% in European studies, palliation is vital because inability to swallow saliva after oesophageal obstruction is a miserable way to die. Carcinoma of the cardia may mimic carcinoma of the lower third oesophagus, or achalasia (p. 74).

Causes

The cause is usually unknown. The importance of different factors varies in different parts of the world. Associations are:

• Alcohol

• Tobacco

• Barrett's oesophagus (p. 66)—the degree of risk is debated. Carcinoma can be the presenting feature of Barrett's oesophagus

• Following corrosive injury (p. 8)

• Achalasia (p. 74)—the risk (< 1%) is less than previously considered

• Iron-deficiency anaemia and postcricoid web, with high oesophageal carcinoma (Patterson–Brown–Kelly or Plummer–Vinson syndrome)—10 times commoner in women, often aged 40–50 years

• Geographical: Caspian littoral (northern Iran: commonest malignancy, although alcohol not consumed); northern China (20 times more common than in Britain); Transkei (South Africa). Molybdenum deficiency, aflatoxin

contamination of cereals and nitrosamines are postulated reasons for this variation
- Familial tylosis (palmar hyperkeratosis) is exceedingly rare

Clinical features

Progressive dysphagia and weight loss are typical, but pain and hoarseness of the voice may occur due to local spread. Patients are usually aged 60–80 years. Rapidly recurrent dysphagia after dilatation should be considered malignant until proven otherwise.

Pathology
- Cervical or mid-thoracic carcinomas are usually squamous
- Dysplasia may precede carcinoma
- Distal oesophageal tumours are often adenocarcinomas due to spread from the gastric fundus, or malignant change in Barrett's oesophagus. The incidence is increasing by 3–4% per year
- Pathology influences adjuvant therapy (see below)

Spread
- Local invasion along sub-mucosal lymphatics, or directly into mediastinal nodes is the rule
- Hiccups or a persistent mid-thoracic ache are ominous, indicating diaphragmatic or mediastinal invasion
- Oesophagobronchial fistula, recurrent laryngeal nerve palsy and atrial fibrillation may occur
- Death usually precedes distant metastases

Investigations

Diagnostic
- Barium swallow (Fig. 2.3, p. 69)
- Endoscopy, biopsy and brushings (98% detection rate), for a tissue diagnosis
- Endoscopists should define the upper and lower limits of macroscopic tumour, but must not dilate malignant oesophageal strictures at the initial endoscopy: this makes them inoperable

Look for complications
- Chest X-ray—mediastinal lymphadenopathy, evidence of aspiration
- ECG—atrial fibrillation

• Other head and neck tumours are common (about 10%) in squamous oesophageal carcinoma

Surgical assessment

• Thoracoabdominal CT scan, with a specific request to look for nodal involvement. It may underestimate mural and lymph node invasion
• Take into account age, cardiorespiratory disease and nutrition
• 'Operability' (patients considered able to survive an operation and live for more than 4 weeks) does not imply resectability
• Lung function tests (including arterial gases), to estimate respiratory reserve
• Endoscopic oesophageal ultrasonography is better than CT scan or MRI for assessing mural invasion and operability, but is not widely available
• The presence of lymph nodes is an indication for adjuvant therapy prior to surgery

Management

The objectives are to relieve dysphagia, prolong survival and to cure a minority. There is no ideal treatment; the site and type of the carcinoma and the general health of the patient determine the approach. Operability is the first decision.

Surgery

• Indicated for fit patients under 70 years without evidence of local invasion, when satisfactory resection can be achieved. This is less than a third of patients with oesophageal cancer
• An experienced oesophageal surgeon, perioperative nutritional support and good physiotherapy are important
• Sub-total oesophagectomy and formation of a gastric tube is usually appropriate, usually requiring separate thoracic and abdominal incisions
• Operative mortality is < 10% in experienced hands
• Surgery alone can only be expected to cure disease confined to the oesophageal wall
• The advent of endoscopically placed self-expanding metal stents has made it difficult to justify surgery for palliation alone

Radical radiotherapy

• Squamous carcinomas that are postcricoid or in the upper third may be radiosensitive
• Commonly converted into palliative therapy because of side-effects

Radiotherapy alone relieves dysphagia in < 50%, so continued endoscopic dilatation is necessary

Palliation

- For most (70%) patients
- Endoscopic dilatation should be performed initially for unresectable tumours, to allow patients to swallow food and saliva
- Surgical palliation is effective in experienced hands, but morbidity is much higher than endoscopic placement of a self-expanding metal stent
- Obstructing tumours are most effectively relieved by endoscopic laser therapy, although this is not always available. Alcohol injection into the tumour through a sclerotherapy needle is cheaper and safe, but less effective
- Intubation—with a self-expanding metal stent has become the procedure of choice for palliation. Swallowing is far better than with traditional plastic (e.g. Celestin) tubes. Covered metal stents are the tube of choice for palliation of perforated oesophageal tumours, which are usually caused by endoscopic dilation. Perforation, tube migration, blockage and persistent discomfort from proximal tubes are disadvantages
- Palliative radiotherapy may relieve pain, but is ineffective for long tumours or adenocarcinomas
- Neoadjuvant chemotherapy is showing encouraging results, especially with epirubicin and 5-fluorouracil. Specialist advice should be sought

Terminal care (p. 149)

Treatment should be carefully considered after assessing the patient, seeing the family and discussion with senior colleagues. Hydration, but not alimentation or antibiotics, is usually appropriate. Good mouth care, pharyngeal suction and liaison with the nursing staff are vital. Aspiration pneumonia is the usual cause of death.

Prognosis

- Mean survival is 10 months after diagnosis
- Overall 5-year survival is about 5%, which has changed little in the last 40 years
- In the minority (30%) who are selected for 'curative' surgery, 5-year survival is up to 25%. This is similar to the results of radical radiotherapy, but there are no direct comparative trials for equivalent stages of disease

2.5) **Achalasia**

Achalasia is a motility disorder characterized by absent peristalsis in the body of the oesophagus, increased lower oesophageal sphincter pressure (> 40 mmHg) and failure of sphincter relaxation during swallowing. It is due to degeneration of the myenteric plexus of unknown cause. Carcinoma of the cardia must be excluded.

Clinical features

- Occurs at any age
- Dysphagia—all patients. Unlike a stricture, dysphagia for liquids as well as solids occurs early (Fig. 2.1, p. 60). Slowly progressive; swallowing may be helped by a trick movement of the head, or Valsalva manoeuvre
- Regurgitation—70%; undigested food, with aspiration
- Weight loss—quite common
- Pain—sub-sternal cramps may be severe and precede dysphagia
- Symptoms for < 1 year and age > 50 years, with weight loss, suggest carcinoma
- Achalasia may present at an advanced stage. Megaoesophagus is a late manifestation that has been reported to cause respiratory obstruction (stridor). The risk of oesophageal carcinoma is increased in megaoesophagus
- Carcinoma of the cardia, gastric lymphoma, diffuse spasm, systemic sclerosis, Chagas' disease (South American trypanosomiasis) and amyloidosis can simulate achalasia

Investigations

- Chest X-ray—an oesophageal fluid level at the aortic knuckle and right lower lobe consolidation, or fibrosis may be present. The gastric air bubble is characteristically absent
- Barium swallow—food debris in the oesphagus with a smooth, tapered distal narrowing and aperistaltic contractions when recumbent are characteristic. Oesophageal dilatation develops later. A video or bread–barium swallow may elucidate difficult cases (Fig. 2.4)
- Endoscopy must always be performed to exclude a stricture and to examine the cardia for carcinoma. Once food debris is negotiated the endoscope easily passes the lower oesophageal sphincter
- Manometry (p. 465) may be the only way to distinguish oesophageal spasm from achalasia and should be performed if dysphagia persists despite a normal barium swallow (p. 82)

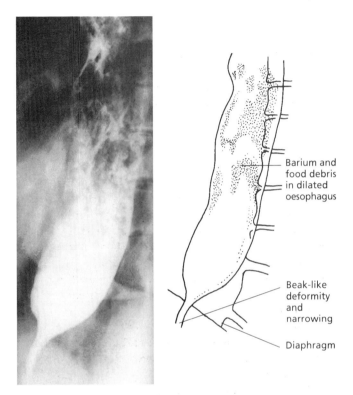

Fig. 2.4 Radiological appearance of achalasia. Barium swallow showing achalasia with dilatation of the oesophagus. Barium is mixing with food residue in the oesophagus. The oesophagus narrows to a typical beak-like deformity at the level of the cardia.

Management

The choice is between endoscopic dilatation and surgery (Heller's cardiomyotomy). Dilatation is often preferred by the patient, with surgery reserved for recurrent symptoms. Drugs have little role, but 5–10 mg sub-lingual dinitrate before meals may provide transient relief.

Botulinum toxin
• Intrasphincteric injections of botulinum toxin, using an endoscope and sclerotherapy needle, paralyse the hypertensive sphincter and abolish dysphagia in most patients
• The toxin is expensive and sphincter tone returns with time, with recurrence of dysphagia, but the risk of perforation with pneumatic dilatation is avoided

• This treatment is best performed in specialist units, but should be considered if there is recurrence or incomplete relief after pneumatic dilatation

Dilatation

• Pneumatic balloon dilatation with X-ray screening is effective in 70%, but repeat dilatations are often required
• Dilatation should only be performed by experienced endoscopists and the patient should be admitted overnight
• A chest X-ray in expiration is necessary 1 h after dilatation, before the patient eats, to look for mediastinal gas or pneumothorax. Perforation occurs in 2%

Surgery

• Indicated when symptoms recur after three attempts at dilatation, or if the patient prefers a definitive procedure at the outset
• Cardiomyotomy is effective in 90% and gives long-term relief. Thoracoscopic cardiomyotomy is being developed, but is still under evaluation

Complications

1 Megaoesophagus is now rare
2 Aspiration pneumonia can be chronic, or the presenting feature
3 Carcinoma may occur in untreated achalasia, but probably not after treatment. It is less common (< 5%) than previously thought
4 Treatment (dilatation or surgical) may lead to:
   • reflux
   • stricture
   • failure to relieve symptoms (reassess the diagnosis)
   • persistent pain, even after apparent relief of obstruction

2.6 **Other conditions** (Fig. 2.5)

Oesophageal dysmotility

Accounts for many patients referred with oesophageal symptoms. Chest pain or dysphagia for liquids and solids are the presenting features. Diffuse oesophageal spasm is the best characterized motility disorder other than achalasia, but is rare in its classical form. Symptoms are caused by high-amplitude, aperistaltic oesophageal contractions without a demonstrable

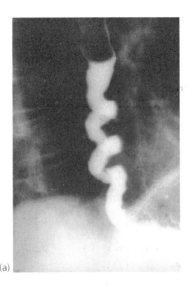

(a)

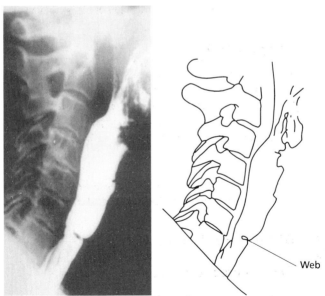

(b)

Web

Fig. 2.5 Radiological appearances of unusual causes of dysphagia.
(a) Barium swallow showing diffuse oesophageal spasm with a typical 'corkscrew' deformity. (b) Barium swallow showing a clearly defined web arising from the anterior wall of the oesophagus and partly encircling it. A jet of barium is passing through the narrowed lumen at the level of the web. (*Continued* on p. 78)

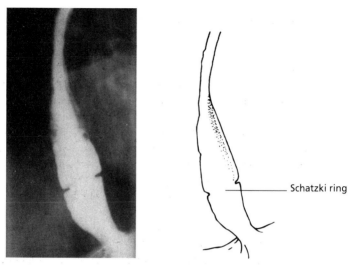

Schatzki ring

Fig. 2.5 (*continued*) (c) Barium swallow showing a narrow ring in the lower oesophagus. This is typical of the appearance of a Schatzki ring. The ring is often visible only when the oesophagus is fully distended by barium.

organic lesion. When symptoms occur without typical manometric or radiological features, the term 'oesophageal dysmotility' is appropriate.

Symptoms
- Dysphagia—intermittent, variable intensity, for both liquids and solids (Fig. 2.1, p. 60)
- Chest pain—may mimic cardiac pain or reflux (p. 81) and be provoked by stress. A persistent ache between severe episodes usually distinguishes it from angina (sometimes termed oesophagodynia)
- Coexistent symptoms of irritable bowel syndrome (p. 367), anxiety or depression are also common
- Weight loss is notably absent

Investigations
- Barium swallow—a corkscrew appearance is classic but unusual. Aperistaltic 'tertiary' contractions are common when recumbent, but stasis does not occur, unlike achalasia (Fig. 2.4, p. 75). Similar asymptomatic changes can occur in the elderly
- Manometry—diagnostic if positive. Repetitive contractions, high-amplitude waves and periods of normal peristalsis are typical, but occur together in a minority (<10%). Negative results do not exclude the diagnosis

• Endoscopy—should be normal, but helps exclude oesophagitis or a stricture

Treatment
• Symptoms are difficult to relieve totally. Reassurance that the pain is not cardiac is essential, also explaining that the drugs prescribed are often used for angina
• A proton-pump inhibitor (lansoprazole 30 mg or omeprazole 20–40 mg daily) should be tried first since dysmotility may be provoked by acid reflux
• Isosorbide dinitrate 5–10 mg sub-lingually four times daily or nifedipine 5–10mg three times daily are adjunctive treatments, but response is unpredictable and side-effects (i.e. headache) are common
• Prokinetic agents often make symptoms worse
• Empirical treatment with amitriptyline in low dose (10–30 mg daily) or Motival (1–3 tablets daily) can help
• Pneumatic dilatation should be reserved for the most severe cases because the outcome is unpredictable

Oesophageal webs

• Not circumferential, unlike rings (Fig. 2.5, p. 78)
• Demonstrated radiologically, but difficult to see at endoscopy
• May be associated with mucocutaneous disorders such as epidermolysis bullosa
• Check for iron-deficiency anaemia, associated with a postcricoid web and high oesophageal carcinoma (Plummer–Vinson syndrome)
• Exclude carcinoma of the upper third of the oesophagus by careful radiology and endoscopy. ENT advice may be necessary

Schatzki's ring

• Circumferential contraction in the middle or lower third, usually diagnosed radiologically rather than by endoscopy (Fig. 2.5, p. 77)
• Typically causes intermittent dysphagia for solids over a long period, but often asymptomatic and of no significance
• If dysphagia is present, dilatation is justified after biopsy. Occasionally pneumatic dilatation is necessary

Diverticula

• Pharyngeal pouches (Zenker's diverticulum) present with intermittent dysphagia and regurgitation in the elderly. Regurgitation of fluid when recumbent may lead to aspiration

- An ENT opinion is advisable after diagnosis by barium swallow taking care to show the upper oesophagus
- Routine endoscopy is not indicated and may be dangerous
- Surgical excision with cricopharyngeal myotomy is the treatment of choice for symptoms. Endoscopic excision by an experienced ENT surgeon is also effective
- Mid-oesophageal and epiphrenic diverticula are an endoscopic hazard, but of no other consequence

Systemic sclerosis

- Dysphagia and heartburn with Raynaud's phenomenon are characteristic
- Recurrent strictures caused by reflux and stasis are the principal problem
- CREST syndrome (digital calcinosis, Raynaud's phenomenon, dysphagia, sclerodactyly and telangiectasia) should be distinguished clinically from systemic sclerosis, because it has a better prognosis
- Proton-pump inhibitors at full doses (lansoprazole 30 mg/day, or omeprazole up to 60 mg/day or more) are the best treatment, because standard antireflux treatment is ineffective. Cisapride 10–20 mg three times daily may help oesophageal emptying
- Endoscopic dilatation is necessary for strictures
- Antireflux surgery may make the situation worse. Refractory cases should be referred to a specialist unit
- Other gastrointestinal complications (nutritional deficiency, malabsorption due to bacterial overgrowth or constipation) should be treated as well

Oesophageal infections

Oesophageal infections occur in the debilitated and immunocompromised (Section 11.4, p. 393). Underlying disease should be sought and treated.

Candidiasis

- Painful dysphagia (odynophagia) with oral candidiasis is typical
- Barium swallow, blind oesophageal brushings or endoscopy with biopsy are diagnostic
- Nystatin suspension 2 mL four times daily for 10 days is as effective and

has fewer side-effects than amphotericin (20 mg lozenges four times daily for 10 days)
• Oral flucytosine 50 mg/kg four times daily is better for patients with AIDS. Maintenance therapy may be needed
• Fever or neutropenia make systemic invasion likely and intravenous fluconazole is indicated

Cytomegalovirus
• Serpiginous or large ulcers in the mid-oesophagus cause painful dysphagia in the immunocompromised
• Oesophageal biopsy is diagnostic
• Ganciclovir (intravenous 5 mg/kg over 1 h, twice daily) for 14 days is only appropriate for severe infection. Recurrence is common

Herpes simplex
• Small, circumscribed ulcers in the mid-oesophagus are seen endoscopically. Ulcers may coalesce or bleed
• Electron microscopy of brushings transported in 4% glutaraldehyde is diagnostic
• Intravenous acyclovir 5 mg/kg three times daily, until tablets can be swallowed (200 mg five times daily for 5 days)

Rumination and regurgitation

Rumination is the chewing of regurgitated food that is then swallowed or spat out. Regurgitation is effortless and involuntary, although it may be a learned habit or indicate psychiatric disease such as bulimia or an anxiety state. It should be distinguished from recurrent vomiting by the lack of nausea and from gastro-oesophageal reflux in which bitter liquid reaches the mouth. Recognition of the disorder and 'unlearning' the habit through biofeedback techniques may help.

Clinical dilemmas

General advice for diagnostic dilemmas is given in Appendix 4 (p. 491).

Causes of chest pain

40% of patients with chest pain and a normal exercise ECG have an oesophageal disorder. The pain may be severe, wake patients from sleep or occur during emotional stress.

• Confirm the history—especially the duration and type of pain, provoking and relieving factors
• Oesophageal reflux and diffuse oesophageal spasm most commonly mimic angina
• An endoscopy to identify oesophagitis is indicated. Although a therapeutic trial of a proton-pump inhibitor may be appropriate, patients must avoid acid-suppressing medication for 3 weeks prior to endoscopy
• Oesophageal manometry and 24-h pH monitoring with symptom recording should be performed after referral to a specialist centre. Provocation tests (edrophonium for spasm or acid perfusion (Bernstein test) for reflux) occasionally help (p. 465)
• A video barium swallow in the recumbent position is an alternative method of diagnosing dysmotility
• Coronary angiography is indicated if no oesophageal lesion can be demonstrated and symptoms are disabling

Dysphagia with a 'normal' barium swallow

Globus hystericus is not the only cause. Diffuse spasm, achalasia and strictures may be overlooked.
• Confirm the history—especially whether dysphagia is for solids or liquids and the duration of symptoms
• Document the present weight and any loss
• Check the films:
  • Is it the correct patient?
  • Do the films show the entire oesophagus?
• Arrange a bread–barium swallow recorded on video, after discussion with the radiologist
• Referral for manometry (p. 465) is indicated for persistent symptoms. Obscure cases of diffuse spasm or achalasia may be detected

3 Stomach and Duodenum

3.1) **Dyspepsia**

Dyspepsia (indigestion) is a non-specific group of symptoms related to the upper gastrointestinal tract. Organic disease must be detected and distinguished from 'non-ulcer dyspepsia' or 'functional dyspepsia', so that specific treatment can be given. Table 3.1 shows the differential diagnosis of postprandial epigastric pain.

Causes

Clinical features

Common symptoms
- Epigastric, usually central upper abdominal, or retrosternal discomfort related to eating, specific foods, hunger or time of day
- Heaviness, unease, postprandial fullness or early satiety are common descriptive terms, often associated with heartburn, flatulence or borborygmi

Indicators of organic disease
- Age > 45 years (but duodenal ulcers are most common at age 20–40 years)
- Symptoms for > 8 weeks
- Radiation to back
- Weight loss
- Associated anorexia
- Dysphagia
- Gastrointestinal blood loss
- Symptoms in smokers, or those taking NSAIDs
- Symptoms at night

Table 3.1 Differential diagnosis of postprandial epigastric pain.

Common	Uncommon*	Rare
Non-ulcer dyspepsia	Biliary colic	Chronic pancreatitis
Duodenal ulcer	Gastro-oesophageal reflux	Small intestinal stricture
Gastric ulcer	Oesophagitis	Mesenteric ischaemia
Duodenitis		Myocardial ischaemia
Gastric cancer		

*Although these conditions are common, they do not usually present with epigastric pain after meals.

Examination
- Epigastric tenderness is non-specific
- Palpate carefully for an upper abdominal mass
- Feel for supraclavicular nodes and hepatomegaly
- Check for ascites

Investigations

- Not all patients need investigation. A therapeutic trial of antacids is indicated if the patient is aged < 45 years, has negative serology for *Helicobacter pylori*, or a negative ^{13}C- or ^{14}C-urea breath test and symptoms are of < 8 weeks duration. Magnesium trisilicate mixture 20 mL as needed is cheap and as good as any alternative (p. 92)
- However, peptic ulcers uncommonly occur in *H. pylori*-negative patients who are not on ulcerogenic drugs

Indications for investigation
The British Society of Gastroenterology guidelines (Appendix 2, p. 480) refer to 'alarm symptoms or signs', indicating a greater likelihood of organic pathology than in other patients and the need for diagnostic upper gastrointestinal endoscopy:
- Age > 45 years with recent onset dyspepsia
- Age < 45 years with positive *H. pylori* serology
- Ulcerogenic medication (e.g. NSAIDs, steroids)
- Vomiting
- Unintentional weight loss
- Symptoms of gastrointestinal blood loss
- Iron-deficiency anaemia
- Epigastric mass
- Previous gastric ulcer
- Epigastric pain severe enough to hospitalize a patient

Specific investigations
- Blood tests—anaemia, a high platelet count or ESR and abnormal liver function tests indicate an organic cause
- Barium meal or endoscopy (see below)
- Ultrasound of the gall bladder and pancreas, if the endoscopy is normal

Barium meal or endoscopy?

Endoscopy is preferable for the initial investigation of dyspepsia because:

• Mucosal lesions (oesophagitis, gastritis, erosions, duodenitis and superficial ulceration) can be seen
• Biopsies can be taken to exclude malignancy and the identification of *H. pylori*
• It is generally well tolerated, especially by the elderly, with light sedation
• Endoscopy is indicated in all patients with dyspepsia aged > 45 years, and younger patients with positive *H. pylori* serology or urea breath test, or any alarm features (see above), or a history of ulcerogenic medication
   A barium meal is indicated if:
• Endoscopy is difficult or impossible—young drinkers tolerate the procedure poorly
• Oesophagogastric anatomy needs defining—cup and spill deformity or anastomoses can confuse endoscopists (Fig. 3.1). It is often easier to evaluate pyloric stenosis, or tumour infiltrating the stomach wall, by barium meal
• A good barium study will identify motility disorders of the oesophagus, which may be missed endoscopically
• The choice may be determined by local availability

Organic dyspepsia

Dyspepsia due to lesions readily identified on routine investigation:
• Duodenal or gastric ulcer
• Duodenitis—usually part of the duodenal ulcer diathesis (Section 3.7, p. 115)
• Gastric cancer
• Reflux oesophagitis
• Gastritis—this is controversial. It is best considered as a histological diagnosis
• Cholelithiasis—pain is usually severe
• Management of organic disease is discussed in the appropriate sections

Non-ulcer (functional) dyspepsia

Defined as upper abdominal or retrosternal discomfort related to meals, lasting for more than 8 weeks and for which no cause can be found after investigation. Rational investigation and management is helped by identifying one of three symptom patterns: dysmotility, reflux or ulcer type.

Dysmotility type non-ulcer dyspepsia
• Upper abdominal pain:

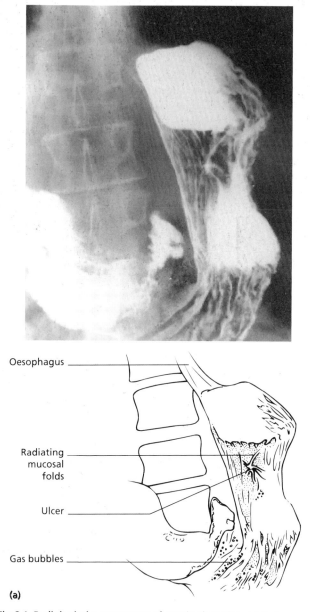

Oesophagus

Radiating mucosal folds

Ulcer

Gas bubbles

(a)

Fig. 3.1 Radiological appearances of peptic ulceration. (a) Barium meal showing a benign gastric ulcer in the body of the stomach, with gastric folds radiating from the edge of the ulcer crater.

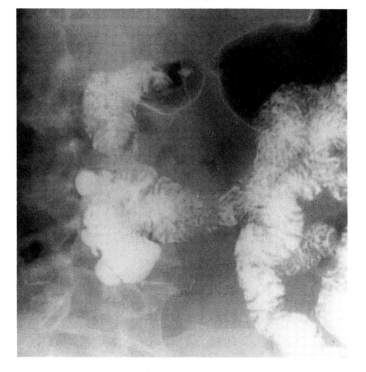

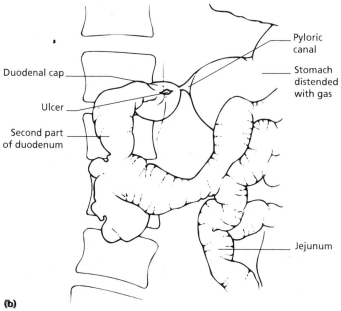

Pyloric canal

Duodenal cap

Stomach distended with gas

Ulcer

Second part of duodenum

Jejunum

(b)

(b) Barium meal showing an ulcer in the first part of the duodenum

- - poorly localized
  - may be several types
  - not at night
  - continuous, rather than periodic
- Abdominal distension
- Premature satiety
- Nausea—but vomiting is unusual
- Food intolerance—variable, but often several types of food

Reflux type non-ulcer dyspepsia
- Retrosternal discomfort:
  - on stooping
  - after large meals
  - on lying flat
  - temporary relief from antacids
- Recent weight gain
- Smoker
- Cyclical severity
- No endoscopic or histological evidence of oesophagitis

Ulcer type non-ulcer dyspepsia
- Epigastric pain:
  - may be described as epigastric burning
  - occasionally at night
- Relieved by antacids or food, or worse after meals; episodic
- No ulcer, past or present

It should be noted that there is often considerable symptom overlap and that many also have symptoms of irritable bowel syndrome (p. 367).

There remain some patients who have upper abdominal pain after meals who do not fit into one of these patterns. Features common to all patients with non-ulcer dyspepsia are:
- The patient remains well
- Weight is steady or fluctuating
- Normal investigations

Treatment of non-ulcer dyspepsia
- Explanation and reassurance are essential
- Lifestyle changes (regular meals, weight loss, less alcohol, stopping smoking) often help
- Drugs should only be used when symptoms are intolerable. Antacids

should always be tried first. The following recommendations are made, but controlled trials have either not shown clear benefits from drug treatments, or have not been performed with some agents

• Dysmotility type—antispasmodic or prokinetic agent (e.g. mebeverine 135 mg or metoclopramide 10 mg three times daily 30 min before meals). Prokinetic drugs such as cisapride have been effective in several trials, including patients with normal gastric motility

• Reflux type—H_2-antagonist or prokinetic agent (e.g. cimetidine 400 mg twice daily, metoclopramide 10 mg three times daily). A therapeutic trial of a proton-pump inhibitor is often difficult to avoid, but if symptoms persist this effectively excludes an acid-related disorder and treatment stopped

• Ulcer type—H_2-antagonist. Eradication of *H. pylori* is indicated. There is evidence that eradication of *H. pylori* relieves symptoms of functional dyspepsia in a small proportion (around 20%), but significantly more than placebo

• Other patients often respond poorly to treatment. An exclusion diet (p. 421) may help

Table 3.2 Recommended treatment options for *Helicobacter pylori*.

Drug	Dose	Frequency	Duration	Cost (NHS, 1998)
PPI	See below	Twice daily ⎫		
Clarithromycin	500 mg*	Twice daily ⎬	1 week	£37.02
Metronidazole	400 mg	Twice daily ⎭		
or				
PPI	See below	Twice daily ⎫		
Amoxycillin	500 mg	Three times daily ⎬	1 week	£20.12
Metronidazole	400 mg	Three times daily ⎭		
or				
PPI	See below	Twice daily ⎫		
Amoxycillin	500 mg	Twice daily ⎬	1 week	£42 approx
Clarithromycin	500 mg	Twice daily ⎭		
Quadruple therapy for initial treatment failure				
Any of triple therapy regimens with DeNol (bismuth subcitrate)	1 tablet	Three times daily	1 week	

Alternative drugs with similar efficacy and cost
PPI = omeprazole 20 mg or lansoprazole 30 mg
Tinidazole 500 mg can be used in place of metronidazole

*Clarithromycin 250 mg is only slightly less effective in this regime.

Which antacid?

There are 70 antacid preparations in the British National Formulary, not all of which are prescribable on the NHS. Efficacy, peripheral effects and cost need to be considered.

Efficacy
- *In vitro* neutralizing capacity is greatest with magnesium hydroxide/ aluminium hydroxide mixtures (Maalox, Mucaine)
- Alginates (Gastrocote, Gaviscon) have low neutralizing capacity but may be better for gastro-oesophageal reflux
- Liquids act more quickly than tablets, but the latter are more convenient

Peripheral effects
- Sodium content is important in patients with cardiovascular, renal or hepatic disease. Magnesium trisilicate mixture has Na 6.3 mmol/10 mL whereas Maalox has 0.1 mmol/10 mL. Gastrocote has half the Na content of Gaviscon
- Aluminium compounds bind bile salts and may be more effective in biliary reflux. They also cause constipation and can be absorbed, which contributes to osteodystrophy and encephalopathy in renal disease
- Magnesium compounds can cause diarrhoea
- Absorption of other drugs (iron, antibiotics, phenothiazines) may be impaired by antacids
- Rebound hyperacidity can occur after regular antacid treatment has been stopped. This can contribute to stress ulcers

Cost
- Magnesium trisilicate, Maalox and aluminium hydroxide tablets are the cheapest (20–30 p for 20 tablets)
- Gaviscon and Gaviscon tablets cost about 75 p for 20 tablets and Gaviscon mixture costs five times as much as magnesium trisilicate mixture

Recommendations
- Magnesium trisilicate tablets or mixture for routine use
- Gaviscon for reflux-type symptoms
- Maalox if a low-sodium antacid is required
- Aluminium hydroxide mixture for biliary reflux
- Acid-suppressing drugs are almost invariably prescribed (H_2-receptor antagonists and some PPIs such as lanzoprazole 15 mg daily are licensed for acid-like dyspepsia), but results are variable

3.2 Nausea and vomiting

The timing, amount and content of the vomitus are important. Associated symptoms often indicate the cause, since isolated nausea or vomiting are rarely organic.

Causes

- Abdominal:
  - gastroenteritis
  - gastric or duodenal ulcer
  - pyloric stenosis
  - ileus
  - intestinal obstruction
  - cholecystitis
  - pancreatitis
  - achalasia
- Metabolic:
  - diabetic ketoacidosis
  - hypercalcaemia
  - hyponatraemia
  - uraemia
- Drugs:
  - opiates, chemotherapy, sulphasalazine, digoxin and many others
  - alcohol
- Cerebral:
  - migraine
  - raised intracranial pressure
  - brain stem lesions
- Vestibular:
  - Menière's disease
  - motion sickness
  - viral (rarely bacterial) labyrinthitis
- Endocrine:
  - pregnancy (easy to miss in the first trimester and patients may not volunteer the presence of amenorrhoea; a tactful direct enquiry will usually produce the true answer)
  - Addison's disease
- Other organic—myocardial infarction
- Non-organic:
  - non-ulcer dyspepsia

- bulimia, anorexia nervosa
- self-induced
- psychogenic

Investigations and management

Assessment
- Look for signs of dehydration
- Listen for a gastric succussion splash and feel for a mass
- Examine the vomitus for volume, blood and bile (the latter indicates patent pylorus)
- Check the urine—osmolality, glucose and a pregnancy test
- Request serum electrolytes, urea, random glucose and calcium
- Metabolic alkalosis (pH > 7.44, $PaCO_2$ > 45 mmHg or 6.0 kPa) only occurs in severe vomiting
- Arrange an endoscopy if vomiting is persistent (p. 95)

Drugs
- Metoclopramide 10 mg three times daily (parenterally) or other prokinetic agent (domperidone, cisapride) for causes other than mechanical obstruction (p. 42)
- Prochlorperazine 25 mg suppository or 12.5 mg intramuscularly, but not intravenously, for metabolic or drug-induced vomiting. A digoxin level within the therapeutic range may still cause vomiting
- Cinnarizine 15 mg or promethazine 25 mg orally for vestibular disorders
- Domperidone 20 mg orally or 60 mg suppository has fewer extrapyramidal side-effects than metoclopramide and is preferable in the elderly and in patients aged < 21 years

Pregnancy
- Avoid all drugs if at all possible
- Promethazine 25 mg oral/injection may be given even in the first trimester, if really necessary

Chemotherapy
- Intravenous dexamethasone 8 mg with lorazepam 2 mg before chemotherapy
- Domperidone 60 mg suppositories four times daily help persistent nausea
- 5-HT$_3$ antagonists (such as ondansetron 8 mg three times daily, oral or parenteral, for a few days) may also be helpful

Persistent vomiting

- Review the diagnosis, especially considering cerebral, brain stem (fourth ventricle), metabolic and mechanical causes
- Arrange an endoscopy if not already performed
- Combination therapy occasionally helps when single drugs fail
- Methotrimeprazine 100 mg by continuous subcutaneous infusion daily is useful in terminal care

3.3 Gastritis

Inflammation of the gastric mucosa (gastritis) represents the stomach's response to infection or injury. Whether gastritis is transient or related to peptic ulcer and gastric cancer depends on the site, type and cause of inflammation.

Classification

Gastritis may be immune or non-immune. The latter is by far the commonest and is usually associated with *H. pylori* colonization of the foregut. Many classifications have been proposed, but the Sydney (1990) system remains the most acceptable, because it combines topographical and morphological details (Table 3.3).

Three types of gastritis are now recognized—acute, chronic and special forms. These are then qualified by site, morphology and associated aetiology, if known.

Site

The stomach is divided into two topographical areas—antrum and body. Gastritis in both sites is termed pangastritis.

Table 3.3 Summary of the Sydney classification of gastritis.

Type	Site	Morphology	Aetiology
Acute	Antrum	Inflammation	Microbial (*H. pylori**)
Chronic	Body	Activity	Non-microbial
Special forms	Pangastritis	Atrophy	autoimmune
granulomatous		Metaplasia	alcohol
eosinophilic		*H. pylori* density	postgastrectomy
lymphocytic			NSAID
hypertrophic			chemical
reactive			Unknown

*Other microbial causes are very rare.

Morphology

The five principal features (inflammation, activity, atrophy, intestinal metaplasia and numbers of *H. pylori*) are graded none, mild, moderate or severe.

- Inflammation reflects the number of chronic inflammatory cells in the lamina propria
- Activity means the presence of neutrophil polymorphs which characterize acute gastritis
- Atrophy evaluates the depth of gastric glands. It is positively related to gastric ulcer, or to cancer and negatively associated with duodenal ulcer
- Intestinal metaplasia is fairly common in chronic gastritis and in association with gastric ulcers or cancer. It may precede early gastric cancer, but is not necessarily premalignant
- Numbers of *H. pylori*, detected by Giemsa or Gram stain (culture and urease techniques only indicate presence or absence of the organism), indicate the density of infection

Other morphological features of gastritis are the presence of erosions (common in acute gastritis), or diagnostic features of special forms (granulomas, eosinophils, cytomegalovirus) which are not graded.

Aetiology

- Microbial—*H. pylori* (see below; Fig. 3.2) causes almost all chronic gastritis (> 95%). *Gastrospirillum hominis* (another spiral bacterium), cytomegalovirus or herpes virus are very rare causes
- Non-microbial causes are listed in Table 3.3. Autoimmune-associated chronic gastritis is largely confined to the body of the stomach, where it causes atrophy, anacidity, B_{12} deficiency and predisposes to cancer

Previous terms for gastritis

- Previous descriptive terms include types A (autoimmune, in the gastric body, associated with atrophy), B (bacterial, in the antrum), AB (pangastritis) or C (chemical, drug-induced)
- Chronic superficial gastritis (acute on chronic gastritis), chronic atrophic gastritis (distinct from gastric atrophy from autoimmune causes) are other terms that have been used

Current aspects of H. pylori

H. pylori is one of the commonest human infections. *H. pylori* is strongly associated with gastritis (which may become atrophic), with gastric and duodenal ulcer, gastric cancer, Ménétrièr's disease and mucosal-associated

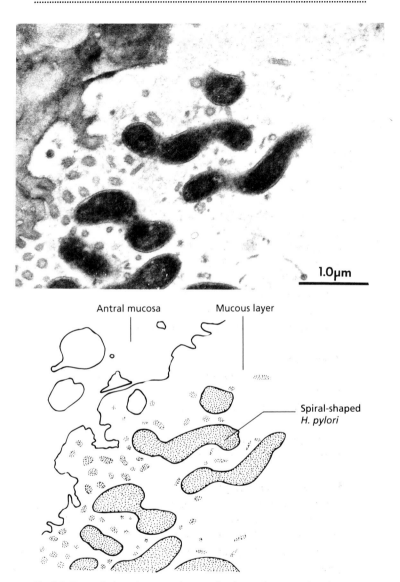

Fig. 3.2 Transmission electron micrograph of antral mucosa in a human patient, illustrating the spiral shape of *Helicobacter pylori*.

lymphoid tissue (MALT) lymphoma. Associations with functional dyspepsia and NSAID-related ulcers are uncertain. However, most individuals come to no harm. There is no recognized association with gastro-oesophageal reflux disease.

Epidemiology

• *H. pylori* has a worldwide distribution, but is much more prevalent in emergent countries, where 80–90% of the population are colonized by the late teens. This has implications for the management of patients born outside the UK

• The route of infection is uncertain. Oro-oral, gastro-oral or faeco-oral routes are possibilities

• *H. pylori* infection can be acquired through inadequately sterilized endoscopes or nasogastric tubes

Pathophysiology

• *H. pylori* can cause inflammation in the antrum (antritis) or body (corpusitis) of the stomach, although these often overlap. Some serotypes, especially those producing Cag A or Vac A cytotoxins, appear to be more pathogenic than others

• Antritis appears to be characterized by hypergastrinaemia and consequently increased acid output and higher risk of duodenal ulcer. Why only a minority of patients with antritis develop duodenal ulceration remains poorly understood. It is likely to be a balance between the pathogenicity of the type of *H. pylori* and other mucosal defence factors (p. 104)

• Duodenitis is caused by *H. pylori* colonization of islands of gastric metaplasia in the duodenal bulb, which are triggered by high acid output

• *H. pylori* corpusitis may lead to gastric mucosal atrophy, decreased acid secretion and increased risk of gastric ulcer or gastric cancer

• Factors determining development of predominant antritis or corpusitis are not clearly understood

Diagnosis of *H. pylori* infection

Non-invasive methods

Serology and breath tests have high sensitivity and specificity.

Serology

• Used for screening and epidemiological studies

• No use for confirming eradication, because antibody titres decline very slowly

• Hospital-based serology is reliable, but 'near-patient' or 'office' kits are less reliable and are best validated for the local population
• Serology is best used for younger patients: false-negative results are more common in patients aged > 50 years, or in children

Urea-breath test (p. 466)
• One of the most reliable methods of detection and ideal for confirming successful eradication
• Depends on detection of urease activity from *H. pylori* by including ^{13}C- or ^{14}C-labelled urea in a test meal. Urea is split by urease into NH_4 and CO_2 and the latter detected in expired air. ^{13}C-labelled urea is increasingly used as it is non-radioactive
• The patient must stop proton-pump inhibitors, antibiotics, prokinetic drugs and bismuth-containing medications for 4 weeks and fast for 6 h before the test
• Any post-treatment test must be delayed for at least 4 weeks after the end of therapy to avoid false-negative results

Invasive methods
These all depend on endoscopic biopsies and are also highly sensitive and specific, although false-negative results can occur with concurrent treatment with proton-pump inhibitors, antibiotics and bismuth-containing medications. They are suitable for diagnosis and for determining the results of treatment, although the same timing as for urea breath test applies.

CLO or urease test
• One or preferably two antral biopsies are placed in a medium containing urea and a pH indicator
• Hydrolysis of urea by urease from *H. pylori* changes the pH with a pink colour developing within a few hours. Commercial kits (CLO test) are available, but test kits costing a few pence can be made by the hospital laboratory, although these need to be locally validated
• Two biopsies from the body of the stomach are also needed if the patient is on PPIs, which may cause migration of *H. pylori* to the corpus

Histology of gastric biopsies
• Stained with Giemsa or even haematoxylin and eosin
• Two juxtapyloric biopsies are needed, as well as two biopsies from the corpus to define the histological type of gastritis (Table 3.3, p. 95)
• Immunohistochemical stains for specific *H. pylori* antigens are also available

Culture of H. pylori

- The gold standard, but is expensive and best reserved for the determination of antibiotic sensitivity when initial treatment has failed
- A proportion of cultures fail to grow, so a negative culture is not proof of successful treatment

Consequences of diagnosis

Once infection has been diagnosed, it is almost impossible to avoid treatment. This should be borne in mind.

Indications for treatment of H. pylori

- Only three indications are fully supported by evidence-based medicine: duodenal ulcer, gastric ulcer and MALT lymphoma
- Patients with uncomplicated duodenal or gastric ulcers should have eradication therapy (Table 3.2, p. 91) at the time of diagnosis
- There is no need for additional acid suppression, except in special circumstances (complicated ulcers (see below), gastro-oesophageal reflux, treatment failure)
- It is strongly recommended that patients with MALT lymphomas are managed at tertiary referral centres
- Patients with duodenitis who are *H. pylori*-positive should be considered as part of the duodenal ulcer diathesis and are probably best given eradication treatment at diagnosis
- Other conditions in which *H. pylori* colonization can be present and may be causally associated are gastritis, drug-induced ulcers, functional dyspepsia, Ménétrièr's disease, gastric cancer and gastric lymphoma (see below)

Treatment of *H. pylori* infection

- The aim of treatment is eradication of the bacterium from the foregut, defined by negative urea/breath test or endoscopic biopsies (not serology or culture), performed at least 4 weeks after the end of treatment
- Treatment fails most often because of poor compliance, or bacterial resistance
- Good compliance can be ensured by counselling the patient regarding the reason for treatment, need for compliance, explanation of dosage schedule, post-treatment tests, possible side-effects, etc.
- The most common (and increasing) bacterial resistance is to metronidazole and if this is likely (e.g. ethnic communities, previous treatment with metronidazole or tinidazole, female) non-metronidazole regimens should be used

• Clarithromycin-resistant strains of *H. pylori* are less common (although said to be increasing). Amoxycillin resistance is exceptional
• Monotherapy regimens must not be used, as they are ineffective and promote resistance
• Dual therapy (usually a proton-pump inhibitor or ranitidine bismuth citrate (RBC) with clarithromycin for 2 weeks) is expensive and the results can be variable. Results of 1 week with RBC and clarithromycin look more promising
• Short-course triple (or quadruple) therapy administered for 1 week forms the basis of European guidelines (Table 3.2, p. 91). Triple therapy regimens consist of a PPI combined with two of amoxycillin, clarithromycin or metronidazole (or tinidazole)
• Quadruple therapy regimens contain bismuth in addition to triple therapy. Whilst these can be used for first-line treatment, compliance is likely to be less good and they are most often reserved for failures of triple therapy
• Triple or quadruple therapy regimens successfully eradicate *H. pylori* in around 90% of patients

Testing after treatment
• Testing by urea/breath test or endoscopic biopsy must be performed at least 4 weeks after treatment has been completed and drugs stopped
• Symptomatic recurrence in an uncomplicated duodenal ulcer is a good predictor of treatment failure
• Confirming eradication is not necessary in every patient if cost is a problem, but is essential in:
  • complicated duodenal ulcers (e.g. after haemorrhage)
  • all gastric ulcers
  • treatment of MALT lymphoma (p. 114)
• Retesting is also helpful in patients with persistent symptoms in spite of eradication therapy for duodenal ulceration, or dyspepsia in the presence of *H. pylori*. However, patients with duodenal ulcers may develop reflux symptoms after eradication and these must be distinguished from ulcer recurrence

Results of eradication and further treatment of ulcers
• Simple duodenal and gastric ulcers will heal after eradication of *H. pylori* without any further acid-suppressive treatment
• Complicated ulcers (e.g. after a bleed) need acid suppression with a PPI or H_2-receptor antagonist until complete ulcer healing. This should always be confirmed endoscopically in gastric ulcers 8–12 weeks after the

presenting episode, and is also best management for complicated duodenal ulcers. However, some gastroenterologists eradicate $H.$ $pylori$, continue treatment with a PPI for 4 weeks and check eradication with a breath test at 8 weeks

• Tests for $H.$ $pylori$ should be done at the following endoscopy, but if the patient is still taking PPIs or H_2-receptor antagonists, then mucosal biopsies must be taken from the body as well as the antrum and sent for histology

• Perforated ulcers and NSAID-associated ulceration are best treated with long-term acid suppression, since these are weakly associated with $H.$ $pylori$. Either PPIs (omeprazole 10 mg, lansoprazole 15 mg daily) or H_2-receptor antagonist (e.g. cimetidine 400 mg or ranitidine 150 mg) can be used post-perforation, but PPIs at full dose are probably preferable in NSAID ulcers and should be given for the duration of NSAID treatment, especially in elderly patients. It is often difficult to stop NSAIDs, and PPIs are better than misoprostol for prophylaxis after an ulcer has occurred

Reinfection after eradication
Reinfection in adults living in the West is low, around 1–3%. Reinfection in children is more common.

Clinical features and investigations

Gastritis can only be reliably diagnosed by histology and can only be adequately classified when biopsies have been taken from both the body and antrum of the stomach. Histological gastritis does not always correlate with either endoscopic appearances or symptoms, and consequently does not always need treatment.

Acute gastritis
• Caused by drugs (salicylates), alcohol, or trauma (stress erosions). $H.$ $pylori$-associated acute gastritis is rarely seen, because infection is usually acquired in early childhood. Infection can also be iatrogenic, transmitted through inadequately sterilized endoscopes or nasogastric tubes

• Often asymptomatic, but dyspepsia, retching, halitosis or haematemesis may occur

• Endoscopic appearances range from normal to erythema or erosions which may be obscured by haemorrhagic oozing (Section 1.5, p. 19)

Chronic gastritis

• Common worldwide, especially in developing countries, or in patients of low socioeconomic status. Prevalence increases with age (in the West about 50% have some chronic gastritis when aged >60 years)

• Almost always caused by *H. pylori*, and only very occasionally auto-immune (p. 104)

• Often antral, asymptomatic and stable for many years

• *H. pylori*-positive antritis predisposes to duodenal ulceration (2–20%)

• Corpusitis predisposes to gastric ulcers. A small proportion (about 3% at each stage) develop intestinal metaplasia, progress to atrophy and then to cancer

• Parietal cell antibodies occur in 10% of patients with chronic gastritis. Pernicious anaemia (in about 10% of those with antibodies, but up to 80% when titre > 1:40) is associated with autoimmune thyroiditis, adrenalitis, vitiligo and insulin-dependent diabetes mellitus

Special forms

• Granulomatous gastritis is a rare feature of sarcoidosis or Crohn's disease

• Eosinophilic gastritis is extremely rare and may indicate vasculitis

• Hypertrophic gastritis (Ménétrièr's disease) is a rare condition that may cause weight loss and diarrhoea due to protein-losing enteropathy. It is strongly associated with *H. pylori*, which should be eradicated. Hypertrophic mucosal folds at endoscopy must be distinguished from lymphoma

• Lymphocytic gastritis causes a varioliform pattern in the fundus

• Reactive gastritis refers to duodenogastric reflux (postgastrectomy) or drugs

Management

• Asymptomatic gastritis does not need treatment, but see Sections 3.1 (p. 91)

• General measures such as avoiding provoking factors (alcohol, NSAIDs and smoking, although the latter is not proven) are appropriate for all symptomatic patients

• Symptomatic treatment with antacids or drugs for non-ulcer dyspepsia (p. 90) are suitable when a specific cause cannot be identified

• In reality, *H. pylori*-positive gastritis is almost invariably treated with eradication therapy (Table 3.2, p. 91), although there is only preliminary evidence for this. Perhaps treatment can be justified on the grounds that it is not possible to predict the ultimate outcome of gastritis in any individual

Specific treatment for other types of gastritis

- Acute gastritis, with bleeding from erosions, is treated with a PPI (omeprazole, lansoprazole, or pantoprazole, p. 20). Sucralfate 1 g four times daily is also used in an intensive care unit context
- Autoimmune-associated gastritis—serum B_{12} should be measured and if <150 ng/L, intramuscular hydroxycobalamin 1000 µg is needed every 3 months for life
- Intestinal metaplasia alone is not an indication for treatment, or repeat endoscopy, unless associated with a gastric ulcer

3.4) Gastric ulcer

Benign gastric ulcers on the lesser curve (Fig. 3.1 p. 88) occur predominantly in the elderly. Ulcers on the greater curve, fundus and in the antrum are more commonly malignant. Gastric ulcers are less common than duodenal ulcers before the age of 40 years, but become more common in the elderly. Features and treatment for gastric and duodenal ulcers are compared in Table 3.5 (p. 119).

Causes

- More than 90% of benign, non-NSAID gastric ulcers are associated with *H. pylori*. Infection is characterized by chronic corpusitis, as opposed to antritis in duodenal ulcers
- Drug-related ulcers (NSAIDs, steroids) are the next most common cause, but may be a separate entity. There are often few symptoms before a complication occurs. The risk of ulceration in patients on steroids has probably been exaggerated
- Chronic, benign ulceration is more strongly associated with smoking than alcohol. Environmental stress may be weakly associated
- Acute ulcers or 'erosions' (small, superficial ulcers) are a separate entity and are related to stress (Cushing's or Curling's ulcers, after neurosurgery or burns, respectively)
- Additional proposed mechanisms include impairment of the mucus–bicarbonate barrier, deficient gastric mucosal blood flow (possibly related to PGE_2) and acid–pepsin damage. Duodenogastric reflux of bile may also damage the mucosa. Although the dictum 'no acid, no ulcer' is valid, acid secretion in patients with chronic gastric ulcers is frequently in the low to normal range

Clinical features

• Ulcers cannot be diagnosed by history or physical examination, nor can gastric or duodenal ulcers be differentiated on clinical grounds. 'Typical' ulcer pain (epigastric, related to meals and relieved by antacids) is non-specific (Table 3.1, p. 85)

• Vomiting, weight loss or unremitting pain sometimes predominate in elderly patients with a gastric ulcer, but malignancy must be excluded by multiple targeted biopsy and brush cytology. Some may be asymptomatic, especially NSAID-associated ulcers, perhaps because of the analgesic effect of the drug

• Complications (haematemesis or perforation, p. 20) may be the presenting feature

Investigations

Blood tests

• Serum ferritin (or iron and total iron binding capacity) should be measured if the patient is anaemic. A microcytic anaemia can also be caused by chronic disease, thalassaemia trait or sideroblastic anaemia, as well as iron deficiency (p. 359)

Endoscopy

• Multiple targeted rim and crater biopsies as well as brush cytology are mandatory, except for gastric ulcers that have recently bled

• When gastric ulcers are diagnosed at emergency endoscopy for bleeding, a further endoscopy should be arranged after the bleeding has stopped, to allow biopsies and brushings to be taken

• Repeat endoscopy after 8–12 weeks of treatment should be booked at the time of diagnosis, to confirm healing. The ulcer site must be biopsied, even if the ulcer has healed. Further endoscopies, with more brushings and biopsies, are necessary for persistent ulcers until complete healing has occurred

• Symptomatic relapse after a gastric ulcer has been diagnosed is an indication for repeat endoscopy

Barium meal

When a gastric ulcer is shown on a barium meal (Fig. 3.1, p. 88), endoscopy should be arranged for biopsies and brushings.

Management

General

• *H. pylori* eradication is the first line of treatment for uncomplicated gastric ulcers (Table 3.2, p. 91). In complicated or *H. pylori*-negative gastric ulcers, additional acid suppression is needed

• Stop smoking—this increases the healing rate and decreases relapse rate

• Alcohol intake—should be curtailed if excessive (this means > 21 units/ week for women, > 28 units/week for men), but abstinence is unnecessary

Which acid suppressant?

• Acid suppression is unnecessary in uncomplicated gastric (and duodenal) ulceration associated with *H. pylori*

• All PPIs heal 90% benign gastric ulcers in 4–6 weeks

• H_2-receptor antagonists remain highly effective (up to 90% healing), but take longer to work (6–12 weeks)

• Cost is a major consideration, but shorter courses of PPIs are less expensive than proprietary H_2-receptor antagonist; however, now that generic H_2-receptor antagonists at a fraction of the cost are available, the cost balance will change

• Generic cimetidine or ranitidine have similar efficacy, although ranitidine may be preferable in those with liver disease or those taking anticonvulsants or anticoagulants, since it does not interfere with hepatic metabolism. A single dose at 6 p.m. is as effective for healing ulcers as divided doses

• In reality, a PPI is now usually prescribed because it is conveniently part of the *H. pylori* eradication and compliance is likely to be improved

• Lansoprazole 30 mg daily may be slightly more effective and cheaper than omeprazole 20 mg daily, but is best taken without food. It may be as effective as omeprazole 40 mg daily. Omeprazole could be more effective than lansoprazole for preventing recurrent peptic strictures. Pantoprazole 40 mg daily has similar efficacy and is competitively priced, but also does not induce hepatic metabolism. This may be an advantage since it should have fewer drug interactions, but it is not yet licensed in the UK for eradication therapy or longer term use

• NSAID-associated gastric ulcers are best healed by PPIs, but H_2-receptor antagonists are also effective, even if NSAIDs have to be continued. Maintenance treatment is recommended if NSAIDs cannot be stopped (see above). Misoprostol 200 µg twice daily can be used for healing NSAID-related gastric ulcers, but diarrhoea occurs in about 20% of patients

Maintenance treatment

• Indicated for patients with cardiorespiratory disease, or any disorder that would affect survival in the event of developing complications of a recurrent ulcer

• Indicated for patients on NSAIDs with a history of ulceration. Many prefer PPIs for the maintenance of NSAID-related ulcers. Omeprazole 10–20 mg daily is currently the only PPI licensed for this indication and may safely be given long term in elderly patients. It should be continued for the duration of NSAID therapy. Misoprostol 200 µg twice daily may also prevent gastric ulcers in patients on NSAIDs, but there are no indications for prescribing this drug routinely and side-effects are more common than with PPIs

Resistant ulcers

• Ulcers that have not healed after 8 weeks of treatment must be rebiopsied and brushed for cytology, as well as taking biopsies from the antrum and corpus to check for *H. pylori* eradication

• In unhealed ulcers, prescribe quadruple therapy (Table 3.2, p. 91) if *H. pylori* has not been eradicated, then double the dose of PPI for a further 8 weeks and arrange a repeat endoscopy

• Poor compliance is probably the commonest cause of failure to heal

• Persistent failure of a gastric ulcer to heal after 12–16 weeks of treatment may be due to malignancy (which can be missed, even with biopsies and brushings), and is often an indication for surgery. Endoscopic ultrasound, if available, can discriminate between benign and malignant ulceration

• Long-term PPIs are appropriate in those unfit for surgery

Indications for surgery

• Complications—bleeding (but also eradicate *H. pylori*, p. 100); perforation (but then continue PPIs, p. 31)

• Failure to heal after 12–16 weeks of treatment, unless the risks of operation are very high

• Relapse on maintenance therapy

• A Billroth partial gastrectomy is the standard operation, carrying a <2% operative mortality and 10–30% incidence of long-term sequelae (p. 122)

Special categories

• Giant ulcers (>2.5 cm diameter)—carry no special risk of malignancy

• Antral ulcers—20% are malignant

• Prepyloric ulcers—behave like duodenal ulcers

• Pyloric canal ulcers—vomiting and weight loss are common; if ulceration extends through to the duodenum, consider lymphoma

• Combined gastric and duodenal ulcers—bleeding and obstruction are said to be more common

Complications

• Complications of gastric ulcers may occur without any preceding symptoms, especially in those taking NSAIDs or steroids

• 50% recur without *H. pylori* eradication therapy

• 25% bleed (Section 1.5, p. 10)

• 10% perforate (p. 31)

• Fibrosis causing deformity ('hour-glass' or 'tea-pot' stomach) is rare. Pyloric stenosis may complicate prepyloric ulceration

• Carcinoma at the site of a 'benign' ulcer is the result of an initial misdiagnosis, rather than malignant transformation, even if the ulcer has responded to conventional treatment

3.5) Gastric carcinoma

Gastric cancer is the fourth most common cause of cancer deaths. There is widespread geographical variation in incidence and prognosis, but the incidence of cancer of the antrum and body (corpus) of the stomach is falling in the West, presumably because of falling prevalence of *H. pylori* infection. This tumour is twice as common in men as in women. In contrast, the incidence of cancer of the cardia is rising. The reason is unknown.

Causes

• No single factor can be implicated, but there is a very significant association between gastric cancer, atrophic gastritis and *H. pylori*. *H. pylori* has been classified by the World Health Organization as a class 1 (definite) carcinogen. The estimated lifetime risk of gastric cancer in a person infected with *H. pylori* is 1%

• Chronic benign gastric ulcers do not predispose to cancer

• Well-differentiated early gastric cancer may develop at sites of intestinal metaplasia, but metaplasia is not definitely premalignant, nor is it an indication for repeat endoscopy and biopsy unless an ulcer is present

• Gastric adenomatous polyps are unusual, but have the same malignant potential as in the colon (p. 333)

- Diet—may explain the high incidence in Japan, China and Central America, since the incidence declines in migrant populations. N-nitrosamines have been implicated. The prevalence of H. pylori is also high in these populations
- Genetic—blood group A is associated with a 20% increase in risk; patients with familial adenomatous polyposis (Section 9.2) have an increased risk of upper gastrointestinal malignancy
- Low socioeconomic class—the incidence is five times higher in labourers than professionals. There is also a high prevalence of H. pylori infection, acquired at a young age, in this group
- Gastric surgery—the increased incidence 15 years after partial gastrectomy is small, but probably real; it may subsequently be explained by the prevalence of H. pylori in this group of patients
- Pernicious anaemia—the risk (about 1%) is increased

Clinical features

General
- Dyspepsia is usual, but is non-specific, poorly related to meals and relief by simple antacids is common
- Anorexia and weight loss are common presenting features and often indicate incurable disease
- Haematemesis is an unusual presentation
- Signs are absent until incurable disease exists
- Metastases to the lungs (lymphangitis carcinomatosa), bone or brain may be the presenting feature. A supraclavicular node (Virchow's node, Troissier's sign), or migratory phlebothrombosis (Trousseau's sign) are uncommon
- Dermatomyositis and acanthosis nigricans are most frequently associated with gastric carcinoma, but are rare
- H_2-receptor antagonist or PPIs can temporarily relieve symptoms and heal malignant ulcers, which can be a diagnostic pitfall

Pathology
- No classification is satisfactory, but there is a spectrum from polypoid lesions through ulcers to diffuse infiltrating cancer (linitis plastica). All types are adenocarcinomas
- The degree of differentiation, local and remote spread affect the prognosis, but not histological type (mucinous, signet ring). Tumours are multiple in 10%

....

Early gastric cancer

• Early gastric cancer is distinguished by an excellent prognosis (90% 5-year survival) after resection. Early gastric cancer is recognized endoscopically at a curable stage, and is probably a distinct entity rather than an early stage of the more common variety. It is often asymptomatic unless the lesion ulcerates, when dyspepsia occurs

• Endoscopy shows a superficial excavated or slightly protuberant lesion which may look insignificant. Biopsy of any gastric lesion is therefore essential if early gastric cancer is to be diagnosed. Local venous or lymphatic metastases are sometimes present, but the prognosis can still be good

Investigations

Dyspepsia lasting more than 8 weeks after the age of 45 years demands investigation (p. 86). Once the diagnosis has been made, a search for clinically silent metastases is indicated, before a decision about treatment is made.

Diagnostic

• Endoscopy—antral ulcers, or rolled and irregular edges of an ulcer crater favour malignancy, but multiple biopsies and brushings must be taken from all gastric ulcers

• Barium meal—blunting, fusion and tapering of mucosal folds radiating from the ulcer favour malignancy (Fig. 3.3). Endoscopy, biopsy and brush cytology are always indicated after radiological diagnosis of a gastric ulcer

Looking for metastases

• Chest X-ray—look for a pleural effusion, solitary metastasis or reticular shadowing from lymphangitis

• Blood tests—leucoerythroblastic anaemia or abnormal liver function tests suggest incurable disease. Elevated alkaline phosphatase may be due to bony metastases if the γ-glutamyltransferase is normal

• An abdominal CT scan is useful in assessing local or hepatic metastases

• Endoscopic ultrasound is a better technique than CT scan for identifying enlarged coeliac axis nodes, but is operator-dependent and likely only to be available at specialist centres

• Laparoscopy is performed by some surgeons, because this is the only way that peritoneal seedlings will be identified prior to full laparotomy. 40% of patients who are found to have peritoneal spread at an 'open and close' laparotomy die within 12 weeks

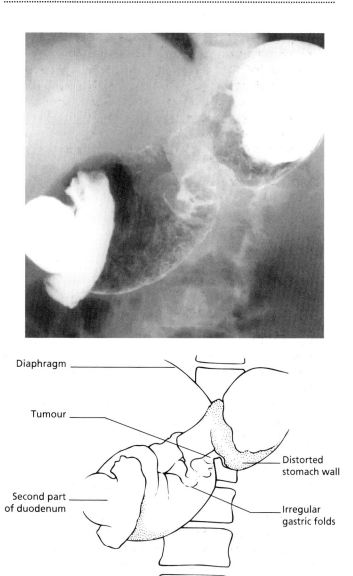

Fig. 3.3 Radiological appearances of gastric cancer. Barium meal showing a large cancer arising from the greater curve and distorting the stomach wall. The abnormal, irregular folds often do not reach the edge of the cancer.

Early diagnosis

An early diagnosis programme is part of the reason for the better outcome in Japan (25% overall 5-year survival). Public awareness and early investigation of dyspeptic symptoms in patients aged >45 years are essential to early diagnosis. Screening asymptomatic individuals (even those with pernicious anaemia or previous gastric surgery) is not justified in the UK.

Management

Curative surgery

• Indicated for patients aged <75 years with no signs of metastases and otherwise in good health—about a third of all patients
• Radical surgery ('R2 resection') has a mortality of 10%, but postgastrectomy sequelae are more common
• The operation rate, curative resection rate and survival are appreciably higher in Japan than the UK, probably as a result of population screening and more aggressive surgery

Palliative surgery

Indicated for obstruction, pain or bleeding.

Adjuvant therapy

Chemotherapy based on 5-fluorouracil remains under evaluation. Specialist oncological advice is appropriate.

Supportive therapy

• Pain can be relieved by omeprazole 20 mg daily, unless it is due to infiltration, when opiates are usually necessary. It is important to ensure adequate pain control, using opiates
• Explanation to the family, home support and liaison with the general practitioner are vital aspects of terminal care (p. 122)

Prognosis

• Local recurrence is the main cause of failure. The prognosis will only be improved by earlier detection followed by effective surgery
• The 5-year survival for all patients is 9%
• Following curative surgery the 5-year survival in the UK is 23%
• Median survival for inoperable disease is 4 months

3.6 Other gastric tumours

Lymphoma

The stomach is the most common extranodal site for lymphoma, but it remains rare. Prognosis is much better than for gastric cancer.

Clinical features
- Gastric lymphoma cannot be distinguished clinically from a benign ulcer or gastric cancer
- Weight loss, nausea and vomiting are said to occur earlier than in gastric cancer and haematemesis may be more common
- An epigastric mass is palpable in about 30%, but splenomegaly and peripheral lymphadenopathy are unusual
- Patients are usually aged 50–70 years

Diagnostic investigations
- Blood tests—a microcytic anaemia and raised ESR are common
- Endoscopy—appearances may be similar to a carcinoma. Multiple ulcerated nodules, transpyloric infiltration and giant rugae favour lymphoma. Deep, multiple biopsies (best performed by snaring a mucosal fold) are necessary, but still may not be positive. Diagnostic laparotomy and frozen section biopsies may then be needed
- Barium meal—polypoid ulcerated lesions on the greater curve and extension into the duodenum favour lymphoma, but none are specific

Further investigations
- Bone marrow—infiltration indicates stage IV disease
- Abdominal CT scan—for staging (Table 3.4)

Table 3.4   Staging of intestinal lymphoma.

Stage*	Interpretation
I	Disease in a single extralymphatic organ
II	Localized involvement of an extralymphatic organ as well as lymph nodes on the same side of the diaphragm
III	Localized involvement of an extralymphatic organ and lymph nodes on both sides of the diaphragm
IV	Diffuse or disseminated involvement of more than one extralymphatic organ, with or without lymph node involvement

*The suffix 'E' may be used to denote extralymphatic lymphoma.

- Histological type—the distinction between 'high' and 'low' grade is more helpful than the type of malignant cell when planning treatment
- Frozen sections (as well as formalin-fixed biopsies) are helpful for immunohistochemistry, and need to be planned with the pathologist before surgery

Treatment

Regimens are complex and evolving. Specialist oncological advice is recommended. General guidelines are as follows:
- Surgery for:
  - stage I disease
  - complications (haemorrhage or obstruction)
- Radiotherapy for stage II disease, often with chemotherapy
- Chemotherapy for stage III or stage IV disease

MALT lymphoma

- *H. pylori* is causally associated with this rare low-grade B-cell lymphoma and successful eradication is followed by remission in some 80% of patients
- It is strongly recommended that, after diagnosis, patients are referred for management to a centre where clinical trials of MALT lymphoma treatment are in progress
- Awareness of this type of lymphoma is important to avoid unnecessary radical surgery or chemotherapy

Polyps

- Hyperplastic polyps are regenerative and the commonest epithelial lesions (70%). They are of no significance. It is good endoscopic practice, however, to biopsy all mucosal lesions, because early gastric cancer may look insignificant (p. 110).
- True adenomatous polyps are unusual but have the same malignant potential as colonic adenomatous polyps. Endoscopic removal or resection is indicated. They may be associated with colonic polyps, so check for large bowel symptoms or blood loss

Leiomyoma

Account for 50% of benign gastric tumours. Haemorrhage due to ulceration at the apex is the main clinical problem. Because they arise from the muscle of the gastric wall they cannot be removed endoscopically, so surgery (wedge resection) is indicated. Leiomyosarcomas probably arise *de novo* rather than from an existing leiomyoma.

Other tumours

- Sub-mucosal lipomas may reach a large size and bleed. Carcinoid tumours are more common in patients with pernicious anaemia. Secondary deposits and heterotropic pancreas are extremely rare
- 'Microcarcinoids' are a histological description of collections of neuroendocrine cells which occur in some patients on long-term treatment with PPIs. They are unrelated to carcinoid tumours and have no clinical significance other than being a trap for the unwary

3.7 Duodenitis

Duodenitis is an endoscopic diagnosis and it can be difficult to determine whether it is causing the patient's symptoms. If the patient is *H. pylori*-positive, as is commonly the case, it is best regarded as an expression of duodenal ulcer disease.

Causes

- Almost always caused by *H. pylori* colonizing islands of gastric metaplasia in the duodenal bulb
- Very rarely caused by Crohn's disease, cytomegalovirus, ectopic pancreatic tissue, nematodes or sarcoidosis

Clinical features

- Duodenitis causes variable symptoms which may be provoked by alcohol or drugs. Ulcer-type pain, dysmotility symptoms (p. 87) or no symptoms may be present. Duodenitis never causes anaemia, but is sometimes the only abnormality found at endoscopy for haematemesis
- Duodenal inflammation is recognized endoscopically as patchy erythema or superficial erosions (salt-and-pepper duodenitis) in the first part of the duodenum. The mucosa can be nodular and the second part of the duodenum is usually normal
- Histology does not always correlate with the endoscopic appearance, but biopsies may show *H. pylori*

Management

- *H. pylori*-positive duodenitis should be treated with eradication therapy (Table 3.2, p. 91)

- Treatment of *H. pylori*-negative duodenitis is empirical and frequently disappointing. It depends on the characteristics of the symptoms (Section 3.1, p. 85)

3.8) **Duodenal ulcer**

Duodenal ulcers are four times more common than gastric ulcers below the age of 40 years and are more common in men. Although the overall incidence is falling due to better living standards and the consequently decreased prevalence of *H. pylori*, the incidence in women is increasing. The natural history of ulcers is a relapsing one: 80% relapse within 1 year of spontaneous healing or after acid-suppressive treatment. Symptoms are said to remit after 10 years, but little is known about the long-term pattern of duodenal ulceration.

Causes

H. pylori

- More than 90% of non-drug related duodenal ulcers are secondary to *H. pylori* antritis, which is followed by hypergastrinaemia and high acid secretion. The latter increases the chance of gastric metaplasia in the duodenal cap, forming a potential habitat for *H. pylori*
- There is a small population of *H. pylori*-negative, non-NSAID duodenal ulcer patients. Some may have a genetically caused high acid output; other rare causes are mentioned on p. 120

Acid and pepsin

- Basal, stimulated and nocturnal acid secretion are increased in most patients
- Pepsinogen (precursor of pepsin) secretion is increased
- The number and sensitivity of parietal cells influence the tendency to hypersecretion of acid
- Faster gastric emptying in duodenal ulcer patients may decrease duodenal pH
- All abnormalities of gastric function, apart from the increased sensitivity of the parietal cell mass to gastrin, return to normal within 6–12 months of eradicating *H. pylori*

Ulcerogenic drugs

- Drugs (NSAIDs, aspirin and possibly steroids) are associated with bleeding

and perforation, but not necessarily with uncomplicated ulcers (Section 1.5, p. 21)
- The elderly are more at risk and may be asymptomatic before presenting with a complication

Other factors
- Blood group O (relative risk 1.25) and non-secretion of blood group substances in saliva are weakly associated with duodenal ulceration
- First-degree relatives are affected in about 20%, compared to a 10% prevalence of duodenal ulcers in the UK, but this may be due to a similar environment and *H. pylori* infection
- Smoking retards healing and increases the likelihood of relapse
- Stress is often said to be related to duodenal ulceration, but this cannot be quantified. It may contribute to the non-specific association with chronic renal failure, lung disease and cirrhosis

Clinical features
- Young men are most often affected. Incidence increases in postmenopausal women
- Epigastric pain classically occurs before meals (hunger pain), wakes the patient at night and recurs several times a year for a few weeks. It may radiate to the back
- Vomiting and weight loss may indicate pyloric stenosis
- Examination, apart from epigastric tenderness, is unremarkable in the absence of complications
- Symptoms frequently fail to fit this pattern and all conditions that may cause dyspepsia (Table 3.1, p. 85) are included in the differential diagnosis

Investigations
Initial presentation
- Endoscopy is the most appropriate method of diagnosis (p. 86) because it can be difficult on a barium meal to distinguish active from past ulceration causing distortion of the duodenal cap
- Biopsies should routinely be taken from the antrum for the diagnosis of *H. pylori* infection, and from the ulcer if unusual causes are suspected (Crohn's disease, lymphoma, ectopic pancreatic tissue)
- Blood tests to detect anaemia or hepatic dysfunction should be performed. An elevated ESR does not occur in uncomplicated ulceration and raises the possibility of Crohn's or other disease elsewhere

Subsequent presentations

• The first recurrence of the same symptoms, in a patient who has had an endoscopically diagnosed duodenal ulcer in the previous 2 years, can be treated without further investigation

• Further recurrence or persistent pain are indications for repeat endoscopy and biopsies to exclude unusual causes

• Fasting serum gastrin concentrations (p. 468) should be measured while the patient is off acid-suppressive treatment if ulcers are postbulbar (p. 120), recurrent, resistant to treatment, or recur after surgery, to establish whether hypergastrinaemia, possibly due to a tumour, is present

Management

H. pylori eradication

• All *H. pylori*-positive duodenal ulcer patients need eradication therapy as outlined above (Table 3.2, p. 91)

• Eradication therapy should be prescribed at diagnosis, or at presentation due to a relapse, or complication

• Simple duodenal ulcers need no additional acid-suppressive treatment

• In complicated ulcers (e.g. after a bleed), acid suppression with a PPI or H_2-receptor antagonist (Section 3.4, p. 106) should be continued for 4–8 weeks. Some gastroenterologists advise continuing treatment until ulcer healing has been confirmed by repeat endoscopy in these patients

• The guidelines for gastric ulcers (stopping smoking, reducing alcohol intake, regular meals, p. 106) apply equally to duodenal ulcers. A summary of the differences between gastric and duodenal ulcers is shown in Table 3.5 (p. 119)

Resistant ulcers

• Patients with persistent symptoms after *H. pylori* eradication, or after 6 weeks of acid suppression if initially *H. pylori*-negative, should be reviewed. Drug compliance, smoking habits or alternative causes of dyspepsia (Table 3.1, p. 85) should be considered

• Repeat endoscopy is necessary to diagnose a resistant ulcer, but a urea-breath test performed >4 weeks after eradication therapy will determine whether treatment has worked (p. 99)

• If there is any doubt about the duodenal ulcer, biopsies must be taken from the ulcer at the repeat endoscopy and fasting gastrin concentrations checked. Acid suppression causes hypergastrinaemia and such drugs should be stopped for 2 weeks before the test if clinically possible

Table 3.5 Practical differences between duodenal and gastric ulcers.

	Duodenal	Gastric
Clinical*		
age	Mainly young	Mainly elderly
gender	Male	Either
pain	Nocturnal or before meals	Soon after eating
vomiting	Unusual	Common
appetite	Normal, increased or afraid to eat	Anorexia
weight	Stable	Loss
Endoscopy	Only for diagnosis	Repeat until healing confirmed
Biopsies	Antral for *H. pylori*	Multiple biopsies and brushings
Treatment	*H. pylori* eradication (Table 3.2)	Acid suppression if *H. pylori*-negative or on NSAIDs
Relapse	Endoscopy only if clinically indicated or to *H. pylori* status	Endoscopy essential Consider surgery
Maintenance	Failed *H. pylori* eradication complications, NSAIDs, aspirin	Failed *H. pylori* eradication NSAIDs, unacceptable operative risk
Surgery	Intractable haemorrhage, perforation, pyloric stenosis	Failure to heal, or persistent suspicion of malignancy

*None of the differences are diagnostic without endoscopy.

- In ulcers colonized by resistant strains of *H. pylori*, or in drug-related ulcers, PPIs (e.g. lansoprazole 30 mg, omeprazole 20 mg/day or pantoprazole 40 mg/day) will heal most ulcers that are resistant to H_2-receptor antagonists
- Failure to heal on PPIs suggests poor compliance, or an unusual cause (such as Crohn's disease or lymphoma)

Relapse
- Eradication of *H. pylori* (p. 91) cures duodenal ulcers and dramatically decreases the incidence of relapse to <5% per year
- Relapses may be due to recrudescence or, rarely, reinfection with *H. pylori*
- Some patients with a cured ulcer may experience reflux symptoms with endoscopic oesophagitis. This has to be distinguished from ulcer relapse. Symptoms are usually mild and respond to alginates

Maintenance treatment

- Maintenance therapy with H_2-receptor antagonists or PPIs is needed in drug-related ulcers, in *H. pylori*-negative ulcers and in those in whom eradication treatment has failed due to resistant strains
- Patients with severe symptoms and recurrent ulceration sometimes request surgery, but the chance of postoperative sequelae (Section 3.9, p. 122) including recurrent ulceration, must be considered

Indications for surgery

The incidence of surgery for duodenal ulceration has declined dramatically. It is still necessary for:

- Continuing, recurrent or major haemorrhage (p. 15)
- Perforation (p. 31)
- Pyloric stenosis (but sometimes symptoms remit after medical treatment; endoscopic balloon dilatation of the stenosis may also be possible)
- Resistant ulcers
- Ulcers causing severe symptoms that persist despite aggressive medical treatment with PPIs
- Frequent relapse, or relapse during maintenance treatment (see above for indications), if the patient prefers surgery to vigorous medical treatment (p. 100). Other pathology (such as Zollinger–Ellison syndrome) must first be excluded

Type of operation

- Vagotomy and pyloroplasty are safer than partial gastrectomy, but the recurrence rate is higher (p. 124). Highly selective vagotomy is an alternative, but results depend on the experience of the surgeon
- Risks of recurrent ulceration (1–10%), unwanted sequelae (10–15%), (p. 122) and mortality (1%) should be discussed with the patient

Postbulbar ulcers

Ulcers more than 3 cm beyond the pylorus are atypical (< 2%) and require a search for underlying disease. Crohn's disease, Zollinger–Ellison syndrome, carcinoma, ectopic pancreatic tissue, lymphoma and tuberculosis are differentiated by biopsies and measurement of fasting plasma gastrin concentration.

Complications

- Relapse—80% after 1 year, 90% after 2 years if untreated, or after a course of acid-suppressive treatment. Asymptomatic relapse occurs in 25%, but does not require treatment unless the patient is taking NSAIDs or is due for major surgery
- Haemorrhage—20% over 5–10 years (p. 12)
- Perforation—10% over 5–10 years (p. 31)
- Pancreatitis and aortoenteric fistula (p. 22)—very rare sequelae
- Pyloric stenosis—profuse postprandial vomiting is characteristic, with an audible succussion splash, but is rare in the UK (1% over 5–10 years). Metabolic alkalosis and uraemia are less common than hypokalaemia. Antral malignancy must be excluded by endoscopic biopsies. Intravenous fluids and nasogastric suction before surgery is the standard approach. Endoscopic balloon dilatation for benign pyloric stenosis works in experienced hands, but stenosis may recur

Gastrinoma (Zollinger–Ellison syndrome)

- Gastrin-secreting neuroendocrine tumours present with recurrent severe duodenal ulceration and diarrhoea, due to excess acid and inactivation of pancreatic lipase; 25% have other endocrine tumours (p. 146)
- Gastrin concentrations (p. 468) are high. H_2-receptor antagonists, PPIs and hypochlorhydria may also cause hypergastrinaemia. The secretin test (> 100% rise in gastrin with a gastrinoma) is not always reliable and gastric acid studies (increased basal and peak acid output) can also give false-positive results
- Localization is difficult because multiple tumours, sometimes in the duodenal sub-mucosa, and metastases are common. Endoscopic ultrasound, pancreatic MRI, or selective angiography may be needed
- Referral to a specialist centre is strongly advised, where treatment with PPIs in a sufficient dose to keep basal acid output < 10 mmol/h is appropriate
- Resection of the tumour is the usual practice
- Octreotide is reserved for advanced malignancy. Streptozotocin is now rarely used
- Outpatients should have their BP, calcium, electrolytes and liver function checked regularly to detect associated endocrinopathies. Gastrin levels are uninterpretable in those on PPIs
- Gastrinomas grow very slowly and prolonged survival is possible even after hepatic metastases have occurred

3.9 Sequelae of gastric surgery

Anatomy of gastric operations

The incidence of gastric surgery was declining before the introduction of H_2-antagonists, and has declined further since. Indications for gastric surgery are given in the appropriate sections (pp. 15, 107, 120).

Derangement of gastric function causes symptoms in nearly all patients after surgery, but adaptation occurs within weeks. After 6 months only 10–15% have persistent symptoms (Table 3.6). A combination of problems is common in those affected and few are specific to the type of surgery.

Vagotomy and antrectomy have the lowest risk of recurrent ulcers, but other complications are commoner after drainage, or resection and total vagotomy. Highly selective vagotomy has the lowest rate of complications but a higher incidence of recurrent ulceration (Fig. 3.4).

Diarrhoea

- More common after truncal vagotomy than after gastric resection
- Rapid gastric emptying and fast intestinal transit are the usual mechanisms, but coeliac disease, immunoglobulin deficiency and bacterial overgrowth should also be considered
- Treatment with smaller, more frequent meals, codeine phosphate up to 120 mg/day or loperamide up to 16 mg/day in divided doses is indicated

Gastric stasis

- Persistent postoperative nasogastric drainage, or later postprandial

Table 3.6 Unwanted sequelae of gastric surgery.

Common	Less common
Diarrhoea	Late dumping
Gastric stasis	Malabsorption
Early dumping	Reflux oesophagitis
Recurrent dyspepsia	Afferent loop syndrome*
Bilious vomiting	Small reservoir*
Weight loss	Retained antrum*
	Carcinoma
	Dysphagia (transient)†

*Specifically after partial gastrectomy.
†Specifically after vagotomy.

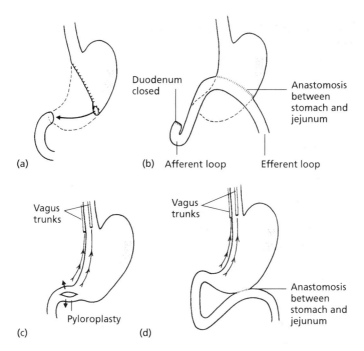

Fig. 3.4 Anatomy of gastric operations. (a) Billroth I partial gastrectomy. (b) Polyp gastrectomy. (c) Vagotomy and pyloroplasty. (d) Vagotomy and gastroenterostomy.

vomiting, may be due to mechanical obstruction or disordered motility
• A barium meal will confirm stasis and may give more information than endoscopy, but both investigations are often needed to demonstrate patency of the anastomosis and to exclude a stomal ulcer
• A prokinetic agent (such as cisapride 10 mg orally or 30 mg rectally three times daily) is worth trying for gastric stasis without mechanical obstruction
• Surgical revision is necessary for outlet obstruction

Dumping

Early dumping
• Rapid gastric evacuation results in a hypertonic load to the small intestine, triggering autonomic reflexes and vasoactive peptide release
• Characteristic symptoms are epigastric fullness, sweating, faintness and palpitations 30 min after eating, and avoided by fasting

- Helpful advice includes eating smaller meals that are low in sugar and high in fibre, to decrease the osmotic load and slow gastric emptying. Drinking before or after, rather than during, meals may help
- Surgical revision is a last resort

Late dumping
- Rebound hypoglycaemia 2–3 h after eating is the cause, because rapid carbohydrate absorption releases excessive insulin
- Relief by eating and the timing of symptoms, are the main differences between late and early dumping: symptoms can be similar

Recurrent dyspepsia

Endoscopy is the first investigation, to determine if the dyspepsia is associated with recurrence of the ulcer.

Recurrent ulcer present
- Recurrent ulcers are not always near the stoma
- All ulcers should be biopsied
- Gastrin concentrations need checking, but very few recurrent ulcers are due to the Zollinger–Ellison syndrome (p. 121)
- Acid suppression with H_2-receptor antagonists or PPIs followed by maintenance treatment are generally appropriate. Sucralfate may be used in this situation. Smoking and NSAIDs should be avoided
- Ulceration may be due to the effect of bile or pancreatic enzymes rather than acid damage
- Surgical revision should not be attempted until fasting gastrin concentrations have been measured. Unfortunately vagotomy, H_2-receptor antagonists and PPIs all cause hypergastrinaemia and results must be discussed with the laboratory. The completeness of vagotomy should be checked by cephalic stimulated acid secretion studies (p. 463), but may also be difficult to interpret due to alkaline reflux

No recurrent ulcer
- Exclude cholelithiasis (ultrasound) and consider early dumping or bilious vomiting as a cause of pain
- Treat for non-ulcer dyspepsia (p. 90) if no cause is found

Bilious vomiting

- Free biliary reflux into the stomach is usually asymptomatic

- Burning discomfort with morning bile-stained vomiting can be treated with a prokinetic agent (such as metoclopramide or cisapride 10 mg three times daily), cholestyramine 4–12 g/day, or aluminium-containing antacids (aluminium hydroxide mixture, 10–20 mL as needed)
- Severe bilious vomiting may be an indication for surgical revision

Miscellaneous problems after gastrectomy

Anaemia
- Inadequate dietary intake or a bleeding recurrent ulcer are the most common causes of iron deficiency after gastric surgery. Malabsorption of iron should only be diagnosed after other (colonic) causes have been excluded by barium enema or colonoscopy, which is mandatory to exclude a colonic neoplasm, especially in those aged >45 years
- Vitamin B_{12} deficiency after partial gastrectomy (usually presenting as macrocytosis) is due to bacterial overgrowth, ileal malabsorption or autoimmune gastritis, since sufficient parietal cells usually remain to produce intrinsic factor
- Osteomalacia due to mild steatorrhoea and calcium chelation is very rare. Steatorrhoea is probably due to rapid transit in the upper gut and poor mixing of food with pancreatic enzymes

Afferent loop syndrome
- Rapid emptying of a kinked afferent loop after a meal causes sudden vomiting. Treatment is surgical after radiological demonstration
- Bacterial overgrowth in the loop after a Polya gastrectomy is rare. Metronidazole 400 mg three times daily is indicated for 1 week, but repeated courses of antibiotics or surgical revision to decrease stasis are often needed

Cancer
- The incidence of gastric cancer 15–25 years after resection (but not vagotomy) is increased about fourfold
- Prospective endoscopic surveillance is not indicated, but postoperative dyspepsia needs investigating

Retained antrum
A very rare cause of recurrent ulceration and hypergastrinaemia, which has to be distinguished from the Zollinger–Ellison syndrome.

Postvagotomy dysphagia
Dysphagia is transient (lasting a few days or weeks) and due to trauma and oedema rather than denervation. No special treatment is needed.

3.10 Clinical dilemmas

Persistent dyspepsia despite treatment

Persistent dyspepsia after an identifiable cause has been treated is usually due to concomitant motility disorder (non-ulcer or functional dyspepsia). A definitive diagnosis of non-ulcer dyspepsia and explanation assists management (p. 90). Treatment aims to provide symptomatic relief.

First steps
• Careful history and re-examination
• Repeat endoscopy to confirm healing of the original lesion

Subsequent investigations
• If the endoscopy, full blood count, ESR and liver function tests are normal, further investigations are not indicated in most patients
• Abdominal ultrasound to exclude gall stones and pancreatic lesions, or small bowel radiology to exclude Crohn's disease, are necessary in a minority
• Outpatient review after 3 months is often better than further invasive investigations if the pain persists without other signs
• Oesophageal pH monitoring, or mesenteric angiography (if there is postprandial pain and weight loss), occasionally allow a diagnosis of reflux or mesenteric ischaemia (very rare) to be made in difficult cases

Dyspepsia and NSAIDs

NSAIDs should be taken with milk or meals. Dyspepsia is a common side-effect, but dyspepsia is a poor guide to the presence or absence of an ulcer, especially in elderly patients taking NSAIDs. Identification of high-risk groups is therefore difficult. Furthermore, ulcers may bleed or perforate without causing preceding symptoms and elderly women taking NSAIDs seem particularly vulnerable. The development of cyclo-oxygenase type 2 (COX-2) inhibitors, which selectively inhibit proinflammatory eicosanoids rather than the synthesis of cytoprotective eicosanoids, appears likely to reduce gastrointestinal toxicity by NSAIDs.

The following approach is suggested.

Initially

• Critically assess the need for NSAIDs. Stop the drug and substitute paracetamol if possible, or try decreasing the dose of NSAIDs and avoid long-acting preparations if not

• Reassess the symptoms after 2 weeks (a pain and stiffness chart, scored out of 10 each morning, may help)

Continued requirement for NSAIDs

• Arrange an endoscopy if dyspepsia has not resolved on stopping the NSAID, or if dyspepsia persists and NSAIDs cannot be stopped. Biopsies for *H. pylori* should be taken

• Eradicate *H. pylori* if present, although the importance of *H. pylori* in predisposing to NSAID-induced ulceration remains debatable. It is probably sensible to eradicate the bacterium even though this may impair the efficacy of acid suppression with PPIs

• Co-prescribe a PPI with the NSAID. Omeprazole 10 mg daily is the only PPI currently licensed for this indication in the UK. Misoprostol 200 µg twice daily is also effective, but may cause diarrhoea. Misoprostol is more effective at preventing NSAID-associated gastric ulcers than duodenal ulcers, but possibly less effective than PPIs

• Use the smallest effective dose of NSAID and avoid sustained-release formulations

• Apart from newly marketed (and expensive) COX-2 inhibitors, there is some evidence that different NSAIDs (such as piroxicam) are more ulcerogenic than others (such as naproxen, or prodrugs such as nabumetone). There is no convincing evidence that slow-release formulations (such as diclofenac), or rectal administration, reduce the incidence of peptic ulcer complications

• Routine prescription of prostaglandin analogues (such as misoprostol) with NSAIDs are not advisable, even in the elderly

4 Pancreas

4.1 Acute pancreatitis

The distinguishing features of acute pancreatitis, predisposing factors, other causes of a raised serum amylase, complications and management are covered in Section 1.7 (p. 33).

Subsequent investigations

• All patients should have an ultrasound scan within 24 h of the diagnosis, to look for gall stones and to assess pancreatic size, although the pancreas may initially be obscured by bowel gas

• Repeat ultrasound should be performed if the first scan did not clearly visualize the biliary tree, and to exclude a pseudocyst if there is persistent pain or pyrexia, or if the amylase has not returned to normal after 5 days

• An ERCP is indicated urgently if common bile duct stones are detected, or if jaundice or cholangitis occur, so that sphincterotomy can be performed. A dilated common duct can be caused by pancreatic oedema, as well as by obstructing stones

• ERCP is also appropriate if acute pancreatitis recurs without a provoking factor, but is contraindicated in the presence of a pseudocyst. It appears to be safe to obtain a pancreatogram in acute pancreatitis

Pseudocysts

Pseudocysts are not related to the severity of the attack. Persistent pain or elevated serum amylase suggest the diagnosis, but an abdominal mass is palpable in only 50%. Ultrasound is the simplest method of diagnosis, but CT scan (Fig. 4.1) may be needed if the pancreas cannot be clearly seen due to overlying bowel gas.

Management
• Pain control and nutritional support are initially indicated

• Enteral nutrition (p. 406) should replace parenteral feeding, which is usually needed during a severe attack of acute pancreatitis, once ileus resolves

• Cysts < 6 cm diameter measured by ultrasound usually resolve spontaneously, but larger cysts may need surgery or aspiration. Size should be monitored by ultrasound scans every few days during the early stages

• Indications for surgery (usually a cystogastrotomy) are persistent pain after 6 weeks, or the development of complications such as obstructive jaundice

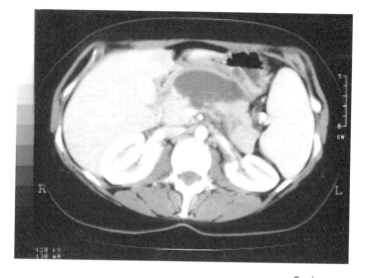

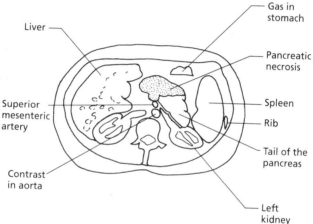

Fig. 4.1 Contrast-enhanced CT scan in a 35-year-old woman showing pancreatic necrosis shortly after developing pancreatitis.

• Endoscopic drainage by inserting a transduodenal or transgastric stent into the cyst to allow internal drainage is effective in experienced hands, but best performed with the assistance of endoscopic ultrasound

• Percutaneous aspiration is rarely appropriate, because recurrence is common

Complications

• Jaundice—due to compression of the bile duct

• Infection—abscess may develop spontaneously, or follow ERCP or aspiration

• Haemorrhage into the cyst—causes collapse with an acute abdomen, but may present with haematemesis if the cyst erodes into the stomach, or if blood enters the duodenum through the ampulla
• Painless ascites—high amylase and protein content, exacerbated by hypoalbuminaemia. Leakage of cystic fluid is occasionally chronic
• Rupture—rare but catastrophic

Recurrence

The first attack of acute pancreatitis is usually the most severe, but 30% of all patients have a recurrent episode. Recurrence is common in alcoholics, or if gall stones have not been treated, but uncommon in idiopathic acute pancreatitis.

Management
• Gall stones should be removed at cholecystectomy, immediately after recovery from the first attack
• An ERCP is indicated to exclude or remove retained stones, and diagnose pancreatic or ampullary tumours
• Consider alcohol and gall stones as the main causes of acute pancreatitis, or occasionally drugs, pancreas divisum, hypercalcaemia or hypertriglyceridaemia (p. 33)
• Counsel absolute abstinence from alcohol, whatever the cause
• Frequent recurrence is almost invariably due to alcohol abuse and progresses to chronic pancreatitis. Recurrent pancreatitis due to very small gall stones very rarely progresses to chronic pancreatitis

Indications for surgery

Early surgery does not increase survival, but surgery is indicated for gall stones, or local complications that fail to resolve.

Gall stones
• Cholecystectomy is indicated immediately after recovery from the acute attack, preferably on the same admission
• Exploration of the common bile duct is not necessary if an ERCP and sphincterotomy have recently been performed. Whilst retained stones are the most common cause of recurrent pancreatitis after cholecystectomy, these can usually be removed at ERCP
• Cholecystectomy should be performed if pancreatitis is diagnosed during

emergency laparotomy for an acute abdomen in the elderly. Peripancreatic drains should be inserted for peritoneal lavage and the abdomen closed

Local complications

• Collections of fluid (pseudocyst), pus (abscess), or necrotic tissue can be visualized by ultrasound and cause persistent pain, elevated amylase, leucocytosis or fever

• Delayed surgical drainage of a collection (6 weeks) is recommended in the absence of fever or jaundice, because 40% resolve and surgery is easier in collections that persist

• Abscesses need early operation if antibiotics (intravenous cefotaxime 1 g and metronidazole 500 mg three times daily) are to be effective

• Cystogastrostomy is most likely to prevent reaccumulation of fluid

4.2 Chronic pancreatitis

Irreversible glandular destruction may follow episodes of acute pancreatitis, or occur without an identifiable attack. The prevalence is increasing in Europe, where it is more common in men and due to alcohol. Acini are replaced by fibrous tissue causing ductular distortion and later atrophy of the islets.

Causes

• Alcohol—commonest factor (80%)
• Gall stones—very rarely cause chronic pancreatitis
• Genetic and congenital—rare hereditary pancreatitis has been linked to a mutation in the cationic trypsinogen gene on chromosome 7q, although how common this is in 'idiopathic' pancreatitis is still uncertain. Pancreas divisum or annular pancreas probably predispose to chronic disease
• Cystic fibrosis (CF; p. 140)
• α_1-protease deficiency
• Malnutrition is no longer thought to be a cause, but the high prevalence among young adults in southern India remains unexplained

Clinical features

Early disease is asymptomatic, but pain, exocrine and endocrine insufficiency supervene in many patients. 90% loss of exocrine function is necessary before steatorrhoea develops. Acute attacks, with attendant complications, may still occur in chronic disease.

Pain

• Frequent abdominal pain, which may be anterior and radiate into the back, or primarily posterior, is characteristic and may be the only feature

• Food or alcohol may exacerbate the pain

• Painful attacks resolve as inflammation is replaced by fibrosis, but this takes many years. The pain sometimes becomes continuous, when it should be distinguished from pancreatic cancer in which symptoms and weight loss are more rapidly progressive

• Painless chronic pancreatitis occurs in a few patients, who present with exocrine insufficiency

Weight loss

Malabsorption and small meals, because of associated pain, lead to malnutrition.

Exocrine insufficiency

• Steatorrhoea (pale, bulky, offensive stools with visible fat globules after flushing) can be massive, but may also be minimal if patients unconsciously reduce fat intake

• Defective secretion of lipase and bicarbonate cause fat malabsorption, but vitamin malabsorption rarely results in clinical osteomalacia or bleeding tendency

• Hypocalcaemia is common, because calcium chelates unabsorbed fat

• Weight loss is exacerbated by protein catabolism, because deficient pancreatic proteases (trypsin) cause protein malabsorption

• Serum B_{12} concentrations are often low because proteases are required to release R-proteins which bind to B_{12}. Pancreatic enzyme supplements are effective and B_{12} replacement is unnecessary

Endocrine insufficiency

• Glucose intolerance and, eventually, frank diabetes occur in 30%

• Insulin requirements are often low due to the lack of glucagon

Miscellaneous

• Jaundice may be caused by distortion of the common bile duct or associated cirrhosis, but pancreatic carcinoma is a more common cause

• Portal hypertension due to splenic or portal vein thrombosis is rare, but needs to be distinguished from associated alcoholic cirrhosis (about 10% of patients with chronic pancreatitis), because surgical decompression occasionally helps

• The risk of cancer is probably not increased, but can be difficult to distinguish from chronic pancreatitis in the early stages. Rapidly progressive symptoms and weight loss are likely to be due to cancer

• Haemorrhage from associated varices, ulcers or periductular vessels is rare

• Pancreatic duct strictures cause stasis and pancreatic calculi. These can cause recurrent acute pancreatitis which is difficult to treat. Endoscopic balloon dilatation of strictures and lithotripsy of calculi are potential alternatives to surgery. Referral is advisable

Investigations

Diagnostic

• Plain abdominal X-ray—30% have pancreatic calcification in the later stages

• Ultrasound—better than a CT scan for detecting tumours, cysts and assessing duct diameter, especially in thin patients

• ERCP—the 'gold standard', revealing duct distortion and side branch dilatation (Fig. 4.2). 'Minimal change pancreatitis' is an indication for repeat ERCP after an interval of 6 months if symptoms persist, or pancreatic function tests (see below)

• MRI—gives excellent images of the pancreas with the appropriate software. Magnetic resonance cholangiopancreatography (MRCP) currently is not as good as ERCP, but may subsequently image the ducts without instrumentation

Blood tests

• Serum amylase may be elevated in acute on chronic episodes of pain, but is often normal in between

• Albumin and clotting studies may be abnormal, due to associated cirrhosis or malabsorption. Low calcium or serum B_{12} suggest malabsorption. Elevated alkaline phosphatase reflects biliary obstruction (if the γ-glutamyltransferase is elevated) or, rarely, osteomalacia

• 2 h postprandial blood glucose > 8 mmol indicates impaired glucose tolerance and > 11 mmol is diagnostic of diabetes

Functional assessment

• Assessment of pancreatic exocrine function is not routinely performed, especially when clinical malabsorption is present because management is rarely altered (p. 465)

• Function tests are indicated to help interpret minimal changes on ERCP and to assist diagnosis when ERCP is not readily available

• Fat globules in stool indicate malabsorption, but·their absence is

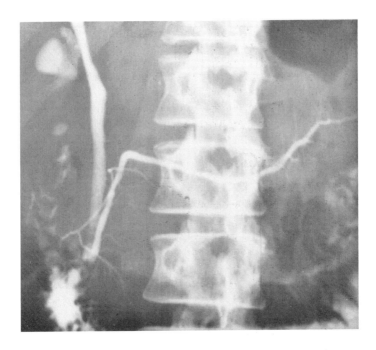

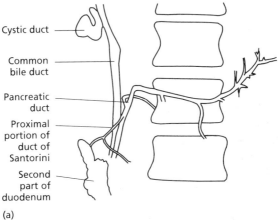

Cystic duct

Common
bile duct

Pancreatic
duct

Proximal
portion of
duct of
Santorini

Second
part of
duodenum

(a)

Fig. 4.2 ERCP in chronic pancreatitis. (a) Normal ERCP showing the pancreatic
duct, duct of Santorini and the common bile duct entering at the papilla.
(*Continued* on p. 138)

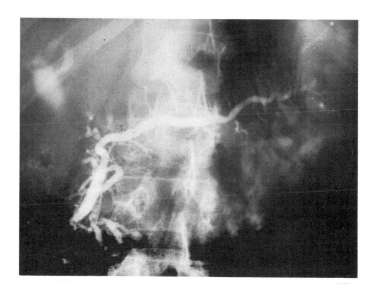

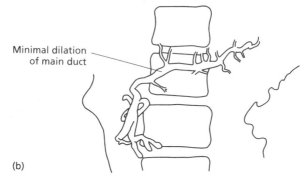

Minimal dilation
of main duct

(b)

Fig. 4.2 (*continued*) (b) ERCP showing moderate chronic pancreatitis (major irregularity of all side branches and minor irregularity of main duct).

unhelpful. Few laboratories quantify faecal fats (normal < 5 g/day), because they do not distinguish pancreatic from intestinal causes

• Direct tests (Lundh test meal with duodenal intubation) are more accurate, but less convenient than indirect tests (such as the fluorescein dilaurate, Pancreolauryl test) which lack specificity (p. 465)

Pain control

- Pancreatic enzyme supplements and avoiding alcohol help alleviate pain
- Dihydrocodeine 60 mg four times daily is sometimes sufficient
- Opiates (pethidine) are often required during severe pain, but dependence is common, possibly because of a susceptible personality in those who also abuse alcohol
- Repeat ultrasound and ERCP are indicated for persistent pain, because duct strictures or calculi may be the cause
- Coeliac plexus block provides temporary relief, sometimes for months. Early hypotension and later impotence or total visceral anaesthesia are potential complications. Recurrent blocks are often necessary, but relief can sometimes be permanent. Coeliac plexus excision by surgery can be valuable in patients who need recurrent anaesthetic blocks
- The assistance of a psychologist to teach coping strategies for pain is helpful for patients with unrealistic expectations
- Referral to a pain clinic helps both patients and physicians
- Surgery is indicated for localized chronic pancreatitis or pancreatic calculi causing severe intractable pain, but should only be performed by an experienced pancreatic surgeon. Total pancreatectomy for diffuse chronic pancreatitis has an unacceptable morbidity and a substantial number still have persistent pain

Exocrine insufficiency

- A low-fat diet (30–40 g/day, p. 419) is important, even with pancreatic supplements. A dietitian's advice is necessary
- Pancreatic enzyme supplements, taken during meals, are a convenient way of replacing deficient enzymes. No one type (Creon, Nutrizym, Pancrease, Pancrex) is of proven superiority to another and anything from 5 to 50 capsules/day may be needed. Enzyme preparations are unpalatable when sprinkled on food
- Creon is convenient, because acid suppression is unnecessary unless steatorrhoea persists despite a low-fat diet
- Persistent steatorrhoea may be due to:
  - poor dietary compliance
  - insufficient enzyme supplements
  - taking the capsules at the wrong time (before or after, rather than during, meals)
  - misdiagnosis (consider Crohn's disease, coeliac disease and thyrotoxicosis)

- Medium-chain triglyceride supplements (Trisorbon) are not very palatable but may help to improve fat absorption if a low-fat diet, enzyme supplements and acid suppression fail to control steatorrhoea

Endocrine insufficiency

- Oral hypoglycaemics are ineffective
- Insulin requirements are usually modest, but control is often difficult. 'Brittle' (labile) diabetes needs careful monitoring of blood sugars and close liaison between patient and diabetic team

Indications for surgery

The decision balancing the quality of life with persistent pain against the complications of surgery is always difficult. Surgery is more likely to be successful when ERCP demonstrates localized chronic pancreatitis or focal lesions such as strictures or calculi, and is rarely indicated when there is diffuse disease. Postoperative steatorrhoea and diabetes which is difficult to control are common, depending on the amount of pancreas resected. An experienced pancreatic surgeon is essential. A joint decision by the physician, surgeons and patient is indicated for:

- Intractable pain
- Pancreatic cysts or pseudocyst
- Recurrent gastrointestinal bleeding

Prognosis

- 80% with alcoholic chronic pancreatitis survive 10 years if drinking stops, but this falls to less than half if drinking continues
- Death occurs from the complications of acute on chronic attacks, the cardiovascular complications of diabetes, associated cirrhosis, drug dependence or suicide

4.3 Cystic fibrosis

CF is the commonest autosomal recessive inherited disorder in Caucasians (1 : 2000 births) and is due to defective regulation of chloride transport. The gene and its product (CF transmembrane regulator) were identified in 1989. Children with CF invariably have bronchiectasis and pancreatic insufficiency, but adults may rarely present with exocrine pancreatic malfunction alone.

Clinical features (Table 4.1)

- Respiratory and pancreatic complications are the most important
- Abdominal pain in adolescents with CF may be due to acute or chronic pancreatitis, intussusception, faecal impaction ('meconium ileus equivalent'), gall stones or duodenal ulceration
- Sufficient pancreatic exocrine function is present in < 10% of adolescents
- Pancreatic exocrine insufficiency causes steatorrhoea, hyperphagia, deficiency of fat-soluble vitamins (A, D, E, K) in children. Malnutrition is less common in adolescents, but steatorrhoea persists
- Impaired glucose tolerance is common (50%), but rarely causes ketoacidosis
- Hepatic disease due to inspissated secretions blocking bile ductules causes pericholangitis, periportal fibrosis or cirrhosis in 5%

Management (for adults)

Diagnosis

- A sweat sodium > 60 mmol/L after pilocarpine iontophoresis is diagnostic in children, but unreliable after adolescence
- There is no reliable test after adolescence, so the diagnosis is usually clinical. DNA analysis was restricted to prenatal diagnosis but is likely to become more widely available

Table 4.1 Clinical features of cystic fibrosis.

Infants	Children	Young adults
Meconium ileus	Bronchiectasis	Bronchiectasis
Rectal prolapse	Cor pulmonale	Chronic pancreatitis
Respiratory infections	Pancreatitis	Cholelithiasis
Failure to thrive	acute	Biliary strictures
Steatorrhoea	chronic	Aspermia
Malnutrition	Diabetes	Biliary cirrhosis
	Gall stones	Duodenal ulcer
	Portal hypertension	Intestinal obstruction
	Hypersplenism	
	Heat exhaustion	
	Colonic strictures	
	(high lipase enzyme	
	supplements)	

Pancreatic malfunction
- Low-fat diet—palatability must be maintained (Section 12.4, p. 419)
- Pancreatic enzyme supplements (p. 139) during meals
- Fat-soluble vitamin supplements are rarely needed if steatorrhoea is controlled
- Nutritional supplements (enteral feeds, medium-chain triglycerides) are prescribable items, but 'ACBS' should be written on NHS prescriptions (see British National Formulary (BNF))

Intestinal obstruction
- Gastrografin enema is diagnostic and may be therapeutic for intussusception. Surgery should only be performed in a specialist unit because of respiratory complications
- Acetylcysteine 200 mg three times daily after recovery stimulates secretions and prevents recurrent pain due to faecal impaction. NHS prescriptions should be endorsed 'S3B' (see BNF)

Other aspects
- Joint management with a respiratory physician is essential
- Genetic counselling for parents and young adults is necessary

Prognosis

- CF used to be a purely paediatric disease, but 80% now live to be older than 20 years, although all have respiratory complications and 90% have pancreatic exocrine insufficiency
- Adults who present with chronic pancreatitis alone probably have a similar prognosis to chronic pancreatitis from other causes

4.4 Pancreatic cancer

The incidence of pancreatic adenocarcinoma is increasing in Europe and does not appear to be due to better diagnosis. Men are more commonly affected than women. Only 1% survive for longer than 5 years. Pancreatic cancer should be distinguished from ampullary carcinoma, which has a much better prognosis (40% 5-year survival).

Causes

The cause is unknown. The following are considered to be risk factors:
- Genetic—hereditary pancreatic cancer is a rare condition, but a mutation

in the DPC-4 gene controlling TGF-β expression on chromosome 18q, has been identified. Studies of this gene in sporadic pancreatic cancer are in progress

- Smoking—occurs at a younger age in smokers
- Alcohol—any association is weak, and chronic pancreatitis not related to alcohol does not increase the risk of pancreatic cancer
- Diabetes—may increase the risk twofold

Clinical features

Tumour site determines the presentation.

- Cancers of the body or tail cause pain, anorexia and weight loss, and have usually disseminated before diagnosis
- Cancers in the head of the pancreas cause jaundice at an earlier stage
- Multifocal tumours are common

Symptoms

- Mean age 66 years
- Epigastric pain is the presenting feature in 75%. It typically radiates to the back, but may be intermittent, provoked by food and relieved by posture
- Painless obstructive jaundice is the other common presenting feature
- Non-specific features, including anorexia, weight loss, depression or lassitude, occur in most patients by the time of diagnosis
- Diabetic patients may present with ketoacidosis
- Recurrent attacks of acute pancreatitis occasionally herald cancer, due to intermittent duct obstruction
- Delayed diagnosis is common because early symptoms are non-specific and weight loss may not have occurred. Chronic pancreatitis is the main differential diagnosis, but rapid progression of symptoms or weight loss indicate carcinoma

Paraneoplastic features

- Rare
- Tender, subcutaneous nodules (like erythema nodosum) and polyarthritis are due to metastatic fat necrosis. Recurrent venous thrombosis (thrombophlebitis migrans), abacterial endocarditis, hypercalcaemia and Cushing's syndrome are other features
- Local spread to the peritoneum causes ascites. Obstruction of the splenic or renal vein can cause portal hypertension, or nephrotic syndrome

Physical signs

- Usually indicate an unresectable tumour
- The exception is isolated jaundice, which may be due to an ampullary carcinoma (p. 144). Courvoisier's 'law' states that jaundice in the presence of a palpable gall bladder is unlikely to be due to stones
- Exceptions to Courvoisier's law are impacted stones in both the cystic and common bile ducts, or a stone in Hartman's pouch causing oedema of the bile duct (Mirizzi's syndrome)
- Hepatomegaly, splenomegaly, ascites, supraclavicular nodes or an abdominal mass are present in 40% at diagnosis

Investigations

The suggested sequence of investigations is shown in Fig. 4.3.
- Percutaneous needle cytology (obtained by an automatic sampling instrument) can be difficult to interpret and is not widely practised. Laparotomy and biopsy may still be required in younger patients to differentiate chronic pancreatitis from cancer, with the option of palliative or radical surgery at the time
- CT scan is only necessary when ultrasound is impracticable (pancreas obscured by bowel gas) or when ERCP fails to provide a definitive diagnosis
- Endoscopic ultrasound may be the most sensitive investigation and provide useful information about resectability, but is not widely available and needs to be performed by a skilled operator

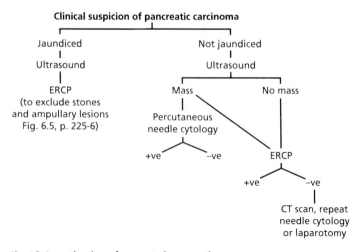

Fig. 4.3 Investigation of suspected pancreatic cancer.

Management

Although a cure is impossible in most patients, it is important not to take a despairing approach. There is much that can be offered by expert palliation. The small proportion (< 10%) who might benefit from radical surgery should be identified first.

Radical surgery

Pancreatoduodenectomy (Whipple's procedure) should only be considered by experienced pancreatic surgeons if:
- The patient is fit
- Tumour < 3 cm
- No metastases detected
  Operative mortality is around 5% in expert hands, but much higher amongst occasional operators. Morbidity after pancreatectomy is substantial.

Palliation of jaundice

- ERCP stent insertion by an experienced endoscopist is preferable in the elderly, because the morbidity is lower and hospital stay substantially shorter than after surgery
- A combined percutaneous radiological and endoscopic approach in difficult cases gives a success rate of up to 90%
- Percutaneous drainage alone is unsatisfactory, because the displacement and infection rates are too high
- Recurrent jaundice after stenting is usually due to obstruction by biliary sludge rather than tumour. The stent should be replaced endoscopically as necessary
- Surgery is indicated if there is evidence of duodenal obstruction or ERCP is unsuccessful. Choledochoduodenostomy and gastroenterostomy are appropriate

Palliation of pain

- Pain can be effectively relieved. It is important to tell this to the patient and family, and to ensure that it is achieved
- Opiate analgesics (start with morphine sulphate Continus (MST) 20 mg twice daily) cannot be introduced too early to relieve pain once the diagnosis is made. The dose is increased by the patient until symptoms are controlled (p. 149)
- Coeliac plexus infiltration with alcohol at the time of palliative surgery

should be considered. Percutaneous coeliac plexus block is more difficult and often needs to be repeated after 2 months

• Radiotherapy can relieve intractable pain

• NSAIDs, benzodiazepines and patient-controlled infusions of opiates also have a place (p. 150)

Ampullary tumours

Any malignant lesion that appears at endoscopy to arise from the ampulla of Vater is called an ampullary tumour, but such tumours are rare. They behave very differently from cancer in the rest of the pancreas because they present earlier, but they have no unique histological features.

• 10 times less common than pancreatic cancer

• 90% present with painless obstructive jaundice

• 80% are resectable by local excision

• 5-year survival after local excision is 40%, with an operative mortality of 7%. Proximal pancreatectomy had a similar mortality and probably improves survival

Prognosis

• Mean survival after diagnosis is < 6 months

• Overall 5-year survival is 0.5–1%

• 5-year survival after pancreatoduodenectomy is 4–15%

4.5) **Neuroendocrine tumours**

Functioning neuroendocrine tumours produce clinically interesting syndromes but are extremely rare. The incidence of all tumours is about 1 per million population. All patients should be referred to a specialist centre for treatment, but outpatient follow-up may be arranged locally. For this reason, management details concentrate on procedure at routine review, rather than definitive treatment. Evidence of recurrent disease is an indication for re-referral. All are rarities, but of these carcinoid tumours, insulinomas and gastrinomas are more likely to be seen.

Carcinoid

45% of carcinoid tumours arise in the appendix, 30% in the small intestine and 20% in the rectum. Metastases must occur before the carcinoid syndrome develops, in 2% of carcinoid tumours. 5-HT (or serotonin) accounts for only some of the effects; kinins, prostaglandins and other vasoactive substances may also be secreted.

Carcinoid syndrome
- Flushing and cyanosis, often provoked by alcohol or food
- Tears, excess nasal secretion
- Diarrhoea, may be episodic
- Hepatomegaly
- Bronchoconstriction
- Cardiac involvement, fibrosis, tricuspid or pulmonary incompetence
- Cutaneous infiltration, often on the lower limbs which become indurated

Diagnosis and treatment
- Clinically silent tumours are often diagnosed incidentally at appendicectomy. Intussusception may occur with ileal tumours
- 24-h urinary 5-hydroxyindoleacetic acid (5-HIAA) excretion > 0.3 mmol/ 24 h. Borderline tests should be repeated after excluding foods rich in 5-HT (walnuts, bananas, avocados)
- Chest X-ray, liver ultrasound, small bowel radiology and echocardiography are necessary to establish the extent of disease. An isotope octreotide scan is useful for detecting metastases if the tumour expresses octreotide receptors, but is expensive and not widely available
- Surgical resection of the primary tumour is curative if the tumour is < 2 cm and has not metastasized. Resection will also decrease systemic effects in metastatic disease. Serotonin antagonists (methysergide, cyproheptadine) have largely been replaced by octreotide (a synthetic analogue of somatostatin). Octreotide, starting at 50 µg subcutaneously twice daily, should be started only by a specialist. A longer acting analogue (alasetron) is being developed

Outpatient checks
- Ask about flushing, diarrhoea and breathlessness
- Palpate for hepatomegaly and record the BP
- Record peak flow rate
- Measure 24-h urinary 5-HIAA and perform a CT scan annually to monitor progress in patients who have had the carcinoid syndrome, but not in other patients unless symptoms develop

Insulinoma

Syndrome

- Spontaneous hypoglycaemia
- Provoked by fasting or exercise and relieved by eating
- Neuroglycopenia may present with confusion, focal neurological deficit or psychiatric abnormalities

Diagnosis and treatment

- 72 h fast under observation in hospital. Blood is taken for glucose, insulin and C-peptide concentrations when symptoms develop. Intravenous glucose must be readily available
- Normal C-peptide concentrations (from the laboratory) exclude exogenous insulin administration, but not sulphonylurea ingestion
- Treatment is surgical because metastases are rare (5%), but localization needs expert imaging

Outpatient checks

- Ask about recurrence of presenting symptoms
- Examine visual fields and check calcium levels annually to detect multiple endocrine adenomatosis (MEA type I; pancreatic endocrine tumour, pituitary tumour and hyperparathyroidism)
- Plasma insulin and C-peptide levels do not need checking unless symptoms recur

Glucagonoma

Syndrome

- Necrotizing migratory erythema (superficial bullous eruption that moves from one area to another)
- Mild diabetes (insulin secretion compensates for excess glucagon)
- Wasting

Diagnosis and treatment

- Elevated plasma glucagon levels are diagnostic
- Initial treatment is surgical if the tumour is localized. Octreotide improves the rash and streptozotocin may be of benefit in metastatic disease

Outpatient checks

- Ask about polyuria, diarrhoea and fatigue

• Examine the skin, check visual fields, serum calcium and glucose (in case of recurrence, or multiple endocrine adenomatosis (MEA) type I)

VIPoma (Werner–Morrison syndrome)

• Watery diarrhoea (profuse, but may be intermittent)
• Hypokalaemia (< 3.0 mmol/L)
• Metabolic acidosis (50% also have gastric anacidity)

Diagnosis and treatment

• Elevated plasma vasoactive intestinal polypeptide (VIP) concentrations may come from a tumour in the pancreas, or rarely from a retroperitoneal neuroma
• Treatment is surgical, but octreotide relieves diarrhoea should the tumour be unresectable

Outpatient checks

• Ask about diarrhoea and fatigue
• Measure serum potassium and VIP levels at annual visits

4.6 Terminal care

Terminal care is an important part of management in patients dying from any disease, but especially in pancreatic cancer when the prognosis is so poor. The essential features are symptom control, communication and supportive care.

Symptom control

Pain

• Best relieved by MST. Start at 20 mg twice daily (20 mg daily is equivalent to eight aspirin/day) and increase by 20 mg/day until symptoms are controlled. The correct dose is that which controls symptoms
• Breakthrough pain between doses can sometimes be treated by increasing the frequency of doses (three or four times a day) rather than the total amount
• Patient-controlled continuous subcutaneous infusions of morphine are useful when pain cannot be effectively controlled by other means
• Benzodiazepines (diazepam 2 mg three times daily) or chlorpromazine (25 mg three times daily) have a synergistic effect with MST for very anxious

patients, but excess sedation must be avoided. Anxiety usually has a cause and is aggravated by ignorance or fear

• Bone pain due to metastases often responds to indomethacin 25 mg three times daily, or slow-release diclofenac 100 mg once daily, with or without MST. Radiotherapy is also effective

• Local pain (arm, leg, chest, abdomen) from metastases may be amenable to anaesthetic nerve blocks, which may need to be repeated

• When oral therapy is no longer possible, subcutaneous morphine by infusion pump (dose/h = oral dose/24) is best combined with methotrimeprazine 100 mg/24 h as an antiemetic. Intramuscular morphine is never justified. Morphine and NSAIDs are available as suppositories

• Fentanyl patches for transdermal delivery are expensive, but are effective and give the patient simple control over their pain

Vomiting

• Consider hypercalcaemia, intestinal obstruction, cerebral metastases and, most important, drug-induced causes

• Standard drugs (p. 94) can be tried. Dexamethasone 2 mg three times daily is frequently helpful

• Methotrimeprazine 100–200 mg/24 h subcutaneous infusion can stop vomiting caused by intestinal obstruction

Irritability

Consider pain, constipation or urinary retention when consciousness is impaired.

Secretions

• Atropine 0.6 mg by intravenous or intramuscular injection (max. 2.4 mg/day) will dry noisy pharyngeal and bronchial secretions

• Hyoscine patches are useful when managing secretions at home, when a trained nurse is not readily available to give subcutaneous injections

Communication

With the patient

• Discussion of the diagnosis should wait until it has been definitely established and a plan of action made

• Delivering bad news should be done sensitively by a senior doctor, if possible in the presence of a relative or friend and a nurse. Patients (and relatives) frequently have little recall of detailed discussion. Try and arrange a quiet place for discussion, undisturbed by bleeps or telephones. The bedside or corridor of an acute medical ward is less than ideal

- Experience indicates that the best approach involves personal introduction, establishing the extent of individual knowledge, a 'warning shot' about news not being as good as hoped for, explanation of the diagnosis with diagrams if necessary, time for the news to be taken in, expression of sympathy or empathy with emotions where necessary, emphasizing what positive features there are, then explanation about the next step

- Not all patients wish to know that they have 'cancer', but the diagnosis should be explained if a direct question is asked

- All patients should be given the opportunity to ask questions, told that symptoms can be treated even if a cure is not possible, and given a contact telephone number (general practitioner, Macmillan nurse, medical secretary) if there are problems

With the family
- May precede or influence discussion with the patient, but it is always useful to talk to both patient and family together. This avoids future confusion about what has been said to individuals and helps cut down communication barriers within the family

- Explain what support is available in the later stages and whom to call

With the general practitioner
- Telephone prior to discharging the patient from hospital
- Say what the patient/family have been told
- Explain what supportive arrangements have been made
- Offer immediate access to hospital if symptoms become intolerable

Supportive care

Home
Liaise with family, general practitioner, district nurse, Macmillan (palliative care) nurses, hospital support team, home help or meals on wheels, as appropriate.

Hospice
- The general practitioner and the patient should agree before a hospice is contacted
- Early referral is advisable. It is poor practice to transfer a patient a few days before death, because the hospice team have no time to apply their skills, or to gain the necessary rapport

5 Liver

Jaundice

Jaundice is clinically detectable when the serum bilirubin is > 50 µmol/L. Classification into three predominant types (prehepatic, hepatocellular and cholestatic) is convenient, but there is considerable overlap in the clinical and biochemical features.

A basic knowledge of bilirubin metabolism is necessary to understand the investigation of jaundice (Fig. 5.1).

Causes (Table 5.1)

- The predominant type of bilirubin must occasionally be identified before a diagnosis is made. A mixed pattern of conjugated and unconjugated bilirubin is usually present, unless there is an enzyme deficiency or transport defect
- Predominant unconjugated hyperbilirubinaemia occurs in:
  - haemolysis
  - Gilbert's syndrome
  - Crigler–Najjar syndrome (children)
  - 'physiological' (neonatal)

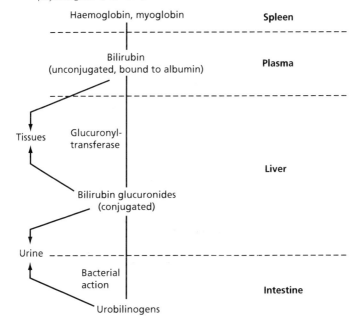

Fig. 5.1 Bilirubin metabolism.

Table 5.1 Causes of jaundice—main types.

	Prehepatic	Hepatocellular	Cholestatic
Common	Neonatal	Viral hepatitis Cirrhosis Alcoholic hepatitis	Common duct stones Pancreatic cancer Primary biliary cirrhosis
Uncommon	Haemolysis Gilbert's syndrome	Hepatic metastases Drug-induced Autoimmune hepatitis Liver abscess Hepatoma	Cholangiocarcinoma Sclerosing cholangitis Benign stricture Pancreatitis

Rare	Crigler–Najjar
	  syndrome
		Lymphoma
		Leptospirosis
		Budd–Chiari
		  syndrome
		Cardiac failure
		Pregnancy
		Postcardiac surgery
		Wilson's disease
		Dubin–Johnson
		  syndrome
		Graft-versus-host disease
			Portal lymphadenopathy
			Chronic pancreatitis
			Choledochal cyst
			Benign recurrent
			AIDS cholangiopathy
			Biliary atresia
			Parenteral nutrition
			Hepatic granulomas

- dyserythropoiesis (such as megaloblastic anaemia) or resorption of a large post-traumatic haematoma may cause an elevated bilirubin, but not clinically detectable jaundice
- Predominant conjugated hyperbilirubinaemia occurs in:
  - cholestasis (intra- or extrahepatic; Tables 6.1 and 6.2)
  - Dubin–Johnson syndrome (without cholestasis)

Table 5.2 Physical signs in hepatic jaundice.

Acute*	Chronic*	Either
Well nourished Tender hepatomegaly	Leuconychia Loss of muscle bulk Telangiectases (spider naevi) Splenomegaly Ascites Peripheral oedema Loss of axilliary/pubic hair Testicular atrophy Dupuytren's contracture	Palmar erythema Bruising Splenomegaly Small or large liver Facial telangiectases

*No clinical sign is invariably associated with either acute or chronic liver disease.

Clinical features

A systematic clinical approach is important.

History
- Occupation (alcohol-related, animal contact, industrial exposure)
- Travel abroad, past or recent (hepatitis-endemic areas, malaria)
- Contact with jaundiced patients
- Injections, especially abroad (drug abuse, transfusions of blood or plasma factors, tattoos)
- Drugs (prescribed, over-the-counter or 'alternative' medicines such as herbal teas, 'Chinese' medicines)
- Sexual relations
- Shellfish consumption (hepatitis A)
- Associated symptoms (the time sequence of symptoms is often helpful in distinguishing hepatitis from cholestatic causes):
  - anorexia, nausea, distaste for cigarettes (hepatitis)
  - right upper quadrant abdominal pain (gall stones)
  - weight loss (malignancy)
  - dark urine, pale stools, pruritus (cholestasis)
  - pyrexia, rigors should always be taken seriously (cholangitis, abscess)

Examination
Good light is essential to detect early jaundice. Icterus is first detectable in the sclerae when the eyes are down-turned (although usually preceded by a change in colour of the urine), but may be visible in the hard palate, especially in patients with discoloured sclerae (elderly, black patients).
- The depth of jaundice is not a reliable indicator of the cause
- Look for signs suggesting acute or chronic liver disease (Table 5.2, p. 156), or cholestasis (Table 6.5, p. 222; Table 6.6, p. 223)
  Other signs to be noted:
- Age—young adults may have Epstein–Barr virus (EBV) hepatitis
- Previous biliary surgery—possible obstructive jaundice
- Fever—suspect cholangitis, although hepatitis may cause a low-grade pyrexia
- Palpable gall bladder—more common in malignant obstruction, but 1 in 4 have obstruction due to common bile duct calculi
- Portosystemic encephalopathy—personality change, confusion
- Fetor—sweet, sickly smell in hepatic failure
- Asterixis—flapping tremor of outstretched hands, with fingers splayed

- Dilated periumbilical veins are rare. They either:
  - flow radiating away from umbilicus (portal hypertension, 'caput medusa'), or
  - flow towards the head only (inferior vena cava obstruction)
- An arterial bruit over the liver is rare—hepatoma or acute alcoholic hepatitis
- Rectal examination for stool colour—pale in cholestatic jaundice

Investigations—all patients

Bloods tests

- Typical values that help distinguish different types of jaundice are given in Table 5.3
- Liver enzymes, aspartate transaminase (AST, previously SGOT) and alkaline phosphatase (ALP) are markers of liver dysfunction rather than 'liver function tests'. Alanine transaminase (ALT, previously SGPT) is more specific than AST, but is not as commonly measured by automated assays
- An AST > 700 is very rare in alcoholic hepatitis and usually indicates coexistent viral infection or drug toxicity (e.g. paracetamol)
- γ-glutamyl transpeptidase (γ-GT) is elevated when a high ALP is of hepatic, rather than bony, origin. It is an unreliable test for alcohol abuse and a raised MCV is more suggestive. Any change in γ-GT does, however, reflect alcohol consumption
- Serum albumin and coagulation (prothrombin time, INR) are better markers of liver function, but serum albumin may also be altered by redistribution of body fluids

Table 5.3 Blood tests in jaundice.

Test	Normal	Prehepatic	Hepatocellular	Extrahepatic
Bilirubin (μmol/L)	3–17	50–150	50–350	100–750
AST (IU/L)	< 35	< 35	300–10 000	35–400
ALP (IU/L)	< 120	< 120	< 120–300	> 300
γ-GT (IU/L)	15–40	15–40	15–200	80–1000
Albumin (g/L)	40–50	40–50	20–50	30–50
Hb (g/dL)	12–16	12–16	12–16	10–16
Reticulocytes (%)	< 1	10–30	< 1	< 1
INR	1.0–1.2	1.0–1.2	1.0–3+	1.0–3.0*
Prothrombin time (s)	13–15	13–15	15–45	15–45*

*Falls in response to parenteral vitamin K 10 mg.

Urine

- Urine testing is less commonly performed now that biochemical tests are readily available, but should not be overlooked
- Bilirubin (tested with Ictotest tablets) is absent in prehepatic causes (the urine is clear, not orange, 'acholuric jaundice')
- Urobilinogen (Dipstix testing), is absent in complete cholestasis

Other tests

- Ultrasound—to look for bile duct dilatation or hepatic metastases. Also helpful to assess hepatic size, splenomegaly, the pancreas, portal blood flow, or lymphadenopathy and ascites. It is not a reliable method of detecting cirrhosis, but much depends on the skill of the operator. Reports commenting on 'increased reflectivity' of the liver are best ignored if liver function tests are normal
- CT scan—in obese patients, or if there are imaging difficulties on ultrasound (usually due to bowel gas)
- Chest X-ray—to look for bronchial carcinoma or metastases
- ERCP (p. 224)

Subsequent investigations

Further investigations depend on the type of jaundice, determined from the results of blood tests and ultrasound. Investigation of extrahepatic and cholestatic jaundice is summarized in Fig. 6.4 (p. 223).

Prehepatic jaundice

- Blood film
- Reticulocyte count
- Direct antihuman globulin (Coombs') test; serum haptoglobins (absent in haemolysis)
- Discuss with haematologists (bone marrow, or Ham's test to exclude paroxysmal nocturnal haemoglobinuria)

Hepatocellular jaundice

- Viral titres—hepatitis B surface antigen (HBsAg), antihepatitis A virus (anti-HAV) IgM, hepatitis C virus (HCV) antibody (Table 5.2, p. 156)
- Paracetamol levels on admission sample if drug toxicity possible
- Antismooth muscle, antinuclear and antimitochondrial antibodies, if viral titres are negative, to look for evidence of autoimmune hepatitis or primary biliary cirrhosis

- Monospot (Paul–Bunnell, for infectious mononucleosis) and serum for 'atypical' infections (e.g. *Leptospira* spp., *Mycoplasma pneumoniae*) if viral serology negative
- Serum iron and iron binding capacity or ferritin (haemochromatosis), α_1-antitrypsin (for protease deficiency), serum copper, caeruloplasmin and 24-h urinary copper (Wilson's disease), if viral titres and autoantibodies are negative
- Liver biopsy if diagnosis remains uncertain, chronic disease is suspected or hepatic enzymes remain abnormal 6 months after acute viral hepatitis. Biopsies should be stained for iron and copper

Cholestatic jaundice
See p. 220.

Drug-induced liver damage

The list of drugs causing jaundice is long, but drug-induced jaundice is not that common. Drug-induced liver damage usually presents as asymptomatic elevation in liver enzymes (p. 207). Hepatotoxic effects (Table 5.4) are divided into those that occur in most patients given a sufficiently high dose of the drug (dose-related), and idiosyncratic (dose-independent) reactions.

The diagnosis is suspected from the history of liver dysfunction or jaundice within 3 months of starting any new drug. Occasionally, liver damage can present a year or more after starting the drug (minocycline, methotrexate, α-methyl dopa). Peripheral eosinophilia is uncommon, although eosinophils in a liver biopsy raise the possibility of drug-induced damage.

Dose-related hepatotoxicity
- Paracetamol (> 10 g/24 h, but less in alcoholics)
- Tetracycline (> 4 g/24 h)
- Anabolic steroids (should only be used by specialists)
- Halothane-induced liver damage is partly related to dose; it should be avoided for anaesthetics < 6 weeks apart
- Methotrexate (usually for psoriasis, rheumatoid arthritis) causes dose-dependent cirrhosis but not jaundice until the terminal stages; liver biopsy is necessary once the total dose exceeds 2 g

Dose-independent hepatotoxicity (Table 5.4, p. 161)
For a complete list of causes, refer to other textbooks (Appendix 2, p. 482).

Table 5.4 Dose-independent hepatotoxicity.

Liver lesion	Common culprits
Hepatitis	Isoniazid
	Sodium valproate
	Rifampicin
	NSAIDs
	Azathioprine
Cholestasis	Co-amoxiclav
	Chlorpromazine
	Prochlorperazine
	Fusidic acid
	Glibenclamide
Chronic hepatitis	Methyldopa
	Nitrofurantoin
	Dantrolene
Alcoholic hepatitis-like	Verapamil
Granulomas	Hydralazine
	Allopurinol
	Phenylbutazone

Management

• Minor elevations in AST (up to threefold) after starting potentially hepatotoxic drugs (especially isoniazid, rifampicin) are not an indication for stopping the drug, since improvement usually occurs
• Stop all possible drugs if enzymes deteriorate or jaundice occurs
• Exclude other causes of jaundice and liver dysfunction (Table 5.1, p. 156)
• Severe, fulminant hepatitis is managed as for other causes (p. 49)
• Monitor liver enzymes until they return to normal—usually over several weeks. Most hepatotoxic effects resolve completely after the drug is withdrawn, unless liver dysfunction is unrecognized for several months (methotrexate, methyldopa)
• Liver biopsy is not necessary if the drug is well known to cause liver dysfunction, unless liver enzymes have not returned to normal after 8 weeks. Liver biopsy is essential if the history is uncertain

Prescribing in liver disease

• Most drugs are safe to prescribe in stable liver disease
• Dose should be decreased by 25–50% of the normal starting dose in patients with hypoalbuminaemia, disordered coagulation or recent encephalopathy

- High-risk drugs are:
  - sedatives (including chlormethiazole and benzodiazepines)
  - opiates (decreased first-pass metabolism enhances the effect)
  - diuretics (overdiuresis can provoke encephalopathy)
  - drugs known to cause dose-related or dose-independent hepatotoxicity (the threshold for hepatotoxicity is decreased)

Postoperative jaundice

Possible causes are:
- Drugs—scrutinize each prescription. Prochlorperazine is often implicated
- Anaesthetic—repeated exposure to halothane within 4–6 weeks. Enflurane is preferable for repeated anaesthetics
- Septicaemia—cholestatic pattern
- Pancreatitis—pancreatic oedema can obstruct the common bile duct
- Latent liver disease—perioperative hypotension may provoke decompensation of cirrhosis
- Hepatitis—transfusion-acquired HCV, or HBV (1–6 months after operation), or operation during the incubation period of hepatitis (shorter interval)
- Benign postoperative cholestasis—self-limiting, 1–2 weeks, especially after cardiac surgery
- Resorption of a large haematoma—jaundice only occurs if there is an associated metabolic disorder, such as Gilbert's syndrome
- Surgical mishap:
  - common bile duct stones overlooked
  - inadvertent ligation of common bile duct
  - oedema, or (later) stricture of the common bile duct
- In liver transplant patients, consider ischaemia, acute rejection, cytomegalovirus (CMV) hepatitis, biliary obstruction and lymphoproliferative disorders

Investigations
- Blood cultures—low-grade sepsis may not cause a fever
- Serology—hepatitis B, C and A, as well as antimitochondrial antibodies, or liver/kidney microsomal antibodies if halothane hepatitis is suspected
- Measure unconjugated bilirubin (> 75% suggests haemolysis, or resorption of a large haematoma)
- Ultrasound—look for dilated bile ducts and at the pancreas. CT scan is better for detecting common bile duct stones, but if the common bile duct is dilated, ERCP is indicated whether a stone is visible or not

• Contact blood transfusion laboratory to trace donors if hepatitis is diagnosed; sexual partners should be traced and offered hepatitis B vaccination if appropriate (p. 184)

Jaundice in pregnancy (p. 428)

Specific conditions related to pregnancy are as follows.

First trimester

Hyperemesis gravidarum—jaundice in 10%, especially in those with Gilbert's syndrome. Self-limiting. Liver failure does not occur.

Third trimester

• Intrahepatic cholestasis of pregnancy—preceded by pruritus. Recurs with subsequent pregnancies. Resolves within 2 weeks of delivery. Self-limiting
• Acute fatty liver of pregnancy—nausea, abdominal pain, encephalopathy. Potentially fatal without prompt delivery
• Pre-eclampsia—often associated with mild changes in transaminases
• HELLP syndrome—potentially severe liver disease associated with pre-eclampsia, haemolysis and thrombocytopenia

Any trimester

Any other cause of jaundice (drugs, viral, common bile duct calculi, etc.).

Jaundice with normal liver enzymes

Bilirubin may be disproportionately elevated compared to the AST or ALP when there is very severe liver disease (acute hepatitis or end-stage cirrhosis), because there are few hepatocytes to produce the enzymes. In these cases the albumin is low and coagulation disordered.

Isolated hyperbilirubinaemia is uncommon. Consider:
• Haemolysis—blood film, reticulocyte count, haptoglobins
• Gilbert's syndrome—unconjugated bilirubin
• Dubin–Johnson or Rotor's syndromes—conjugated bilirubin

Gilbert's syndrome

• Slight elevation of unconjugated bilirubin is common (up to 5% of the population). It is not an indication for ultrasound or other investigations in the absence of symptoms
• Liver enzymes are otherwise normal
• Bilirubin increases on fasting (rarely necessary to establish)

- Jaundice is rare, except in concomitant illness with anorexia
- No treatment other than reassurance is necessary

Crigler–Najjar syndrome
Crigler–Najjar syndrome (glucuronyl transferase deficiency) rarely affects adults, although some with the milder (type II) form survive from childhood.

Dubin–Johnson and Rotor's syndromes
Dubin–Johnson and Rotor's syndromes are very rare causes of isolated conjugated hyperbilirubinaemia that can present with jaundice in adults.

Other causes of hyperpigmentation
Very occasionally other causes of diffuse hyperpigmentation (carotenaemia, melanosis) may be confused with jaundice, but these do not cause scleral discoloration and the bilirubin is normal.

Hepatic decompensation

Hepatic decompensation is often reversible in chronic liver disease, except in chronic cholestasis when it marks the terminal phase. An acute exacerbation of chronic hepatic failure is far more common than acute (fulminant) liver failure (p. 49).

Causes

Every patient who presents with decompensation of chronic liver disease should be investigated for a provoking factor:
- Intestinal bleeding from:
  - varices
  - ulcer
  - erosions
- Infection:
  - urinary tract
  - chest
  - spontaneous bacterial peritonitis (usually *Escherichia coli*, now less often pneumococcal) in ascites
- Drugs:
  - excess diuretics (hypokalaemia, hypomagnesaemia or uraemia)
  - sedatives
  - opiates (including codeine, co-proxamol)
- Alcohol abuse

- Progression of underlying disease
- Excessive dietary protein (only in severe chronic liver disease)
- Hepatocellular carcinoma (p. 203)

Clinical features

Hepatocellular dysfunction
- Jaundice increasing
- Encephalopathy:
  - personality change, inability to draw a five-pointed star
  - drowsiness, inappropriate behaviour
  - stuporous, inarticulate speech
  - coma
  - the changes in mental state are graded 1–5 (grade 5 means no response to painful stimuli), but this is only clinically valuable in fulminant hepatic failure (Table 1.6, p. 50)
- Hepatic fetor:
  - sweet, sickly smell
  - precedes coma
- Asterixis
  - arms outstretched, wrists hyperextended, fingers apart
  - slow (every second), flapping movements at the wrist
- Fever and other signs of infection may be absent

Portal hypertension
- Ascites—develops or increases (p. 167)
- Varices are not a sign of decompensation, but bleeding (p. 15) often triggers acute on chronic hepatic failure
- Venous hum—heard as a buzzing over the liver. It is rare

Child's grading
Child's grading (Table 5.5) may be clinically useful in predicting survival in patients with bleeding oesophageal varices or possibly in patients with cirrhosis undergoing surgery. Mortality from variceal bleeding in grade A is 5%, grade B is 20% and grade C is 40%.

Investigations

- Rectal examination for melaena
- Culture urine, blood and sputum if available
- Ascitic tap and urgent Gram stain on admission. Neutrophil count in

Table 5.5 Child's grades.

Feature	A	B	C
Bilirubin (μmol/L)	< 35	35–51	> 51 (i.e. jaundiced)
Albumin (g/L)	> 35	30–35	< 30
Ascites	None	Controlled	Poorly controlled
Encephalopathy	None	Minimal	Advanced
Nutrition	Excellent	Good	Poor

ascitic fluid > 250/mL is an indication for antibiotics, even if no organisms are seen
- Electrolytes, urea, full blood count, coagulation studies
- α-fetoprotein (AFP) for hepatoma
- EEG is the most reliable method of detecting encephalopathy and can be used for monitoring progress, but repeated clinical examination is sufficient for most patients

Management

Acute episode
- Identify and treat the provoking factor, especially infection—intravenous cefotaxime 1 g three times daily is appropriate until the organism is identified
- Dietary protein and salt restriction:
  - protein < 40–60 g/day (p. 420)
  - no salt added to food
- Lactulose starting at 90 mL/day until mild diarrhoea develops and then reduced, but not stopped (more effective than neomycin 4 g/day, which is now rarely used)
- Magnesium sulphate enema—if constipation is present when starting treatment or unable to tolerate oral lactulose
- Vitamin K 10 mg for 3 days should be given by slow intravenous injection if the prothrombin time > 22 s (INR > 1.5), although coagulation rarely returns to normal. Intramuscular injection is probably safe if the prothrombin time is < 45 s, but less pleasant for the patient
- FFP is only indicated if there is active bleeding (2–4 units rapidly, repeated after 8 h if bleeding continues)
- Intravenous saline must be avoided, especially in the presence of oedema or hyponatraemia due to liver disease, because salt (and water) are avidly

retained due to secondary hyperaldosteronism. Added salt on food and sodium-containing drugs (many antacids, p. 92) should also be avoided

• B vitamins (such as intravenous Pabrinex 1 + 2 vials for 3 days) should be given to alcoholics, who often have dietary deficiency

• Omeprazole 20 mg daily may decrease the risk of stress-induced gastric erosions, but this is debatable

• Monitor:
  • clinical state (encephalopathy) daily
  • daily weight (more accurate than a fluid balance chart)
  • daily electrolytes, INR and full blood count
  • twice weekly bilirubin, AST, ALP and albumin

• Patients aged < 60 years with acute on chronic liver failure not due to alcohol may be suitable for a liver transplant, although this is best deferred until after recovery from the acute episode (p. 53; Appendix 1, p. 477)

After recovery

• Discharge the patient only when the weight, diuretic dose and mental state are stable

• Normal dietary protein intake can be resumed when the encephalopathy resolves. Protein restriction should be avoided if possible, because patients are protein-depleted and the diet is unpleasant

• Continue dietary salt restriction (no salt added to food or cooking) to delay reaccumulation of ascites

• Lactulose can be decreased to 10–30 mL at night, before discharge and discontinued in outpatients

• In a few patients encephalopathy returns when dietary protein intake is normal. These will continue to need lactulose as well as continued protein restriction

5.3) Ascites

Ascites means free fluid in the peritoneal cavity. It is thought that peripheral vasodilatation is the initial event, possibly due to impaired hepatic metabolism of endogenous vasodilators. This decreases renal blood flow, which stimulates the renin–angiotensin–aldosterone axis, leading to salt and water retention. Portal venous hypertension is then the driving force that causes fluid to accumulate in the peritoneal cavity. This theory does not readily explain ascites in malignant disease, which also responds to aldosterone antagonists.

Table 5.6 Causes of ascites.

Common	Uncommon	Rare
Cirrhosis	Nephrotic syndrome	Budd–Chiari syndrome
Carcinomatosis	Cardiac failure	Portal vein thrombosis
		Tuberculous peritonitis
		Chylous ascites
		Pancreatitis
		Biliary ascites
		Constrictive pericarditis
		Meig's syndrome
		Pseudomyxoma peritonei
		Ovarian hyperstimulation syndrome
		Peritoneal mesothelioma

Causes

Most cases (90%) are due either to chronic liver disease or carcinomatosis with peritoneal seedlings (Table 5.6).

• Rapid onset of ascites is a feature of decompensated cirrhosis, malignancy (including hepatoma), portal or splenic vein thrombosis, or Budd–Chiari syndrome

• Ascites in an alcoholic cirrhotic with pancreatitis may be due to hepatic decompensation or pancreatitis. High ascitic amylase distinguishes pancreatic ascites, but measurement needs discussion with the biochemist

• Severe right heart failure, constrictive pericarditis, or Budd–Chiari syndrome can be confused with cirrhosis. The clinical signs (hepatomegaly, elevated jugular venous pressure and ascites) are the same, so a high index of suspicion and echocardiography are indicated if cirrhosis has not been proven by liver biopsy. Cirrhosis secondary to cardiac failure is extremely rare and if the two conditions coexist, alcohol or haemochromatosis should be considered. A large ovarian cyst can occasionally simulate ascites, but unlike ascites, the centre of the abdomen is dullest to percussion

Investigations

Examination of ascitic fluid is essential when ascites is first diagnosed, or if the clinical condition changes. The colour, protein content, results of microscopy and culture should be recorded on every sample; other tests are performed as indicated (Tables 5.7, 5.8). Investigation of the underlying cause is then appropriate.

Consider non-hepatic causes of ascites if liver enzymes and coagulation studies are normal. Pay particular attention to:

Table 5.7 Ascitic fluid investigations.

Condition	Investigation	Interpretation
All ascitic fluid	Colour	Table 5.8
	Protein*	< 25 g/L, transudate (cirrhosis, or hypoalbuminaemia)
		> 30 g/L, exudate (malignancy, or inflammation), but there is substantial overlap between the two groups
	Culture	Any growth is abnormal
Patient unwell	Gram stain	> 1 bacterium/mL or > 250 polymorphs/mL indicate bacterial peritonitis
	Ziehl–Nielsen	If tuberculosis is suspected
Malignancy	Cytology	Large volume (20–50 mL), fresh specimen necessary. Malignant cells are diagnostic
Pancreatitis	Amylase	Varies between laboratories
Milky (chylous) ascites	Triglyceride	> 5 mmol/L is abnormal; normal in pseudochylous ascites
Ascites from a biliary leak	Bilirubin	Ascitic fluid/serum bilirubin (ratio > 1.0 is abnormal)

*The serum–ascites protein gradient (serum albumin–ascitic albumin) is more accurate than the ascitic protein content alone for identifying the cause of ascites. An exudate (such as malignancy) has a protein gradient < 11 g/L, and a transudate (such as portal hypertension) has a gradient > 11 g/L.

- serum albumin (consider intestinal, as well as urinary loss)
- urine protein (24-h collection)
- echocardiography (to exclude cardiac causes)

Management

The aim is a gradual, controlled loss of ascitic fluid. Diuretics are usually adequate, supplemented by fluid restriction and a low-sodium diet if ascites becomes refractory. Rigid insistence on fluid and salt restriction at too early a stage merely make the patient's life miserable, but views vary.

Table 5.8 Colour of ascitic fluid.

Pale straw	Haemorrhagic	Turbid	Milky
Cirrhosis	Carcinomatosis	Infection	Chylous
Nephrotic	Pancreatitis	Pancreatitis	Pseudochylous
Cardiac failure	Tuberculous		

Paracentesis with colloid replacement has regained favour for refractory ascites, but diuretic treatment remains the initial approach.

• Fluid loss > 500 mL (0.5 kg) each day exceeds the capacity of the peritoneum to absorb ascites and results in hypovolaemia, unless peripheral oedema is present

• Other drugs should be reviewed and NSAIDs stopped because they cause fluid retention with deterioration in renal function

Small or moderate amounts of ascites

• Treated as an outpatient, starting with spironolactone 100 mg/day and no salt added to the food, rather than a low-sodium diet. Amiloride (5–15 mg/day) is an alternative if side-effects of spironolactone (e.g. gynaecomastia) are unacceptable

• Loop diuretics are less potent in ascites, although they are used to augment response to aldosterone antagonists (Fig. 5.2, p. 171)

• Review and weigh every week (aim for 2–4 kg/week) until ascites disappears

• Increase spironolactone by 100 mg/day every 3–5 days if ascites persists. The half-life of spironolactone is increased in liver disease: more frequent dose increases do not allow a steady state to be achieved

• Admit to hospital if spironolactone 200–300 mg/day at home are ineffective (Fig. 5.2, p. 171)

Refractory ascites

• Ensure that all specimens (Table 5.7, p. 169) have been taken and that the cause of ascites has been established

• Start a low-sodium diet (p. 421) and fluid restriction (1000–1500 mL/day)

• Indications for paracentesis include tense ascites causing respiratory distress or discomfort and ascites that persists despite treatment as in Fig. 5.2 (p. 171)

• Start therapeutic paracentesis, with intravenous colloid replacement (40 g albumin/5 L removed). This means 200 mL 20% salt-poor albumin, which is expensive. Some units use 1000 mL synthetic polymerized gelatins (e.g. Haemaccel or Gelofusin)

• Remove up to 5000 mL ascites/day for 3 days

• Colloid replacement is essential to avoid hypotension and the hepatorenal syndrome

• Diuretic therapy may then prevent reaccumulation of ascites

• Paracentesis with colloid replacement is appropriate as the initial approach for tense ascites because it provides rapid relief. The risks of infection or rapid drainage causing renal impairment are probably no

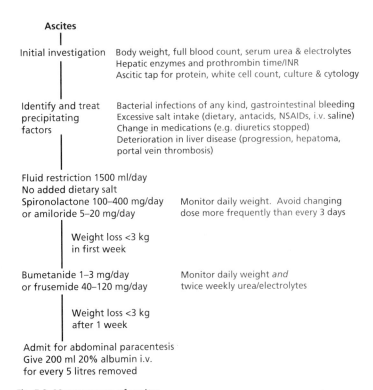

Fig. 5.2 Management of ascites.

greater than the hazards of high-dose diuretics (20–70%, including renal impairment, hyponatraemia and encephalopathy)
• TIPSS has been used with limited success. Referral to a specialist centre is necessary
• Surgical insertion of a peritoneovenous (LeVeen) shunt is only occasionally justified by the underlying condition—infection or blockage of the shunt are common

Hepatorenal syndrome

Functional renal failure without any other demonstrable cause in the context of advanced liver disease is intimately related to the renal circulatory changes in cirrhosis and the management of ascites. Renal cortical hypoperfusion appear to be the key event, but renal blood flow and glomerular filtration rate do not correlate with the severity of ascites. A separate defect in tubular sodium handling is likely and hepatovascular natriuretic peptides may play a role.

Features

- Precipitated by excessive diuretic therapy, paracentesis without adequate colloid replacement, hypotension during surgery, and aggravated by sepsis
- Hyponatraemia and a high urea are invariable. Urine sodium is low (< 10 mmol/L), but there is little response to fluid challenge
- Sodium is avidly reabsorbed, water retained and ascites becomes refractory, whilst cortical hypoperfusion leads to renal failure
- Hyponatraemia, uraemia and hepatic failure contribute to terminal coma

Management

- Recognize the signs at the earliest stage—increasing urea or creatinine (bilirubin may interfere with assays), especially with hyponatraemia—and reduce the dose or stop diuretics
- Correct intravascular hypovolaemia with intravenous colloid (200 mL 20% salt-poor albumin daily for 3 days) whilst maintaining fluid restriction (1000 mL/day)
- Low-dose dopamine (3 µg/kg/min) may improve renal blood flow, but not glomerular filtration rate and the response is usually disappointing
- Haemodialysis or haemofiltration are ineffective and have no impact on survival
- Liver transplantation is the only treatment to affect survival, but is usually inappropriate by the time hepatorenal syndrome is established
- Prevention is the key, because mortality approaches 100% once hepatorenal syndrome is established. The following decrease the risk:
  - avoid hypotension, inadequate biochemical monitoring of diuretic therapy, excessive paracentesis and nephrotoxic drugs (aminoglycosides) (p. 164)
  - recognize and treat sepsis promptly
  - mannitol 10% 20 mL/h intravenous infusion before and during surgery, helps maintain a diuresis
- Active measures are inappropriate if the underlying disease cannot be treated

Malignant ascites

The response to aldosterone antagonists, fluid and salt restriction is similar to cirrhotic ascites, but tense ascites is common and best managed by paracentesis. This may need to be repeated frequently. Instillation of cytotoxic drugs into the peritoneum is rarely effective and illogical if chemotherapy has not affected metastatic disease. Specialist advice should be sought. A peritoneovenous shunt may provide relief for some months before it blocks.

Chylous ascites

Chylous ascites is caused by lymphoma obstructing lymphatics, surgical transection of lymphatics during aortic aneurysmectomy, lymphangiectasia, or occasionally the nephrotic syndrome. Pseudochylous ascites, caused by malignancy or infection, looks the same but has a normal triglyceride content (Table 5.7, p. 169).

Treatment is with diuretics, salt restriction and dietary fat substitution with medium-chain triglycerides. Resection of a localized area of lymphangiectasia may be possible.

5.4 Portal hypertension

Portal hypertension usually arises from postsinusoidal obliteration due to cirrhosis. Obstruction of the hepatic, portal or splenic veins (Fig. 5.3) may also raise portal venous pressure and cause collateral venous dilatation (varices).

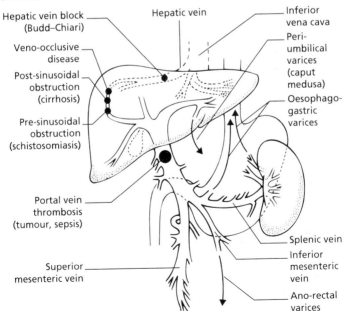

Fig. 5.3 Sites of obstruction causing portal hypertension and varices.

Causes

Three main groups exist; presinusoidal, hepatic (sinusoidal) and venous outflow obstruction (postsinusoidal) (Table 5.9). The distinction is practical because presinusoidal causes have relatively normal hepatocellular function, which means that encephalopathy after a gastrointestinal bleed is less common and the results of surgical decompression are better. Hepatic causes are commonest in the West, but schistosomiasis is commonest worldwide.

Clinical features

The consequences of chronically raised portal venous pressure are varices, ascites, splenomegaly, hypersplenism, or portal hypertensive enteropathy.
• Varices—oesophageal varices are common, gastric and anorectal varices are less common. Umbilical varices (caput medusae) only occur if the umbilical vein remains patent after birth, and are very rare
• Ascites (p. 167)
• Hypersplenism—recognized by splenomegaly, anaemia, thrombo-cytopenia and leucopenia. It indicates severe, long-standing portal hypertension and is a bad prognostic sign
• Portal hypertensive enteropathy may cause mucosal congestion and bleeding from the stomach, small bowel or occasionally the colon. Gastropathy is by far the commonest site and may be becoming more common, due to variceal sclerotherapy (p. 19). Enteropathy is usually detected when there is recurrent bleeding of uncertain origin in a patient with portal hypertension who does not have obvious varices

Table 5.9 Causes of portal hypertension.

Presinusoidal	Sinusoidal	Venous outflow obstruction
Extrahepatic	Cirrhosis*	Budd–Chiari syndrome
portal vein thrombosis	Congenital hepatic	Veno-occlusive disease
splenic vein thrombosis	fibrosis	
Intrahepatic		
schistosomiasis		
primary biliary cirrhosis*		
sarcoidosis		
myeloproliferative disease		

*Portal hypertension in cirrhosis is complex and partly due to postsinusoidal obliteration.

Investigations

The diagnosis is made by finding splenomegaly or varices in the presence of chronic liver disease. Spleen size, however, does not correlate with the degree of portal hypertension and a normal spleen size does not exclude the diagnosis.

• Liver biopsy—histological proof of chronic liver disease should always be established if possible

• Endoscopy is best for detecting oesophageal and gastric varices. Asymptomatic patients with cirrhosis need not be endoscoped, because bleeding only occurs in 30% of patients with known varices and the benefit of treating varices prophylactically is inconclusive

Difficulty arises when liver histology is apparently normal in the presence of varices and splenomegaly. This is an indication for:

• Ultrasound—with hepatic and portal vein Doppler studies to look for venous obstruction

• Portal, splenic and hepatic venography—largely replaced by Doppler ultrasound, but may be needed if transplant is being considered. Best performed at a specialist referral centre, together with review of liver histology

Management

Treatment of portal hypertension is directed at the complications of bleeding varices (p. 15) or ascites (p. 170). Specific treatment of the underlying disease (such as abstinence in alcoholic cirrhosis, venesection in haemochromatosis or anticoagulation in coagulopathies) is also appropriate.

Variceal prophylaxis

• Sclerotherapy or banding (p. 16) is not indicated unless bleeding has occurred. It must be systematic and done repeatedly to be of value. The highest risk of rebleeding is in the first 6 weeks after the initial bleed

• Varices recur after obliteration in about 40%

• Propranolol 20–40 mg three times daily decreases the risk of bleeding and is indicated if it can be tolerated. It is the treatment of choice for portal hypertensive gastropathy

• Nitrates (isosorbide mononitrate 30–60 mg daily) also reduce portal venous pressure and are indicated if propranolol cannot be tolerated, or if a patient rebleeds whilst taking propranolol

TIPSS

Radiological insertion of a stent has transformed the management of refractory variceal bleeding. The technique is demanding and only available at specialist centres.

• Principal indication is active or recurrent, especially gastric, variceal bleeding in spite of sclerotherapy, banding or other medical intervention. It effectively controls bleeding, but is best considered a temporizing measure pending transplantation

• There has been limited success in managing refractory ascites (p. 171)

• Early complications relate to insertion, but late complications include occlusion (40% at 1 year) and chronic encephalopathy (around 25%). Monitoring patency by Doppler ultrasound is necessary

Indications for surgical decompression

• Surgery (portosystemic shunting, oesophageal stapling or transection) should be considered if a third episode of bleeding varices occur despite sclerotherapy, and liver function is good (albumin normal, no encephalopathy during bleeding). This usually means patients with presinusoidal portal hypertension

• Orthotopic liver transplant is more commonly appropriate

Portal or splenic vein thrombosis

Malignancy, pancreatitis, portal sepsis or haematological disorders (see below) can cause thrombosis of the portal or splenic veins. 50% are idiopathic.

• Rapid development of ascites without deteriorating hepatocellular function is the clue. The possibility should always be considered if refractory ascites develops in cirrhosis

• Treatment is directed at the ascites and underlying cause

• Anticoagulants or thrombolysis are rarely indicated because of the risk of variceal bleeding. Surgery is usually unsatisfactory because the veins used for grafting are blocked

Budd–Chiari syndrome

Hepatic vein obstruction may be caused by haematological disorders (polycythaemia, protein C deficiency, antithrombin III deficiency, paroxysmal nocturnal haemoglobinuria), antiphospholipid syndrome (positive anticardiolipin antibody), malignancy, trauma, or oral contraceptives.

• Abdominal pain, tender hepatomegaly and ascites are variable: it may

present as a severe, acute condition, or as a mild, chronic illness
• Liver biopsy is diagnostic
• Preservation of Reidel's lobe on an isotope liver scan is characteristic but unusual
• Treatment of the underlying disease, anticoagulation or surgical decisions (including transplantation) are best made at a referral centre

Veno-occlusive disease

Non-thrombotic obliteration of intrahepatic venules is diagnosed by liver biopsy, but may be difficult to distinguish from Budd–Chiari syndrome. Pyrrolizidine alkaloids (*Senecio* ragwort, or comfrey herbal teas), irradiation and cytotoxic drugs are possible causes.

5.5 Hepatitis

Hepatitis involves inflammation of the whole liver. Most episodes are subclinical, detected (if at all) by abnormal liver enzymes, but the spectrum extends to subacute hepatic necrosis and fulminant failure. It may be caused by viral or bacterial infections, drugs, chemicals or toxins.

Causes (Table 5.10)

Although identification of hepatotropic viruses appears to be proceeding

Table 5.10 Causes of hepatitis.

Common	Uncommon	Rare
Hepatitis viruses	Hepatitis viruses	Delta virus*
A	C (parenteral non-A, non-B)	CMV
B	E (enteral non-A, non-B)	Hepatitis G
Alcohol	Epstein–Barr virus	Coxsackie A and B
	Drugs (p. 160)	Herpes simplex
	Autoimmune	Echovirus
	Ischaemia	*Mycoplasma*
		Leptospirosis
		Measles
		Arenavirus (Lassa)
		Flavivirus (yellow fever)
		Rickettsia (typhus)
		Chemicals (iron, CCl_4)
		Toxins (mushrooms)

*Only with coexisting hepatitis B infection.

through the alphabet (hepatitis A, B, C, D, E, G), almost all cases of transfusion-associated hepatitis can be accounted for by currently known viruses (including CMV, Herpes simplex virus, etc.). Hepatitis F was described by a French group, but is no longer considered to represent a separate entity.

Clinical features

A high prevalence of asymptomatic hepatitis is suggested by the frequency of patients with antibodies to hepatitis A, B or E without recalling a specific illness.

History
These features are characteristic of viral hepatitis (all types), but are less common in other causes of jaundice.
• Prodrome (2 days to 2 weeks)—malaise, anorexia, distaste for cigarettes, nausea, myalgia, fever
• Jaundice:
  • prodromal symptoms start to resolve
  • itching is rare (except in alcoholic cholestatic hepatitis)
  • dark urine and yellow (not clay-coloured) stools are common
• Associated symptoms can occur in any viral hepatitis although most commonly reported with acute hepatitis B, including arthralgia, arthritis and an urticarial rash. Membranous glomerulonephritis and nephrotic syndrome have been reported in persistent hepatitis B infection
• Resolution is usual, although some forms progress to chronic disease (Table 5.11)
• The most common presentation of hepatitis C is by the blood transfusion service after detection in donors, who are often asymptomatic

Examination
• Jaundice (anicteric cases are detected by liver enzyme tests)
• Tender hepatomegaly
• No signs of chronic liver disease (Table 5.2, p. 156) except in alcoholic hepatitis, when fever is also prominent
• Splenomegaly is commonly present in alcoholic hepatitis, infectious mononucleosis (EBV) or rickettsial infections. It occurs in about 15% of uncomplicated viral hepatitis

Outcome
• Complete recovery may take several weeks, or occasionally months. Lassitude and anorexia are commonly the most persistent symptoms

Table 5.11 Differences between types of viral hepatitis.

	A	B	C	D	E	G
Incubation (weeks)*	2–6	4–26	6–12	3–20	2–9	?
Transmission	Faeces Saliva	Blood Semen Saliva Perinatal	Blood ?Semen	Blood ?Semen	Faeces	?
Epidemic	Yes	No	?Yes	No	Yes	No
Risk factors	Children Institutions Seafood Travel to Middle/Far East Seasonal (winter) Homosexuals	Middle/Far East Drug abuse Homosexuals Haemophiliacs Renal dialysis Neonates of HBV +ve mothers	Drug abuse Haemophiliacs Transfusion	HBV only Drug abuse Homosexuals	Travel to North India/ Middle East/ Mexico	?
Chronic disease	No	5–20%	20–60%	30–50%	No	No
Prevention	Immunoglobulin Vaccination	Immunoglobulin Vaccination	Screen blood products	None	None	None
Carrier	No	Yes (< 10%)	Yes (?50%)	Yes (?5%)	No	? No

*The incubation period varies widely.

• Fulminant hepatic failure (p. 49) hardly ever occurs in hepatitis A and is exceptionally rare in hepatitis C. It develops in about 1% of symptomatic hepatitis B infections, common in hepatitis D and is characteristic of hepatitis E acquired during pregnancy
• Chronic liver disease may follow acute viral hepatitis, but the risk depends on the virus (Table 5.11). This includes all grades and stages of chronic hepatitis (p. 185), cirrhosis (p. 197) and hepatocellular carcinoma (p. 203)
• Relapse, usually with a milder attack, occurs in 2–10%. Recovery may still be complete, or it may indicate progression to chronic liver disease
• Asymptomatic carriers (5–10% following hepatitis B) may have normal liver function or chronic liver disease

Investigations

Liver enzymes
• An AST more than 10 times the upper limit of normal is the hallmark of acute hepatitis (Table 5.3, p. 158). The pattern of change in relation to serological markers is shown in Fig. 5.4
• The AST does not always correlate with the degree of liver damage, especially in severe cases or in chronic hepatitis C infection (p. 189)
• Predominant cholestasis is unusual in acute viral hepatitis, but more common in *Leptospira* and alcoholic hepatitis
• An AST > 700 in alcoholics suggests another aetiological factor, such as paracetamol toxicity or viral illness

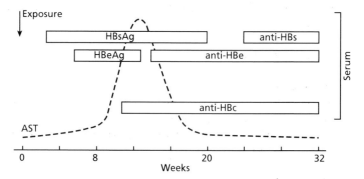

Fig. 5.4 Time course of enzyme and serological changes in acute hepatitis B. Adapted from Weatherall D.J. *et al.* (eds) *Oxford Textbook of Medicine*, 2nd edn, by permission of Oxford University Press.

Other blood tests
- Monospot or Paul–Bunnell test is advisable in young adults who are HAV IgM and hepatitis B-negative. EBV DNA or IgM can be measured if there is doubt about the diagnosis, but also consider *Mycoplasma pneumoniae*
- Neutropenia is common in viral hepatitis before jaundice appears. Atypical monocytes are seen in infectious mononucleosis, and rarely in cytomegalovirus or toxoplasmosis. Haemolytic anaemia is a rare complication of hepatitis B

Serology
- Hepatitis A IgM (anti-HAV IgM) and HBsAg should always be checked
- Hepatitis B e antigen (HBeAg) should be checked if HBsAg-positive, to assess infectivity
- δ-antigen should be checked if the patient is HBsAg-positive and a drug abuser, homosexual, or unwell
- Antibody tests for hepatitis C are appropriate if anti-HAV IgM and HBsAg are negative
- Autoantibodies (antismooth muscle and antinuclear antigen) should always be checked if tests for hepatitis A, B and C are negative

Polymerase chain reaction (PCR)
- PCR detects viral DNA (hepatitis B) or RNA (hepatitis C), indicating the presence of active viral infection and replication
- Its main role is in confirming the presence of hepatitis C viral RNA when an HCV antibody test is positive, so that decisions can be made about interferon therapy for chronic hepatitis (p. 185) and the response can be monitored
- Serotype identification of hepatitis C is also important when deciding about treatment (p. 190)

Meaning of markers

Hepatitis A
- Anti-HAV IgM antibody indicates recent infection (within 8 weeks) and disappears soon after jaundice appears
- Anti-HAV IgG antibody indicates immunity, appears within 2 weeks of infection and persists for years

Hepatitis B (Table 5.12)
- Occasionally infection without detectable HBsAg occurs, or hepatitis B surface antigen can disappear on recovery

Table 5.12 Serological markers in hepatitis B.

Stage	HBsAg	HBeAg	Anti-HBs	Anti-HBe	IgM	IgG	Anti-HBc
Incubation	+	+	−	−	−	−
Acute hepatitis	+	+	−	−	+	+
Carrier	+	±	−	±	±	+
Convalescence	−	−	+	+	±	+
Recovery	−	−	+	−	−	+
Vaccination	−	−	+	−	−	−

- Persistence of HBsAg for more than 6 months defines a carrier
- About 2% per year will subsequently develop antibodies
- The complete virus is called the Dane particle. Antihepatitis B core antigen (anti-HBcAg) acts against the core, which is formed in the hepatocyte nucleus

Hepatitis C

- First-generation ELISA tests for HCV antibody (against C100-3 antigen) gave false-positive results, especially in autoimmune chronic hepatitis and alcoholics
- Second-generation ELISA or radioimmunoblot assay (RIBA, 'third generation') against a range of HCV epitopes are more reliable, approaching over 95% positive predictive value
- PCR (p. 181) is the only absolute confirmatory test
- HCV antibody develops in 85% within 9 months of infection and disappears in about 50% within 10 years

Management

Acute attack

- No specific treatment is available and most patients will settle with symptomatic treatment
- General or specific immunoglobulin does not alter the outcome of severe hepatitis A or B
- Bed rest is unnecessary. Exercise has no effect on the severity of the attack or relapse rate, but most patients with hepatitis prefer to avoid exercise
- Careful hand washing and a high standard of personal hygiene are essential to prevent transmission. Cups, eating utensils and towels are

traditionally not shared until the jaundice resolves, if the diagnosis is hepatitis A, but this is unnecessary

• Admission to hospital is only necessary for severe attacks or if the patient is unwell and lives alone. Isolation is unnecessary, but gloves should be worn when handling all excreta (urine, faeces, vomit) or when taking blood

• It is essential to withdraw drugs or alcohol if these are the causative agent

• Patient preference is the best guide to diet. A low-fat diet is often preferred by patients, but otherwise has no special value

• Every case of hepatitis must be notified to the Medical Officer of Environmental Health (p. 398)

Contacts

• It is usually too late to treat close contacts of hepatitis A (shared bathrooms or kitchens and physical contact) with human normal immunoglobulin (5 mL intramuscular injection), but this should be discussed with a consultant in communicable diseases if more than one case occurs

• Sexual partners of hepatitis B patients should be tested for HBsAg and if not immune given recombinant vaccine (p. 184). Hyperimmune HBV immunoglobulin can be given as well if abstinence is impracticable whilst active immunity develops (2–4 weeks)

• Sexual partners of hepatitis C patients should be tested and may be advised to use barrier methods of contraception, although in one study of 44 patients with HCV chronic hepatitis, none of 42 sexual partners or 20 non-sexual contacts had detectable HCV antibody

Follow-up

• Abstinence from alcohol is often recommended until liver function has returned to normal, but moderate drinking (4–8 units/week) is not harmful

• Normal activity, including work, can be resumed as soon as the patient feels ready, but this often takes 2–6 weeks

• Liver enzymes should be checked after 6 weeks and again after 6 months if they have not returned to normal

• Abnormal liver enzymes elevated over twofold after 6 months are an indication for further investigation, including ultrasound and liver biopsy. Minor abnormalities can be observed with repeat blood tests every few months, and only investigated if there is an increasing trend

• Chronic hepatitis (see p. 185)

Immunization

Hepatitis A

Active immunization

Active immunization with live attenuated and killed vaccines have largely been replaced by recombinant vaccines. It is indicated for:
• Travellers to highly endemic areas (Indian subcontinent, Middle East, South America, Mexico), who will not be staying in hotels
• Close contacts (family, institutional members) of patients with acute HAV who have not previously been exposed, given in a different site to immune globulin

Passive immunization

Passive immunization with intramuscular human normal immunoglobulin 5 mL is effective for about 4 months. In many cases it suppresses the clinical manifestations rather than preventing infection. It is indicated for:
• Close contacts of patients with acute HAV (infection risk is 45% in children, 5–20% in adults)
• Travellers to endemic areas leaving too soon to complete a course of active immunization. It is cheaper to test travellers for antibodies to HAV rather than to give immunoglobulin indiscriminately

Hepatitis B

Active immunization

Active immunization with recombinant HBV vaccine (three doses, 0, 1 and 6 months apart) is indicated for:
• HBsAg-negative close contacts of patients with acute HBV
• Haemophiliacs
• Renal dialysis patients
• Patients requiring repeated transfusion
• Staff of institutions for mentally retarded
• Prisoners and prison staff
• Laboratory staff
• Health-care personnel (including doctors, dentists, nurses and students)
• People working abroad in highly endemic areas
• Drug abusers, prostitutes and homosexuals are not readily vaccinated, but should be offered vaccination if the opportunity arises
• Booster doses are needed every 5–10 years at present

Passive immunization

Passive immunization with two doses of intramuscular hyperimmune HBV immunoglobulin 500 IU 1 month apart should be given to:

- Non-immune staff with needle-stick injuries from HBV-infected patients, within 1–7 days, followed by active immunization after 7 days. For needle-stick injuries from HBV-negative patients, active immunization should be commenced and policy procedures reviewed
- Close contacts of patients with acute HBV
- Neonates born to HBV-positive mothers (200 IU within 12 h of birth and 0.5 mL (10 µg) recombinant HBV vaccine at separate sites. Second and third doses of recombinant vaccine at 1 and 6 months)

Hepatitis C, D, E, G

Neither passive nor active immunization are currently effective.

5.6 Progressive liver disease

Classification of chronic hepatitis

Chronic hepatitis is defined as hepatic inflammation continuing for more than 6 months. This time limit needs modification in individual cases, especially those of autoimmune aetiology. It is a histological diagnosis and, like cirrhosis, is a stage in the progression of many liver diseases of different aetiology (p. 188). The old terms of chronic persistent, lobular and active hepatitis have been largely abandoned in favour of a more structured approach defining the grade of hepatic inflammation, the stage of fibrosis (Fig. 5.5) and the cause of the liver disease (Table 5.13).

- This classification caters for patients with very active inflammation (grades 3 or 4) who may not yet have developed any fibrosis (stage 0 or 1), and for patients with end-stage, inactive cirrhosis (grade 0 or 1, stage 4)
- Treatment decisions depend primarily on the cause, but grading and staging provide a logical foundation. Patients with minimal activity but extensive fibrosis (e.g. grade 1, stage 4) cannot reasonably be expected to respond to any current medical treatment whatever the cause

Causes

- A specific cause can be identified for most (70–85%) of cases of chronic hepatitis (Table 5.14, p. 188)
- Table 5.14 emphasizes the detail and different investigations necessary

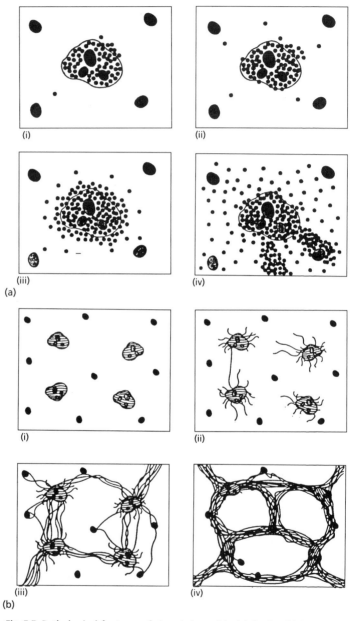

Fig. 5.5 Pathological features of chronic hepatitis. (a) Grades. (b) Stages as explained in Table 5.13. Adapted from Batts and Ludwig *American Journal of Surgical Pathology* 1995; **19:** 1409–17.

Table 5.13 Histological classification of chronic hepatitis.

Grade	Lymphocytic piecemeal necrosis	Lobular inflammation and necrosis
0	None	None
1	Minimal, patchy	Occasional spotty necrosis
2	Mild, involving some or all portal tracts	Little hepatocellular damage
3	Involving all portal tracts	Noticeable hepatocellular change
4	Severe, may have bridging necrosis	Prominent and diffuse hepatocellular damage

Stage	Descriptive	Criteria
0	No fibrosis	Normal connective tissue
1	Portal fibrosis	Fibrous portal expansion
2	Periportal fibrosis	Periportal or rare portal septa
3	Septal fibrosis	Fibrous septa with distortion of architecture; no obvious cirrhosis
4	Cirrhosis	Cirrhosis

for a specific diagnosis. It is always best to have complementary discriminating investigations that confirm the diagnosis, rather than to depend on a single result. Otherwise the unwary will fall into traps such as confusing autoimmune chronic hepatitis with primary sclerosing cholangitis, or missing concomitant haemochromatosis or hepatitis C infection in an alcoholic

• Essential investigations for all patients with progressive liver disease include a meticulous history, hepatitis serology (B, C), autoantibodies, serum ferritin or iron/total iron binding capacity ratio, and liver biopsy with iron, copper and PAS stains

Viral chronic hepatitis

Hepatitis B
• Chronic infection is more common in men, infection at a young age, haemophiliacs, black people and Asians. Up to 60% of chronic HBsAg carriers have little or no hepatic inflammation
• The clinical picture varies from mild non-specific symptoms to evidence of severe chronic liver disease. Arthralgia and an urticarial rash can occur, as in acute HBV infection
• Spontaneous improvement occurs in up to 30%
• Patients with minimal or mild inflammation on biopsy (grade 1 or 2, broadly consistent with previous 'chronic persistent' and 'chronic lobular'

....

Table 5.14 Diagnosis of specific causes of chronic hepatitis.

Viral hepatitis*	
B	HBsAg and HBeAg positive. Viral DNA by PCR rarely indicated. Orcein stain positive on liver biospy
C	HCV antibody by ELISA or RIBA, confirmed by PCR for HCV RNA. Lymphoid follicles characteristic on biopsy
B and D	Antibody to δ virus
Autoimmune	Antismooth muscle antibody titre > 1:80, antinuclear antibody > 1:80. Elevated IgG titre, female predominance (8:1), associated thyroiditis
Metabolic Haemochromatosis	Serum ferritin > 1000 µg/L or Fe/TIBC ratio > 80%. HLA-A3 positive. PCR positive (see text) Perl's stain positive on biopsy
Wilson's	Serum caeruloplasmin < 0.2 g/L. Increased urinary copper (> 0.1 mg/24 h). Increased liver copper
α_1-antitrypsin deficiency	Serum α_1-antitrypsin < 0.2 g/L, PiZZ phenotype on electrophoresis. PAS-positive globules on biopsy
Alcohol	History, random alcohol, γ-GT, raised MCV, elevated IgA. Fatty infiltration, megamitochondria, Mallory's hyaline on biopsy
Drugs	History. Amiodarone, methotrexate, nitrofurantoin, α-methyl dopa, etc. Wide variety of features on biopsy, especially eosinophil infiltrate
Biliary Primary biliary cirrhosis	Antimitochondrial antibody titre > 1:250, M2 antigen specific. Elevated serum IgM. Bile duct proliferation, lymphoid aggregates and granulomas on biopsy
Primary sclerosing cholangitis	ERCP. Sigmoidoscopy and biopsy (80% associated with ulcerative colitis)
Autoimmune cholangitis	Cholestatic LFTs. Negative AMAb. Pericanalicular inflammation on biopsy (p. 192)
Cryptogenic	All other causes excluded (15–30%)

*Hepatitis A and other hepatotropic viruses (e.g. Epstein–Barr virus, herpesvirus, arboviruses) cause acute, but not chronic, liver disease. Fe/TIBC, iron/total iron binding capacity.

patterns) have an excellent outlook. No treatment is indicated and annual liver function test monitoring can be performed by the family doctor, with referral for review (and possible rebiopsy) if there is a twofold increase in AST or symptomatic deterioration

• Patients who are HBeAg-positive (marker of continued viral replication) who have marked activity on liver biopsy (grade 3 or 4) should be considered for interferon and specialist advice sought. Treatment is expensive and local protocols may exist

• Intramuscular α-interferon 5 MU three times weekly for at least 3 months reduces the AST level in up to 70% and a sustained loss of viral replication in 30% (becoming HBeAg- and HBsAg-negative). Side-effects (malaise, headache, nausea) are almost universal, but usually tolerable. Women and patients with high transaminases (> 200 IU/L) respond more readily, but there is limited evidence yet that interferon either prevents progression to cirrhosis or improves mortality

• Adjunctive therapy with other antiviral agents is being examined. Liver transplantation in active HBV infection is usually contraindicated

• Prognosis is variable. Patients with inactive cirrhosis do well, but in cirrhosis with marked inflammation, 5-year survival is around 50%. Hepatocellular carcinoma occurs in a small minority (although HBV is the principal risk factor for hepatocellular carcinoma) and is most common in HBeAg patients. Surveillance with ultrasound and AFP measurements every 3–12 months does not alter outcome

Hepatitis C

• Up to 70% develop chronic hepatitis, but only 20–40% develop cirrhosis, often decades after infection

• Symptoms, management and outlook of mild degrees of inflammation are as for HBV (see above). However, transaminases are an inaccurate measure of the degree of inflammation in HCV and cirrhosis may be present with normal liver function tests

• Detection of HCV antibodies should be performed or confirmed with RIBA. Biopsy is usually appropriate when antibodies are detected, but if available PCR for HCV RNA (p. 181) should be checked first: biopsy and treatment can be avoided in those with no detectable viral RNA

• When there is active inflammation (grade 3 or 4, although some hepatologists prefer the more detailed Knodell score), treatment with interferon should be considered

• Response to interferon, however, is generally poor even compared with HBV. Higher doses (5–10 MU three or more times weekly) for longer periods (up to 12 months) leads to sustained loss of viral replication (monitored by PCR for HCV RNA) in 5–30%. Response measured by normalization of AST is more common (up to 50%), but histological severity is not accurately reflected. Serotype 3 (more common in Europe) responds better than types 1 or 2 (prevalent in the Far East)

Autoimmune chronic hepatitis

- Classically divided into two types, although the type does not alter treatment and has little influence on prognosis
- Type 1 is the most common form, identified by antinuclear or antismooth muscle antibodies (70–100%); 10% also have weakly positive antimitochondrial antibodies
- Type 2 show antiliver kidney microsomal antibodies (100%) and may more commonly progress to cirrhosis
- A minority only have antibodies to soluble liver antigens or characteristic histology and no identifiable autoantibody. The term 'lupoid' hepatitis has been abandoned and has nothing to do with systemic lupus erythematosus.

Clinical features
- 80% women, most commonly aged 10–30 or > 50 years (men are usually in the older age group)
- Malaise, arthralgia, anorexia or an urticarial rash may precede jaundice by several months. Onset is abrupt in a third, but others may have mild symptoms and be identified on investigation of abnormal liver function tests
- A minority (up to 30%) have associated autoimmune thyroiditis, diabetes, pleurisy/pericarditis, glomerulonephritis, ulcerative colitis or haemolytic anaemia
- Signs of chronic liver disease (Table 5.2, p. 156) are common, but patients often look remarkably well. Cushingoid features may reflect steroid treatment

Investigations
- AST is elevated 2–20 times and accurately reflects the degree of hepatic inflammation. Albumin is normal or low. Leucopenia and thrombocytopenia, due to hypersplenism, indicate severe disease. Serum IgG is usually elevated
- HLA-B8 is present in 30–80%, being more common in younger patients and those with more aggressive disease. Tissue typing is indicated if there are unusual features (e.g. males, or outside normal age range)

• Autoantibody tests (see above) and liver biopsy are diagnostic, but confidence in the diagnosis is increased if the IgG is also elevated
• Histology shows a mononuclear infiltrate of the portal and periportal areas, piecemeal necrosis and fibrosis, or cirrhosis. Iron and copper stains should always be performed and be negative
• ERCP is indicated if the ALP is disproportionately elevated (> threefold), because the histology of primary sclerosing cholangitis can occasionally be mistaken for chronic active hepatitis

Treatment
• Treatment is with prednisolone 30 mg daily. Response is monitored by serial AST measurements and the dose decreased by 5 mg daily every 2–4 weeks once the AST has been less than twofold elevated for 4 weeks. A dose of 5–10 mg daily is usually necessary indefinitely
• If steroid-induced side-effects are prominent azathioprine should be introduced at an early stage. Some do this routinely within 4 weeks and rapidly reduce the dose of prednisolone to 10 mg daily
• Steroids can sometimes be stopped after 1–2 years, but active disease frequently recurs, sometimes in a fulminating illness
• Repeat liver biopsy to assess progress is not usually justified if the clinical and biochemical response has been good

Prognosis
• In patients without cirrhosis, about a third will develop cirrhosis even with treatment after 5 years
• The 5-year survival rate even after cirrhosis has occurred, however, exceeds 90% and < 10% developed ascites, bleeding varices or encephalopathy
• Liver transplantation is appropriate if decompensation occurs in spite of immunosuppression

Primary biliary cirrhosis

• Interlobular and septal bile ducts are destroyed by chronic granulomatous inflammation of unknown cause
• Increasing cholestasis leads to cirrhosis and the complications of portal hypertension
• Antimitochondrial antibodies are almost invariably present

Clinical features
• 90% women

- Age 40–60 years
- Incidental detection of an elevated ALP is now the commonest presentation. Most (80%) asymptomatic patients have progressive disease and will develop symptoms, although this may take many years
- Pruritus almost always precedes jaundice by 6 months to 2 years and lethargy is common
- Skin pigmentation, xanthelasma, xanthomas, hepatomegaly and a palpable spleen are characteristic signs. Malnutrition and ascites are very late signs because hepatocellular function is relatively preserved, although oesophageal varices are common
- Osteoporosis is common. Fat-soluble vitamin deficiency often causes bone pain (osteomalacia) and disordered coagulation in the later stages

Investigations

- Elevated ALP and γ-GT (5–20 times normal). This is initially the only biochemical abnormality and hepatic origin is confirmed by the elevated γ-glutamyltransferase. AST may be slightly elevated but albumin remains normal until late
- Antimitochondrial (M2) antibodies are present in high titre in 98%. These are specific to primary biliary cirrhosis, although M4 antimitochondrial antibodies may occur in autoimmune chronic hepatitis. Patients with positive antimitochondrial antibodies and normal liver function tests are likely to develop primary biliary cirrhosis over the course of 10 years
- Serum IgM and cholesterol are usually elevated
- Ultrasound (to exclude other causes of cholestasis; Table 5.1, p. 156)
- Liver biopsy demonstrates chronic inflammation around the bile ducts, with granulomas and cirrhosis. In the precirrhotic stage it can occasionally be difficult to distinguish from other forms of chronic hepatitis or primary sclerosing cholangitis, but autoantibodies, other serological tests and ERCP should be discriminating
- Autoimmune cholangitis is a condition with the biochemical and histological features of primary biliary cirrhosis together with high antinuclear antibody titres, but negative antimitochondrial antibodies

Management

- As for other causes of cirrhosis, the aim should be to assess hepatic function, specific treatment, treatment of complications and consideration of liver transplantation
- The results of liver enzymes should be recorded at each outpatient visit
- Treatment with ursodeoxycholic acid 750–1000 mg daily improves ALP and bilirubin, some aspects of liver histology and results in a trend towards

improved survival with a decrease in liver transplantation. Since it is usually well tolerated, treatment should be started early. Other drugs (steroids, azathioprine, penicillamine, colchicine, cyclosporin, methotrexate) have not been shown to work in controlled trials

• Symptoms of pruritus (cholestyramine 4–12 g/day), diarrhoea (low-fat diet) bone pain (1α-cholecalciferol 1 µg daily and oral biphosphonates) are treated as necessary. Fat-soluble vitamins—monthly intramuscular injections of vitamin A 100 000 U and vitamin K 10 mg are indicated for prophylaxis when jaundice develops. Acute vitamin deficiencies need higher doses (Table 12.13, p. 423)

• Complications of portal hypertension are treated in the standard way (ascites—Fig. 5.2, p. 171) and variceal bleeding (p. 15). Encephalopathy is rare

• Patients may want to get in touch with the Primary Biliary Cirrhosis Support Group (Appendix 1, p. 478)

• Hepatic transplantation is curative and should be considered for patients < 60 years, with jaundice (bilirubin 100 µmol/L), uncontrolled pruritus, or complications of portal hypertension. The earlier the referral, the better the results of transplant, and when clotting is disordered or ascites develops, time is short (p. 208)

Prognosis
• Mean survival in asymptomatic patients is 12 years, but some patients have rapidly progressive disease
• Once jaundice develops, survival is < 2 years
• 5-year survival following transplant is 80–90% and improving

Haemochromatosis

• Autosomal recessive metabolic disorder causing inappropriate intestinal iron absorption and tissue damage from iron deposition ('bronze diabetes')

• Uncommon (3–8:1000 population), but increasingly recognized and an iron stain should be performed on all liver biopsies that reveal chronic hepatitis or cirrhosis

• Caused by an amino acid substitution (cysteine for tyrosine) in about 90% of cases. DNA analysis by PCR is both sensitive and specific

• The mechanism of increased iron absorption remains unknown

Clinical features
• Many patients now present as relatives of an index case, during

investigation of an incidental finding of abnormal liver function tests or with elevated ferritin
- Non-specific malaise and abdominal pain are the commonest symptoms

Classical signs
Classical signs include:
- Age 40–60 years, usually male, because menstrual loss protects premenopausal women
- Arthropathy—earliest or only sign, as a symmetrical polyarthropathy in metacarpophalangeal (always look for evidence of arthritis in the first and second metacarpophalangeal joints) and larger joints. Chondrocalcinosis may be visible on X-rays
- Hepatomegaly—with signs of chronic liver disease (Table 5.2, p. 156). The liver may be tender. A bruit suggests a hepatoma, which develops in 10% or more of those with established cirrhosis
- Diabetes—but exocrine pancreatic malfunction is rare
- Pigmentation—from a 'winter tan' to slate-grey
- Testicular atrophy and loss of libido, pubic and axillary hair are due to impaired pituitary function caused by iron deposition, as well as chronic liver disease affecting hormonal metabolism
- Cardiac failure (dilated cardiomyopathy) is now rarely due to iron deposition, but should always be considered in patients who have both cardiomyopathy and cirrhosis. Alcohol usually only affects one organ or the other, but alcohol abuse is also more common in patients with haemochromatosis

Investigations
- Abnormal liver enzymes depend on the amount of liver damage
- Serum iron is high and total iron binding capacity is low, with a high saturation (often > 80%). Ferritin is markedly elevated when cirrhosis is present, but may only be at the upper limit of normal in earlier stages. Ferritin is an acute phase protein and is elevated in inflammatory conditions as well as alcoholics
- Now that PCR for the specific mutation is available, this is likely to become the initial investigation of choice when iron overload is suspected, or in investigating the families of index cases
- Liver biopsy is diagnostic. All biopsies should routinely be stained for iron (Perl's stain). Alcohol, chronic haemolysis (with or without repeated transfusion), hepatic prophyria or excess iron ingestion may cause hepatic siderosis to a lesser degree
- CT scan is not routine and MRI is under trial. Since hepatic density

correlates with iron load, CT scans have been used as an alternative to repeated liver biopsy, but management is possible without repeated scans or biopsies

Management

- Venesection to a haematocrit < 0.50 and total iron binding capacity > 50 µmol/L (saturation < 40%, or ferritin < 100 µg/L) is the best treatment. This initially means twice-weekly venesection and is best arranged with the haematologists
- Outpatient checks:
  - ask about fatigue, dyspnoea, arthritis and control of diabetes
  - record liver and spleen size
  - check liver enzymes, iron and iron binding capacity (if not being measured by the haematologists) and glycosylated haemoglobin (if diabetic)
  - deterioration in liver enzymes despite normal iron studies suggests a hepatoma
- Screen first-degree relatives by PCR analysis if available, or HLA typing if not. If the HLA type (usually A3) is the same as the index case, the risk of haemochromatosis is about 95%. Measuring total iron binding saturation is less sensitive, but substantial iron overload is likely if > 60%
- Homozygote relatives should have a liver biopsy, then be followed up if there is no evidence of haemochromatosis, preferably at a specialist centre, with total iron binding saturation measurements every 6–12 months. Venesection is usually indicated if saturation increases to 40%
- Heterozygote relatives should only have a liver biopsy if liver enzymes are abnormal or iron binding saturation is > 40%. Follow-up is probably unnecessary if enzymes and saturation are normal
- Oral iron chelating agents are not yet available

Prognosis

- Liver histology improves with effective venesection, although cirrhosis is irreversible if present
- Cardiac failure is a poor sign
- Survival is normal if the diagnosis is made before irreversible liver damage or diabetes has occurred
- Once cirrhosis has developed, 10-year survival is around 70% and 20-year survival around 50%
- About a third of those with established cirrhosis will die from hepatocellular carcinoma, sometimes a decade after initial venesection is completed

Wilson's disease

- The metabolic defect of copper metabolism causing copper deposition in the liver and brain (hepatolenticular degeneration) remains unknown
- The prevalence may be as high as 30 per million population

Features

- Neuropsychiatric features usually precede hepatic disease in young adults, although the converse is true in children
- Chronic active hepatitis, cirrhosis or, rarely, fulminant hepatic failure may be the presenting feature
- Kayser–Fleischer rings at the periphery of the cornea are diagnostic, but can only be detected by slit lamp examination and may be absent in fulminant disease
- Haemolytic anaemia may be the presenting feature, with normal LFTs

Management

- Diagnosis is established by the combination of low serum caeruloplasmin (< 0.2 g/L) and low serum copper (reference range from the laboratory), increased urinary copper excretion (> 1.0 μmol/24 h) and excess hepatic copper in a liver biopsy. All young patients with chronic active hepatitis should have these tests
- Penicillamine must be given for life. Referral to a specialist centre is advisable. There is a risk of fulminant failure if penicillamine is stopped suddenly. Trientine or tetrathiomolybdate are alternatives if the patient cannot tolerate penicillamine
- The family should be screened (serum caeruloplasmin, serum copper and 24-h urinary copper), but liver biopsy is not needed if these tests are negative. Genetic counselling should be offered to relatives

Hepatic granulomas

- Granulomas on liver biopsy are usually an unexpected finding and often increase rather than resolve diagnostic confusion (Table 5.15)
- Granulomatous hepatitis is a misnomer, because neither the histological nor biochemical picture is that of hepatitis
- Symptoms are non-specific, or those of the underlying disease

Differential diagnosis

- The usual dilemma is to distinguish sarcoidosis from tuberculosis, because steroids for the former would be totally wrong for the latter.

Table 5.15 Causes of hepatic granulomas.

Common	Uncommon	Rare
Sarcoidosis	Brucellosis	Histoplasmosis
Tuberculosis	Drugs	Coccidioidomycosis
Primary biliary cirrhosis	hydralazine	Blastomycosis
Idiopathic (20–40%)	allopurinol	Berylliosis
	many others	Crohn's disease
	Q fever	Whipple's disease
		Hodgkin's disease
		Syphilis
		Leprosy
		Schistosomiasis
		Ascariasis

Sarcoidosis is usually distinguished by chest X-ray (hilar lymphadenopathy, middle zone infiltrates), elevated serum angiotensin-converting enzyme, negative Mantoux and positive Kveim tests, but these do not always resolve the dilemma. A trial of antituberculous chemotherapy and rebiopsy is then the safest course of action

• Idiopathic hepatic granulomas have a good prognosis. Occasionally there is a prolonged febrile illness, sometimes with acute abdominal pain and arthritis. Prednisolone 30 mg/day is then indicated, but only after investigation has excluded other (particularly infective) causes

5.7 Cirrhosis

Cirrhosis means loss of normal hepatic architecture due to fibrosis, with nodular regeneration. It implies irreversible liver disease and is the final stage of chronic liver disease from a variety of causes (Table 5.14, p. 188).

Causes (Table 5.16)

Most (70%) are due to alcohol, hepatitis B or hepatitis C (Section 5.5). Up to 20% are of unknown cause (cryptogenic).

Clinical features

Presentation varies from asymptomatic abnormal liver function tests to end-stage liver disease. A long period of compensated cirrhosis, when the patient feels well, is common. The equilibrium is easily upset (p. 164) as hepatic reserve dwindles, leading to:

Table 5.16 Causes of cirrhosis.

Common	Uncommon	Rare
Alcohol	Primary biliary	Haemochromatosis
Hepatitis B	Autoimmune	Wilson's disease
Hepatitis C		α_1-protease deficiency
(parenteral non-A, non-B)		Secondary biliary (strictures,
Cryptogenic		sclerosing cholangitis,
		atresia, cystic fibrosis)
		Cardiac (chronic right heart failure)
		Budd–Chiari syndrome
		Drugs
		methotrexate
		others

- Hepatocellular failure (p. 165):
  - encephalopathy
  - bleeding disorder
  - cutaneous signs (Table 5.2, p. 156)
  - altered drug metabolism (p. 161)
  - malnutrition (loss of muscle bulk)
- Ascites (p. 167)
- Portal hypertension (p. 173):
  - splenomegaly
  - hypersplenism
  - bleeding varices
  Other features include:
- Increased risk of hepatocellular carcinoma (p. 203) (largely related to male gender than the cause of cirrhosis)
- Tendency to infections (especially spontaneous bacterial peritonitis)
- Increased frequency of peptic ulceration
- Risk of renal failure following surgery (hepatorenal syndrome, p. 171)

Diagnostic pitfalls
Some of the clinical features of cirrhosis may be simulated by portal or splenic vein thrombosis, Budd–Chiari syndrome, or constrictive pericarditis (p. 168).

Investigations

A clinical diagnosis should usually be confirmed by liver biopsy, because biochemical tests correlate poorly with histological changes and treatable causes may be overlooked, even in alcoholics.

Blood tests

- Liver enzymes may be normal in the compensated phase. Marked elevation of the AST or ALP occur in alcoholic hepatitis or biliary cirrhosis, until the terminal stages when the levels fall (no functioning hepatocytes, no enzymes)
- HBsAg, HCV antibodies, antimitochondrial, antinuclear and antismooth muscle antibodies and serum ferritin should be measured even if the cause appears alcohol-related
- Elevated serum IgA, IgM or IgG are common in alcoholic, primary biliary and autoimmune diseases, respectively, forming part of the pattern of features (including history, other serological tests and liver histology) that confirm a specific diagnosis
- Thrombocytopenia and leucopenia are features of hypersplenism. Coagulation should be normal (INR < 1.3, prothrombin time < 22 s) before percutaneous liver biopsy

Liver biopsy

- Biopsy can usually be delayed until after recovery from an acute presentation
- Ascites and disordered clotting should be treated before biopsy, because the risk of haemorrhage (normally < 1 : 100) is increased. FFP 2 units immediately before biopsy is more effective at correcting disordered coagulation than vitamin K
- Transjugular liver biopsy is safe for decompensated cirrhotics, in experienced hands, if the diagnosis needs to be established despite coagulation that cannot be corrected
- Histological features include fibrosis and nodular regeneration; special stains (such as Perl's for iron, PAS for protease deficiency) contribute to a specific diagnosis

Management

Cirrhosis need not be progressive, even if it is irreversible.

General measures

- Alcohol—complete abstinence is essential if the aetiology is alcoholic, but is otherwise unnecessary, although restricted intake (< 4 units/week) is sensible advice
- Nutrition—a normal diet is possible in compensated cirrhotics. During encephalopathy protein should be restricted (40 g/day) and salt should not be added to food if ascites develops (p. 172)

- Drugs—NSAIDs, sedatives and opiates should be avoided (p. 161)
- Complications (portal hypertension, ascites) are treated in the standard way (pp. 173, 167), whatever the cause

Specific treatment

- Alcoholics—abstinence alters the prognosis from 30% to about 70% survival at 5 years
- Hepatitis B and C—α–interferon improves biochemical liver function, but has not yet been shown to improve mortality (p. 189)
- Primary biliary cirrhosis—ursodeoxycholic acid may be of value (p. 191), pending a decision about transplantation
- Haemochromatosis—venesection may improve liver histology (p. 193), although established cirrhosis is irreversible
- Wilson's disease—penicillamine (p. 196)
- Surgery for extrahepatic biliary strictures or atresia

Alcohol and the liver

- Four pathological types of alcoholic liver disease are recognized: fatty liver, acute hepatitis, chronic hepatitis and cirrhosis
- The reasons why some (especially women, Asians and Afro-Caribbeans) are susceptible to liver disease and others develop cerebral, pancreatic or cardiac disease remain unknown
- The amount of alcohol consumed is not directly related to the degree of damage, but the World Health Organization recommendations are < 28 units/week for men and < 21 units/week for women (1 unit is equivalent to one glass of wine, one pub measure of spirits or half a pint of beer)
- Alcohol abuse does not exclude less common causes of chronic liver disease, including viral or autoimmune chronic hepatitis or haemochromatosis

Fatty liver

- The mechanism is complex. Ethanol oxidation to acetaldehyde increases hydrogenated nicotinamide adenine dinucleotide (NADH), which favours triglyceride accumulation by decreasing fatty acid metabolism
- A palpable liver, increased MCV (> 98 fL) and mildly disordered liver enzymes are usually the only features, but these may also be the only signs of established cirrhosis
- Fatty change is rapidly reversible upon abstinence from alcohol
- Liver biopsy is necessary to confirm the diagnosis and exclude irreversible disease. It may also reinforce the need for abstinence. It is reasonable

to recheck liver enzymes after 2 months of complete abstinence in alcoholic patients without signs of chronic liver disease, and only to biopsy those whose enzymes remain abnormal

• Obesity, diabetes and parenteral nutrition are other causes of fatty liver

Acute hepatitis

• Jaundice, fever, signs of alcohol withdrawal (tremor, agitation, perspiration), tender hepatomegaly and biochemical changes of hepatitis (Table 5.3, p. 158) are characteristic. A cholestatic picture is more common than in viral hepatitis, as is a polymorphonuclear leucocytosis

• A heavy binge is usually the provoking factor, often on top of established liver disease. 30% die

• Fulminant hepatic failure is not uncommon and the risk is increased by even moderate doses of paracetamol

• Steroids (40 mg daily for 6 weeks) have been shown to reduce mortality in one controlled study, excluding patients who were bleeding from varices or septic, but remain controversial

Chronic hepatitis

• The clinical and biochemical features are the same as in other types of chronic hepatitis (p. 185), so other causes should be excluded, even in drinkers

• Progression to cirrhosis is almost certain without abstinence

Cirrhosis

• Telangiectases and Dupuytren's contracture are more common findings in alcoholic cirrhosis than in other types, but other clinical features are similar (Table 5.2, p. 156)

• A micronodular cirrhosis is usual

• Management is directed at complications (ascites, portal hypertension, encephalopathy). Abstinence may still alter the course of end-stage alcoholic cirrhosis: it is never too late to stop drinking

• The risk of hepatoma is increased

General points on management

• Detoxification is trying for everybody. A suggested protocol is shown in Fig. 5.6

• Adequate control of agitation is essential if seizures are to be avoided. Nursing staff must be advised to give 'as required' sedation readily if there are any signs of agitation

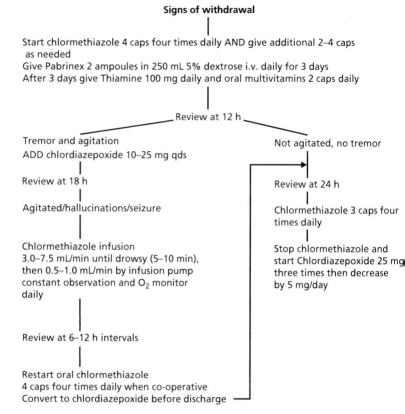

Signs of withdrawal

Start chlormethiazole 4 caps four times daily AND give additional 2–4 caps as needed
Give Pabrinex 2 ampoules in 250 mL 5% dextrose i.v. daily for 3 days
After 3 days give Thiamine 100 mg daily and oral multivitamins 2 caps daily

Review at 12 h

Tremor and agitation
ADD chlordiazepoxide 10–25 mg qds

Review at 18 h

Agitated/hallucinations/seizure

Chlormethiazole infusion
3.0–7.5 mL/min until drowsy (5–10 min),
then 0.5–1.0 mL/min by infusion pump
constant observation and O$_2$ monitor
daily

Review at 6–12 h intervals

Restart oral chlormethiazole
4 caps four times daily when co-operative
Convert to chlordiazepoxide before discharge

Not agitated, no tremor

Review at 24 h

Chlormethiazole 3 caps four
times daily

Stop chlormethiazole and
start Chlordiazepoxide 25 mg
three times then decrease
by 5 mg/day

Fig. 5.6 Detoxification of alcoholics.

- Chlormethiazole is better than chlordiazepoxide for controlling hallucinations
- Vitamins A, C and B$_1$ and folate are commonly deficient. Intravenous vitamins (such as Multibionta 1 + 2 vials in 250 mL 5% dextrose) should be given every day for 3 days to all alcoholic patients admitted to hospital
- Alcoholics with a high MCV (sometimes as high as 115 fL) should still have folate, B$_{12}$ and thyroid function checked
- Careful examination of peripheral nerves, coordination, eye movements, short-term memory and mental state is often rewarding. Wernicke's encephalopathy (confusion, nystagmus, cranial (VI) nerve palsy, ataxia) is a medical emergency and reversible in the early stages with thiamine. The signs of Wernicke's, or those of Korsakoff's psychosis (short-term memory loss and confabulation) can be overlooked by the unwary
- Counselling services and psychiatric intervention have variable results. They should be discussed with the patient and arranged if the patient is willing to cooperate (Appendix 1, p. 471). Whilst there are some striking

successes, there are more recidivists. Family involvement is as important as organized care

• Chlormethiazole should not be prescribed to outpatients, because it is often sold or abused

Prognosis

• 15% of alcoholics develop cirrhosis over 10 years
• The Child's classification (Table 5.5. p. 166) is useful for comparing the outcome of variceal bleeding or surgery in groups of patients with cirrhosis, but not helpful for predicting the course in an individual
• 5-year survival in alcoholic cirrhotics is 50% overall, 30% for continued drinkers and 70% for abstainers

5.8 **Tumours**

Hepatoma

Primary hepatocellular carcinoma is the most common malignant tumour in the world, although rare in the West. The incidence is around 2:100 000 in Europe and 85:100 000 in Taiwan. Eighty per cent of all patients have pre-existing cirrhosis and most are male. All types of cirrhosis predispose to hepatoma, although hepatitis B is the commonest cause worldwide.

Causes
• Hepatitis B or C
• Alcoholic cirrhosis is the commonest predisposing factor in Europe
• Haemochromatosis
• Aflatoxin (fungal infection of ground nuts) and Thorotrast (radiological contrast medium used until 1950) are now rare causes

Clinical features
• Rapid development of ascites, increasing liver size or jaundice in a patient with known cirrhosis should always suggest a hepatoma
• Fever, weight loss and right upper quadrant pain are typical
• A hepatic arterial bruit or rub are highly suggestive but rare. A bruit can also sometimes be heard in acute alcoholic hepatitis

Investigations
• Elevated AFP (> 20 ng/mL) occurs in 80%. Other causes are rare, but include testicular, ovarian or pancreatic tumours, hydatidiform mole and

pregnancy. In patients with an AFP > 100 ng/mL, 97% have a hepatoma

• Ultrasound is as sensitive as CT scanning for detecting hepatic tumours and should be the first imaging technique. CT scanning should be performed if there is doubt, or if anatomical relations of the tumour are not clearly demonstrated by ultrasound

• Liver biopsy should be avoided if the tumour appears confined to one lobe, pending a decision about surgery. Tumour may seed down the biopsy track, rendering the tumour inoperable. However, in multifocal lesions, biopsy under ultrasound control is necessary for a histological diagnosis. A rare, fibrolamellar type of hepatoma occurs in non-cirrhotics and has a better prognosis

• Angiography is indicated if surgery is planned, for therapeutic embolization or intra-arterial chemotherapy. It is unnecessary for planning surgery if ultrasound demonstrates tumour in both lobes of the liver, because this means incurable disease

• Some centres screen cirrhotics for hepatoma by ultrasound or AFP measurement every 6 months, but there is no evidence that this prolongs survival and is not recommended routinely

Management

• Surgical resection may be possible in 20–30%. Tumour must be confined to one lobe of the liver, without extrahepatic spread. Referral to a specialist centre for preoperative assessment is recommended

• Transplant has an unacceptable recurrence rate, except in localized tumours of the fibrolamellar type. The occasional success in hepatocellular carcinoma, however, means that it is worth discussing exceptional cases (young patients, prepared to accept a < 10% chance of cure) with a transplant centre

• Chemotherapy (mitozantrone, adriamycin, or multiple drugs) is unsatisfactory at present. 10–30% respond, but mean survival is only 9 months. Hepatic arterial infusion of drugs and transcatheter arterial chemoembolization (TACE) are under trial

• Angiographic tumour embolization and radiotherapy are useful for relieving pain, but cannot be expected to offer a cure

• Prevention by hepatitis B vaccination is a hope for the future

Prognosis

• Median survival is 12 weeks after diagnosis

• In the minority who have surgical resection, 1-year survival is 60% and 5-year survival is 25–40% in some studies

Metastases

In Europe 90% of liver tumours are metastatic. Colorectal, breast, lung, gastric or pancreatic cancers are the common primary sites. Metastases are said not to occur in cirrhotic livers. Median survival after diagnosis of hepatic metastases is 2–4 months. Earlier diagnosis by ultrasound is increasing this period (the 'lead time'), although prognosis remains unchanged.

Single hepatic metastases from colorectal cancer should be considered for resection at a specialist centre, in patients aged < 50 years. More than 2-year survival has been reported. Chemotherapy or arterial embolization offer no better results than for primary liver tumours.

Benign tumours

Haemangiomas are usually found incidentally on ultrasound or CT scanning. They may be confused with metastases (although the density is different) and present a hazard at liver biopsy, but are otherwise unimportant. Hepatic adenomas are very rarely associated with the oral contraceptive pill and these are best resected.

5.9 **Abscesses and cysts**

Hepatic abscess (often multiple) may be occult and surprisingly difficult to diagnose.

Pyogenic

- Cholangitis, diverticulitis or following abdominal surgery are now the usual causes, as opposed to appendicitis, but often no cause can be found
- Fever (90%), weight loss and malaise are non-specific. Hepatomegaly and right upper quadrant pain occur in about 50%. Jaundice is a bad prognostic sign
- Blood cultures are negative in 50%. If *Streptococcus milleri* is grown, it is almost invariably due to a liver abscess
- Ultrasound of the liver is always indicated for patients with fever and mild derangement of liver enzymes. CT scanning is more sensitive for lesions near the diaphragm
- Needle aspiration under ultrasound control identifies the organism in 90%. Mixed aerobes and anaerobes are usual

• Percutaneous drainage of a single abscess and the one or two largest cavities of multiple abscesses should be performed by a radiologist. Surgical drainage is now rarely indicated

• Intravenous metronidazole 500 mg and cefotaxime 1 g three times daily should be given for 2 weeks, followed by oral antibiotics for 6 weeks, depending on the sensitivity of the organism

Amoebic

• Very rare in those living in Europe, but patients may present years after living in the tropics

• 80% are aged < 40 years

• Pain is more common and systemic features less common than in pyogenic abscesses. Point tenderness is typical and hiccups herald impending rupture, but dysentery is unusual

• Ultrasound and markedly elevated serum antibodies to *Entamoeba histolytica* are diagnostic in > 90%. Hot stools should be examined for trophozoites (p. 388), which are highly suggestive of the diagnosis. Aspiration of thick, pink–brown 'anchovy sauce' pus is characteristic, but not indicated unless the diagnosis cannot be confirmed in other ways

• Metronidazole 800 mg three times daily for 10 days is effective in most patients, but should always be followed by diloxanide 500 mg three times daily for 10 days to prevent recurrent invasive disease.

• Drainage is needed only for impending rupture, indicated by severe pain, pleuritic pain, or hiccups. Recurrent fever may be due to secondary bacterial infection

Hydatid cysts

• Symptomless hepatomegaly in those from the eastern Mediterranean, South America or Welsh farmers is occasionally due to cysts of *Echinococcus granulosus*

• Liver function is usually normal, eosinophilia often absent and serological tests may be only weakly positive. Ultrasound presents a characteristic appearance of multiple 'daughter' cysts, with clearly defined walls. Hydatid complement fixation tests should be checked before aspiration of any hepatic cysts in patients from endemic areas

• Hydatid cysts are often best left alone if asymptomatic. Albendazole (800 mg daily for 28 days) may be effective and is an adjunct to surgery for symptomatic disease. Surgery is indicated for increasing size, complications of local pressure or secondary infection. Liver biopsy is contraindicated because of the risk of anaphylaxis

Polycystic liver disease

Occasional cysts in the liver are a common finding on ultrasound and of no significance, but multiple cysts indicate polycystic liver disease with auto-somal dominant inheritance. Associated polycystic renal disease often dominates the clinical picture, but polycystic liver disease may occur in isolation. Cysts may be massive (> 15 cm diameter) and gross hepatomegaly can cause discomfort. Haemorrhage into a cyst or rupture present as an acute abdomen. Surgical exploration and marsupialization of the affected cyst(s) is then indicated. Portal hypertension or hepatic failure is rare except when polycystic disease presents in childhood. Transplant is then possible. The risk of cholangiocarcinoma (but not hepatoma) may be increased.

5.10 Clinical dilemmas

General advice is given in Appendix 4 (p. 491).

Asymptomatic abnormal liver function tests

Elevated liver enzymes or serum bilirubin are an increasingly common incidental finding due to automated biochemical tests. Normal ranges (Table 5.3, p. 158) represent the 95th centile of a selected healthy population. At best this leads to earlier diagnosis of treatable disease, but at worst it exposes the patient to the complications of ill-advised investigations. The following plan is recommended.
- Ask about:
  - Alcohol intake
  - Drug treatment or abuse
  - Previous jaundice
  - Family history of hepatic or chronic disease
  - Recent viral illness
  - Overseas travel
- Examine for:
  - Hepatomegaly and splenomegaly
  - Signs of chronic liver disease (Table 5.2, p. 156)
  - Lymphadenopathy
  - Urticarial rash or arthritis (associated with chronic hepatitis)
- Then investigate (Fig. 5.7)

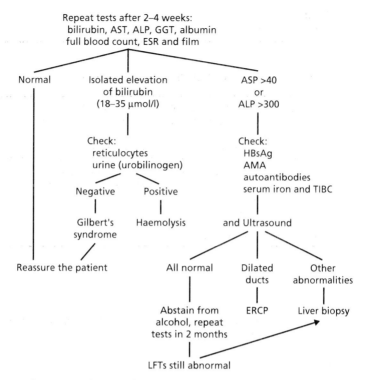

Fig. 5.7 Investigation of asymptomatic abnormal liver function tests.

Liver transplantation (Table 5.17)

Indications for liver transplant in fulminant hepatic failure are given in Table 1.8 and relative contraindications in Table 5.18. The timing of transplant in chronic liver disease is difficult, so early discussion with a referral centre (Appendix 1, p. 477) is advisable.

Table 5.17 Diseases potentially curable by transplant (adults).

Primary biliary cirrhosis
Cryptogenic cirrhosis
Postviral cirrhosis (except those still HBeAg +ve)
Alcoholic cirrhosis (if abstinent)
Autoimmune chronic hepatitis
Primary sclerosing cholangitis
Budd–Chiari syndrome
Fibrolamellar hepatoma
Fulminant hepatic failure (Section 1.10, p. 53)
Metabolic disorders: Wilson's disease, others (usually children)

Table 5.18 Relative contraindications to liver transplant.

Active hepatitis B or C infection (viral DNA or RNA in serum)
Malignancy (although unifocal hepatocellular or fibrolamellar tumours in young
    patients may be an exception)
Recent or continued alcohol abuse (abstinence for < 6 months)
Psychological inability to comply with post-transplant treatment and monitoring
    (involving regular medication, weekly blood tests, and liver biopsies)
Age > 60 years (but carefully selected older patients have done well)
Previous upper abdominal surgery
Portal vein thrombosis
Extrahepatic malignant tumours
Cardiorespiratory or renal disease

The other side of the coin is that every hospital has a responsibility to face the difficult task of finding donors.

Timing
- End-stage liver disease—histological evidence of irreversible liver damage (fibrosis), with
    - jaundice (bilirubin > 100 μmol/L in primary biliary cirrhosis), or
    - ascites refractory to both spironolactone and a loop diuretic, or
    - after two separate episodes of variceal haemorrhage, or
    - recurrent or chronic encephalopathy, or
    - one episode of documented spontaneous bacterial peritonitis
- The timing is simplest in primary biliary cirrhosis, because once the bilirubin is > 100 μmol/L, the prognosis is usually less than 1 year
- The prognosis in the later stages of primary sclerosing cholangitis or other types of cirrhosis is much more difficult to predict
- The patient and family should understand the irreversible nature of the disease, the likely delay of weeks (or months) whilst a matched donor is found, and the prognosis

Postoperative implications
- Hospital stay is usually 4 weeks
- Frequent blood tests are necessary (weekly for several months and then less frequently) to measure cyclosporin levels, biochemical and haematological tests, in addition to outpatient visits
- Drug compliance must be good
- Graft rejection occurs in 25% and retransplant is necessary in 15%

Prognosis

• 80–90% 5-year survival in primary biliary cirrhosis, but results are constantly improving. After 1 year, the outlook is excellent. Primary biliary cirrhosis and autoimmune liver disease have very occasionally recurred in the transplanted liver, although chronic rejection may look histologically similar

• 50–80% 5-year survival in primary sclerosing cholangitis or cryptogenic cirrhosis

6 Gall Bladder and Biliary Tree

6.1) **Clinical anatomy of the biliary tract**

The biliary canaliculi adjacent to each hepatocyte drain into interlobular, then septal, bile ducts which combine to form intrahepatic ducts visible on cholangiography. The right and left hepatic ducts join at the porta hepatis to form the common hepatic duct, which unites with the cystic duct from the gall bladder to form the common bile duct. This enters the duodenum through the head of the pancreas (Fig. 6.1).

Gall bladder contraction is stimulated by cholecystokinin (secretin) after meals. Biliary flow is controlled by a pressure gradient between the common bile duct and duodenum, as well as the peristaltic pump action of the sphincter of Oddi, which is also influenced by cholecystokinin.

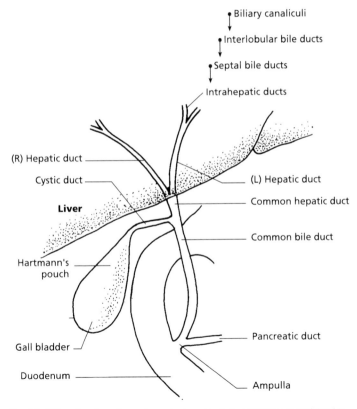

Fig. 6.1 Biliary tract anatomy. Important anatomical variations are explained in the text.

Anatomical anomalies of pathological importance

• Opening of the common bile duct onto a duodenal diverticulum (cannulation of the papilla is difficult and ERCP/sphincterotomy potentially dangerous, due to risk of perforation)

• Accessory artery superior to the ampulla of Vater in 1% (sphincterotomy can lead to major haemorrhage)

• Separate exit points into the duodenum of the common bile duct and main pancreatic duct (endoscopic cannulation is difficult)

• Cystic duct fails to join the common hepatic duct in 20% (both the duct and its union must be identified before ligation or stapling, especially at laparoscopic cholecystectomy)

• Cystic artery may arise from the left hepatic or gastroduodenal arteries, rather than the right hepatic artery

• Choledochal cysts occur in 1 : 15 000 in Western countries (more common in Japan). The commonest type is a fusiform dilation of the common bile duct, usually presenting with jaundice and abdominal pain in children, but sometimes (10–20%) in adults

• Congenital, segmental, saccular dilatation of the intrahepatic bile ducts is termed Caroli's disease. It may be associated with renal tubular ectasia

6.2) Gall stones

Bile is concentrated in the gall bladder, which acts as a reservoir between meals for bile acids (cholic and chenodeoxycholic acid) which are essential for emulsifying lipids prior to digestion and absorption. Bile acids form the outer, hydrophilic layer of micelles which contain lipid-soluble cholesterol in the centre. Phospholipids insert into the micellar wall to increase the micellar capacity for cholesterol.

Insufficient bile acids (e.g. caused by failure of enterohepatic recycling in terminal ileal disease) or imbalance between cholesterol and phospholipid concentrations in bile, will lead to precipitation of cholesterol crystals from the supersaturated bile, which then form the nucleus for gall stone formation (lithogenic bile). Incomplete gall bladder emptying allows crystals to grow into gall stones. There are proteins that either promote or inhibit nucleation and the balance between these factors may be the key determinant in an individual's susceptibility to form gall stones.

Pigment stones are caused by bilirubin forming insoluble calcium precipitates in bile. Black, brittle pure pigment stones account for 70% of radio-opaque gall stones. Brown pigment stones are soft, often intrahepatic and unusual (Fig. 6.2).

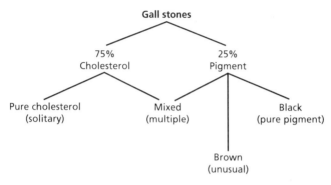

Fig. 6.2 Types of gall stones.

Prevalence

On ultrasound studies of a normal population, 7–15% people have gall stones, which become more common with age. Conditions predisposing to gall stones are shown in Table 6.1.

Symptoms

Most gall stones remain 'silent' in the fundus of the gall bladder. Migration to the cystic duct and impaction causes acute or chronic cholecystitis which resolves when disimpaction occurs, or progresses to complications (Fig. 6.3).
• Silent stones—complications develop in 1–2% per year, or in 3% per year in those with mild symptoms at presentation

Table 6.1 Conditions predisposing to gall stones.

Cholesterol	Black pigment	Brown pigment
Gender (2F:1M)	Chronic haemolysis	Sclerosing cholangitis
Obesity	sickle cell	Oriental
Diet (low fibre)	spherocytosis	biliary parasites
Race (Europe, USA,	prosthetic valve	
American Indians)	Cirrhosis	
Cirrhosis (30%)	Biliary infection	
Terminal ileal	*E. coli*,	
Crohn's	*Clostridium* spp.	
resection		
Drugs		
oral contraceptive		
clofibrate		

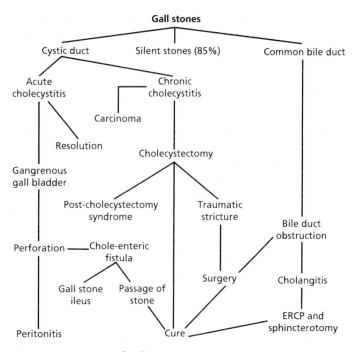

Fig. 6.3 Consequences of gall stones.

- Acute cholecystitis—persistent, severe right upper quadrant pain, fever and leucocytosis (p. 29). Acalculous acute cholecystitis is rare and caused by bacterial infection, polyarteritis or trauma
- Chronic cholecystitis—recurrent biliary colic, dyspepsia, fat intolerance and non-specific features
- Common bile duct stones—jaundice, abdominal pain (p. 221)
- Cholangitis—jaundice, fever, abdominal pain (p. 228), usually due to stones in the common bile duct
- Gangrenous gall bladder and empyema—septic, and severe illness, with local peritonism
- Mirizzi's syndrome—obstructive jaundice due to external compression of the common hepatic duct by a stone impacted in the cystic duct, often associated with cholangitis
- Biliary fistula—from a chronically inflamed gall bladder into the small intestine or colon, resulting in air in the biliary tree, resolution of symptoms or, very rarely, impaction at the ileocaecal valve and gall stone ileus
- Perforation—local or diffuse peritonitis after acute cholecystitis

• Carcinoma of the gall bladder or bile ducts—jaundice, weight loss, pain (p. 230). More common in patients with gall stones, but does not justify prophylactic cholecystectomy

Investigations

Ultrasound
• Most effective non-invasive method of detecting stones, but often finds incidental, silent stones. Stones may occasionally be missed, even in experienced hands. In some patients the gall bladder cannot be identified because of gas, fibrosis or unusual anatomy
• Also useful for diagnosing biliary obstruction, acute or chronic cholecystitis and for assessing gall bladder function when performed before and after a fatty meal (p. 220)
• If the gall bladder wall is of normal thickness, gall stones are likely to be incidental to symptoms of abdominal pain
• CT scan is usually better, but still fallible, at identifying common bile duct stones

Blood tests
• All are normal in chronic cholecystitis or silent stones
• Elevated ALP or γ-GT suggests common duct stones. Leucocytosis occurs in acute cholecystitis or cholangitis
• Serum cholesterol is unrelated to biliary cholesterol, but is elevated in primary biliary cirrhosis

Other tests
• Plain abdominal X-ray—mandatory in acute abdominal pain. May show calcified stones, enlarged liver or air in the biliary tree (chole-enteric fistula, clostridial cholangitis or postintervention)
• Oral cholecystography—indicated for assessing gall bladder function before non-surgical treatment (p. 220)
• Isotope scanning—useful in acute cholecystitis (p. 29)
• ERCP—for diagnosis and treatment of biliary obstruction (p. 224)
• Percutaneous transhepatic cholangiogram (PTC)—indicated when dilated intrahepatic ducts are detected on ultrasound and ERCP is not technically possible or readily available. Complementary to ERCP if proximal biliary anatomy needs clarifying (a cholangiocarcinoma may block the flow of contrast); or for stenting tortuous strictures (p. 224)
• Intravenous cholangiography and the bromsulphthalein (BSP) test for assessing biliary excretory function, are obsolete

Indications for surgery

Most decisions are straightforward. Difficulty arises in deciding whether gall stones in patients with non-specific symptoms are the cause or merely incidental (Table 6.2). Remember that 85% of asymptomatic gall stones remain asymptomatic for over 15 years.

Laparoscopic cholecystectomy

Laparoscopic surgery through a periumbilical incision and two upper quadrant punctures for instrument manipulation is now the commonest technique and safe in experienced hands. Previous upper abdominal surgery or gross obesity make it more difficult and conversion to open cholecystectomy is necessary in 1–5% of all procedures. The risk of bile duct injury is similar (0.25%) to standard cholecystectomy; if a postoperative bile leak occurs from the cystic duct, sphincterotomy or stent placement at ERCP are usually effective. Advantages over standard cholecystectomy are the short hospital stay (< 48 h), limited postoperative pain and early return to work (< 1 week). Unlike non-surgical options (dissolution or lithotripsy), there is no risk of stone recurrence.

Mini-laparotomy cholecystectomy

Surgery through a 4–5 cm incision is an alternative favoured by some surgeons. Standard cholecystectomy is now largely confined to patients in whom laparoscopic surgery is not possible, or when exploration of the common bile duct is necessary, usually for very large calculi that it has not been possible to extract at ERCP.

Table 6.2 Symptomatic or incidental stones?

	Symptomatic	Incidental
Pain	Acute episodes < 60 s	Constant dull ache
	Like labour contractions	Variable
	1–72 h duration	Most days, or continuous
Pain-free interval	Several weeks/months	Rare
Fat intolerance	Common	Common
Flatulence	Common	Common
Bloating	Less common	Common
Physical signs	RUQ tenderness or none	RUQ tenderness or none
Ultrasound	Gall stone(s)	Gall stone(s)
	Thickened wall	Normal gall bladder wall
Oral cholecystogram	Non-functioning	Functioning (may be poor in the elderly)

RUQ, right upper quadrant.

Colour plate section

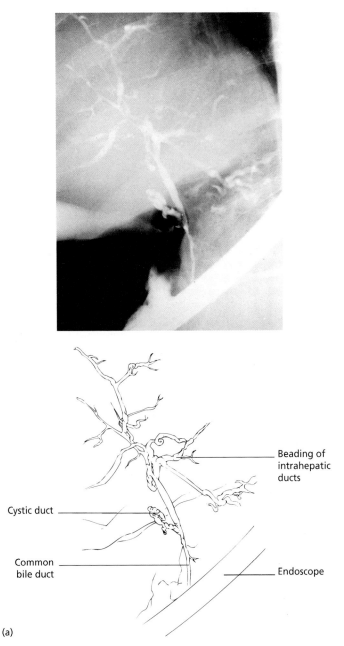

(a)

Plate 6.1 Primary sclerosing cholangitis in an asymptomatic 42-year-old man with quiescent total ulcerative colitis for 18 years
(a) ERCP in primary sclerosing cholangitis.

[Facing p.218]

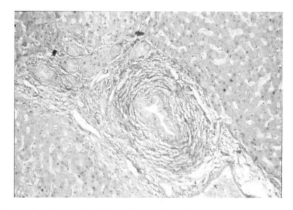

(b)

(b) Liver biopsy showing 'onion skin' peribiliary fibrosis (reticulin stain x 70).

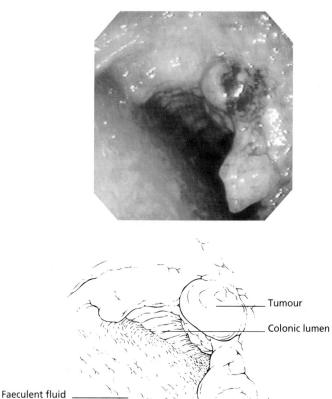

(c)

(c) Coincidental colorectal carcinoma.

Absolute indications for cholecystectomy

- Acute cholecystitis—optimum treatment is surgery during the same admission, on the next available operating list (p. 30)
- Chronic cholecystitis—typical history of biliary colic and a contracted or non-functioning gall bladder shown by ultrasound or cholecystography after a fatty meal
- Common bile duct stones—age < 70 years, after ERCP and sphincterotomy in patients who also need a cholestectomy. In patients > 70 years or those at poor operative risk, endoscopic sphincterotomy alone has a lower mortality, although the risk of recurrent biliary colic remains
- Gangrenous gall bladder—emergency cholecystostomy is often safer than cholecystectomy. Later elective cholecystectomy or spontaneous closure are then possible
- Gall stone ileus—to relieve intestinal obstruction, with later cholecystectomy
- Elective cholecystectomy is indicated if gall stones are considered to be the cause of abdominal pain
- Gall stone pancreatitis—early cholecystectomy after recovery from pancreatitis is essential if recurrent pancreatitis and complications are to be avoided
- Irritable bowel syndrome, peptic ulcer, chronic pancreatitis or renal tract disease may produce similar symptoms to chronic cholecystitis and should be excluded if doubt exists
- Postcholecystectomy syndrome is more common in patients who present with non-specific symptoms (flatulent dyspepsia)

Non-surgical options

These options must be balanced against safe operations (mortality 0.1% age < 50 years, 0.5% > 50 years) which remove all gall stones without recurrence, although retained stones occur in about 2% and other complications (including postcholecystectomy syndrome) in 10%.

Only 10–20% patients with symptomatic gall stones are suitable, and treatment is unsuccessful in up to a third. The risk of recurrent stones is the main drawback of all techniques that leave the gall bladder *in situ*. Symptoms should be present before any treatment is contemplated.

Indications for non-surgical management

- Patient declines surgery
- When the surgical risk is unacceptable

- Functioning gall bladder demonstrated by oral cholecystography, isotope (HIDA) scan, or ultrasound before and after a fatty meal
- Non-calcified gall stones on abdominal X-ray or ultrasound. CT scan is needed to assess the degree of calcification in solitary calculi
- Solitary stones must be < 1 cm for reasonable success, although larger stones can be fragmented by lithotripsy
- Patient understands the risk of recurrence and need for long-term treatment

Ursodeoxycholic acid (UDCA)

A single dose of 10–13 mg/kg/day for 4 months (50% dissolution rate) and continued for up to 2 years achieves optimum success (80–90% after 1 year) in patients with radiolucent stones < 5 mm in diameter that float on oral cholecystography. Diarrhoea is the main side-effect, but is less common than with chenodeoxycholic acid. Treatment (750 mg/day) for each year costs over £550. Recurrence after successful treatment is 10% per year for 5 years, then plateaus (50% at 10 years), so maintenance treatment may be indicated, similar to lithotripsy.

External shock-wave lithotripsy (ESWL)

General, epidural or spinal anaesthesia is needed, although immersion is no longer necessary. Most effective for solitary stones 15–20 mm in diameter, when the cystic duct is patent (70% success by 8 months). ESWL is usually inappropriate when there are more than three calculi. Transient biliary colic occurs in about 35% and 3–5% develop pancreatitis or cholecystitis. UDCA (500–750 mg/day) is needed after ESWL and up to 90% are reported free of stones after 1 year. Recurrence without continued UDCA is 50% at 5 years.

Other approaches

These techniques are not yet established and for the main part remain experimental.

- Contact dissolution—methyl-*tert*-butyl ether (MTBE) via percutaneous cholecystotomy is invasive and associated with bile leakage needing cholecystectomy in 5%
- Percutaneous cystolithotomy—puncture of the gall bladder with gall bladder drainage for up to 10 days

6.3 Cholestatic jaundice

Cholestatic jaundice is due to interruption of bile flow anywhere in the biliary tree. The site of obstruction is either extrahepatic, when there is mechanical obstruction to the main bile ducts, or intrahepatic when the obstructing lesion is usually not visible (except with intrahepatic strictures, stones or tumour). 'Obstructive jaundice' usually applies to extrahepatic causes. About 20% of patients with clinical or biochemical features of cholestasis have hepatocellular disease.

Causes

Extrahepatic obstruction (Table 6.3)
About 70% of cholestatic jaundice is due to extrahepatic obstruction. Extrahepatic ducts dilate in distal obstruction, as caused by pancreatic carcinoma, before intrahepatic duct dilatation, which occurs early in high obstruction (at the porta hepatis), and is readily detected by ultrasound.

Table 6.3 Causes of extrahepatic cholestasis.

Common	Uncommon	Rare
Common duct stones	Portal lymph nodes	Pseudocyst
Panceatic cancer	Pancreatitis	Choledochal cyst
	acute	
	chronic	
	Post-traumatic stricture	
	Cholangiocarcinoma	
	Ampullary carcinoma	

Intrahepatic obstruction (Table 6.4)
• Drug-induced cholestasis and primary biliary cirrhosis are the commonest causes
• Benign recurrent cholestasis presents as recurrent cholestatic jaundice lasting for several weeks, for which no cause can be found

Table 6.4 Causes of intrahepatic cholestasis.

Common	Uncommon	Rare
Drugs	Viral hepatitis	Benign recurrent
phenothiazines	Alcoholic hepatitis	Hodgkin's disease
many others	Primary sclerosing cholangitis	Intrahepatic stones
Primary biliary cirrhosis	Cirrhosis	Hepatic granulomas
	Metastases	
	Septicaemia	
	Cholangiocarcinoma	

- Jaundice in Hodgkin's disease is usually extrahepatic, due to lymph nodes obstructing the porta hepatis. Intrahepatic cholestasis is usually preterminal
- Septicaemia or total parenteral nutrition occasionally cause cholestatic jaundice, usually in a patient with multiorgan failure

Clinical features

- Jaundice appears slowly, often preceded by pruritus
- Itching and pale stools are characteristic of both intra- and extrahepatic cholestasis (Table 6.5)
- Dark urine also occurs in hepatocellular (but not prehepatic) jaundice, but urobilinogen is only absent in complete bile duct obstruction
- Extrahepatic cholestasis may be associated with pain and fever, indicating cholangitis (Table 6.6). Urgent culture, antibiotics and drainage are then indicated (p. 228). This is rare in intrahepatic cholestasis
- If the gall bladder is palpable in the right upper quadrant, then jaundice is unlikely to be due to stones (Courvoisier's sign). By implication, it is more likely to be due to malignancy

Investigations

Confirmation of cholestasis

- ALP is markedly elevated (> three times, often 10 times, normal), associated with an elevated γ-GT
- Bilirubin concentrations reflect the duration of cholestasis. The highest levels are reached in complete obstruction by carcinoma or end-stage intrahepatic disease such as primary biliary cirrhosis
- An isolated high ALP without elevated bilirubin suggests intrahepatic disease (primary biliary cirrhosis or primary sclerosing cholangitis)—as long as Paget's disease is excluded!

Table 6.5 Physical signs in cholestatic jaundice.

Pale stools
Dark orange urine
Scratch marks (excoriation)
Polished nails (itching)
Finger clubbing
Xanthelasma (eyelids)
Xanthomas (rarely palmar creases, tendons)
Hepatomegaly
Palpable gall bladder (especially carcinoma)

Table 6.6 Differences between extrahepatic and intrahepatic cholestasis.

	Extrahepatic	Intrahepatic
History	Abdominal pain Fever Middle age/elderly Previous biliary surgery	Anorexia, malaise Contact/blood transfusion Drug exposure or abuse
Examination	Fever Abdominal tenderness Palpable gall bladder	Ascites Stigmata of liver disease (Table 5.2, p. 156) Encephalopathy

Biochemistry	Concomitant elevation of
	   bilirubin and alkaline
	   phosphatase
	Prothromin time corrects
	   with vitamin K
		High alkaline phosphatase
		   without elevated bilirubin
		
		Concomitant elevation of
		   transaminases

- ALP isoenzymes are very rarely indicated and only when there is real doubt about the origin of the ALP

Identifying the cause

The main aim is to distinguish intra- from extrahepatic cholestasis. The sequence of investigations is shown in Fig. 6.4.

Ultrasound

Ultrasound is not good at identifying common bile duct stones, although it will detect a dilated common bile duct (diameter > 7 mm).

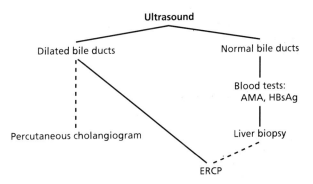

Fig. 6.4 Sequence of investigations in cholestatic jaundice.

ERCP

- ERCP should be rapidly arranged if intrahepatic ducts are dilated
- A dilated common bile duct *without* an obstructing lesion occurs shortly after an obstructing stone has passed (air may also be seen in the biliary tree)
- Or after cholecystectomy (persists for years, but rarely > 9 mm diameter)

PTC

PTC is now rarely indicated and only if:
- ERCP is not readily available
- ERCP does not opacify all of the biliary tree (cholangiocarcinomas can obstruct flow)
- Therapeutic stenting of a high, tortuous stricture is necessary (performed in conjunction with ERCP, or by percutaneous insertion of a self-expanding metal stent)

Indications for ERCP

Diagnostic

- Jaundice with dilated intrahepatic ducts
- Cholangitis (urgently, within 48 h)
- Jaundice or elevated ALP with normal calibre intrahepatic ducts, when liver biopsy does not establish a diagnosis and especially if the patient has ulcerative colitis (high chance of primary sclerosing cholangitis)
- Recurrent acute or chronic pancreatitis (Fig. 4.2, p. 138)
- Postcholecystectomy pain (p. 232)

Therapeutic

- Sphincterotomy for common bile duct stones (Fig. 6.5)
- Stenting of malignant strictures (Fig. 6.5)
- Acute pancreatitis if ultrasound identifies stones in the gall bladder

Management

Jaundice due to extrahepatic obstruction can usually be relieved by sphincterotomy and stone extraction or stent insertion at the time of ERCP. A joint decision with the surgeons can then be made about further procedures (such as cholecystectomy, Whipple's procedure, choledochojejunostomy or segment III biliary diversion).

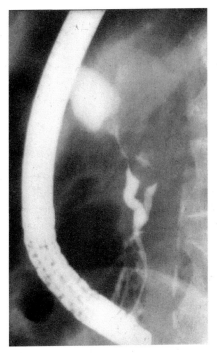

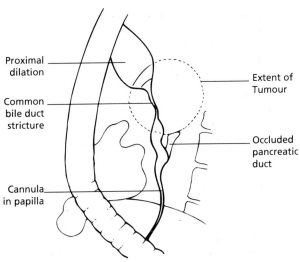

Proximal dilation

Extent of Tumour

Common bile duct stricture

Occluded pancreatic duct

Cannula in papilla

(a)

Fig. 6.5 ERCP in biliary obstruction. (a) ERCP demonstrating a blocked pancreatic duct due to a carcinoma which has caused stricturing of the common bile duct (CBD) leading to dilatation of the proximal biliary tree. (Continued on p. 226)

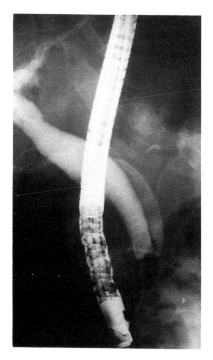

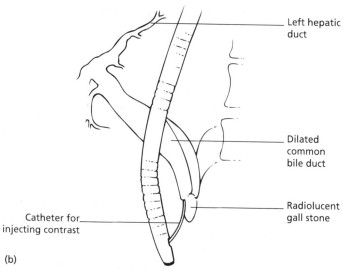

Left hepatic
duct

Dilated
common
bile duct

Radiolucent
gall stone

Catheter for
injecting contrast

(b)

Fig. 6.5 *(continued)* (b) ERCP in a patient with obstructive jaundice due to gall
stone impacted in the csommon bile duct.

Common bile duct stones

Patients > 70 years
- Endoscopic sphincterotomy (8–15 mm incision through the ampulla) allows the stones to be extracted by trawling the common bile duct with a balloon cannula or basket. It may be possible to crush large calculi with a lithotripter to aid extraction. Whilst duct clearance at the initial ERCP is optimal, small residual stones can be allowed to pass spontaneously, often with some further pain
- Subsequent cholecystectomy is not required in 90%
- If large calculi cannot be extracted, or if the patient is very frail or sick, insertion of a large (11 French gauge) stent is effective at preventing recurrent jaundice or cholangitis

Fit patients < 70 years
- Endoscopic sphincterotomy is usually performed first
- Early cholecystectomy with peroperative cholangiography is then necessary, to remove the source of stones and confirm clearance of the bile ducts. Some surgeons prefer to perform cholecystectomy and exploration of the bile ducts as a single procedure, without first doing an endoscopic sphincterotomy

Retained stones after cholecystectomy
- ERCP is diagnostic and therapeutic (sphincterotomy)
- Acute cholangitis or acute pancreatitis with common bile duct stones at any age are indications for urgent sphincterotomy within 48 h

Malignant biliary strictures
- Endoscopic insertion of a stent is indicated, pending a decision about surgery. Brushings for cytology and sometimes biopsies can be taken at ERCP to confirm malignancy, although false-negative results are common
- Curative surgery should be considered if the patient is young (< 60 years) and fit, with a pancreatic tumour < 2 cm on CT scan. Palliative surgery is indicated if there are signs of duodenal infiltration
- The success rate of stent insertion (85%) is similar to palliative surgery, but complications and hospital stay are appreciably reduced
- Duodenal obstruction by tumour following stent insertion (which might have been avoided by surgery) is unusual (17% in one controlled trial)
- Repeat ERCP for blocked stents is required in 20% with malignant obstruction, after 3 months. Most stents block in time and replacement is usually straightforward when recurrent jaundice develops

• High or tortuous strictures are best stented by percutaneous radiological insertion of a self-expanding metal stent or joint percutaneous and endoscopic procedure. If this fails, jaundice can sometimes be relieved by segment III biliary diversion in expert hands

Benign biliary strictures

• Single benign strictures (often post-traumatic) are best treated surgically at a specialist referral centre, although balloon dilatation at ERCP may be possible

• Surgical treatment usually involves biliary drainage through a Roux loop. A loop of jejunum leading to the anastomosis can be left with a radio-opaque marker, so that percutaneous dilatation under fluoroscopy can be performed if the stricture recurs

Surgery in cholestatic jaundice

• Mortality and complications are common—up to 50% if the patient has underlying cirrhosis

• Contributing factors are the age of the patient (often elderly), sepsis (especially cholangitis), cause of jaundice (cirrhosis or malignancy) and predisposition to renal failure (hepatorenal syndrome, p. 171)

6.4 Cholangitis

Bacterial cholangitis

Ascending infection in the biliary tree occurs when the main bile ducts are obstructed, usually by stones. Surgery or endoscopic procedures can introduce infection.

Features (Charcot's triad)
• Jaundice
• Pain—usually central, severe and colicky, but may also be minimal
• Fever—may be minimal in the elderly, those on steroids and the immunosuppressed
• A high index of suspicion is needed in any patient with fever and cholestatic liver function tests

Management
• General—blood cultures, intravenous fluids, pethidine
• Antibiotics—intravenous piperacillin 4 g four times daily is more effective than ampicillin and metronidazole

- Ultrasound—to look for a dilated common duct (> 7 mm), although obstructing stones are rarely seen
- Drainage—urgent (< 48 h) ERCP and sphincterotomy if common bile duct stones are present, whatever the age. Mortality is 5–10%
- Emergency surgery and exploration of the common duct has a mortality of 30% in poor-risk patients

Primary sclerosing cholangitis

All parts of the biliary tract may be involved in a fibrosing process that ultimately leads to biliary cirrhosis. The cause is unknown. 75% have associated ulcerative colitis and 20–30% subsequently develop cholangiocarcinoma.

Clinical features
- 70% are male
- Asymptomatic elevation of ALP in a patient with ulcerative colitis (rarely Crohn's disease) is highly suggestive. Patients usually have a quiescent pancolitis
- Pruritus, jaundice, right upper quadrant pain and weight loss occur in 75%
- Bacterial cholangitis and oesophageal varices due to portal hypertension occur less commonly than in other types of progressive liver disease
- Rapid deterioration may be due to a cholangiocarcinoma in later stages, which is more common in those with ulcerative colitis

Investigations
- ALP is elevated together with γ-GT. Antimitochondrial antibodies are negative
- Ultrasound excludes other causes of cholestasis (gall stones are also more common in ulcerative colitis)
- ERCP is diagnostic. It demonstrates irregular stricturing and dilatation (beading) of intrahepatic ducts. 30% have a stricture of an extrahepatic bile duct. Diffuse cholangiocarcinoma can rarely cause this appearance
- Liver biopsy may be characteristic, but the diagnosis must be confirmed by ERCP. Histological appearances can be confused with autoimmune chronic hepatitis, but an unusually high ALP in these patients is an indication for ERCP (p. 229)
- Sigmoidoscopy and rectal biopsy should be performed in patients who have not previously been diagnosed as having ulcerative colitis

Management

- There is no specific treatment, although ursodeoxycholic acid 500 mg twice daily is under trial. Symptomatic treatment is the same as for primary biliary cirrhosis (p. 192)
- Colonoscopy and serial biopsies are appropriate to exclude colonic dysplasia, since colorectal cancer complicating ulcerative colitis appears to be more common (Plate 6.1, facing p. 218)
- Colectomy does not alter the course of primary sclerosing cholangitis in ulcerative colitis
- Hepatic transplantation should be considered in patients with end-stage disease (jaundice, ascites), although the timing is more difficult and the outcome less good than for primary biliary cirrhosis (p. 208)

Prognosis

- Mean duration from the onset of symptoms to death is 7 years, but the time is very variable and most are now detected at the asymptomatic stage during investigation of cholestatic liver function tests
- 5-year survival after transplantation is 50–70% and improving

Secondary and autoimmune cholangitis

- Very rarely, an identical picture to primary sclerosing cholangitis can be caused by long-standing biliary obstruction due to a benign stricture or common duct stones
- Autoimmune cholangitis is a recently described entity with cholestasis, high titres of antinuclear and antismooth muscle antibodies, but negative antimitochondrial antibodies. The clinical features and histological appearance are similar to primary biliary cirrhosis

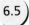

Cholangiocarcinoma

Carcinoma may arise anywhere in the biliary tree. The site determines the presentation—distal tumours obstruct main ducts and present early; intrahepatic tumours present late and may be mistaken for hepatomas. There is a high prevalence in Thailand and the Far East, possibly due to liver fluke (*Clonorchis sinensis*) infection.

Clinical features

- Age > 60 years

- Associated with:
  - primary sclerosing cholangitis
  - biliary cirrhosis (primary or secondary)
  - ulcerative colitis
- Jaundice, followed by pruritus (pruritus precedes jaundice in primary biliary cirrhosis or primary sclerosing cholangitis). Carcinoma of the pancreas or ampulla are more common causes. The jaundice occasionally fluctuates, which can be deceptive
- Pain—epigastric and mild
- Weight loss and diarrhoea, due to fat malabsorption
- Rapid deterioration in a patient with primary sclerosing cholangitis or primary biliary cirrhosis
- Hepatomegaly or a palpable gall bladder are quite common, but splenomegaly and ascites are rare

Diagnosis

- Investigations for cholestatic jaundice (ultrasound and ERCP; Fig. 6.5, p. 225) will suggest the diagnosis
- Blood tests show a cholestatic picture. AFP is normal
- Ultrasound identifies dilated ducts, but only occasionally detects a tumour mass
- CT scan more often shows a tumour, but magnetic resonance cholangiography is under trial and may prove the most reliable imaging technique
- ERCP shows an abrupt or irregular obstruction to contrast, usually at the hilum. A percutaneous transhepatic cholangiogram is then indicated to define the extent, if intervention to relieve jaundice is considered feasible

Difficulties

- Histological confirmation. Liver biopsy rarely shows tumour even in intrahepatic lesions
- Brush or bile cytology, which should be obtained at ERCP, is not easy to interpret (30% positive)
- Distinguishing distal lesions from pancreatic cancer. CT scan may show the site of the main bulk of the tumour
- Widespread intrahepatic cholangiocarcinoma looks like primary sclerosing cholangitis. The clinical course over a few weeks indicates the diagnosis
- There are rare but well-documented cases of intraductal hepatocellular carcinoma

Management

Cure is rarely possible unless a tumour is found incidentally at hepatic transplant for primary biliary cirrhosis or primary sclerosing cholangitis.

Resection

Surgery should be considered for distal, localized tumours in young patients who present with jaundice early. Referral to a specialist centre is advisable.

Symptomatic treatment

* Endoscopic stenting of distal strictures to relieve jaundice and itching. This may be difficult, because most tumours are at the porta hepatis (p. 224)
* Cholestyramine 4–12 g/day, or oxymetholone 100–150 mg/day, for pruritus
* Analgesics for pain
* Low-fat diet for diarrhoea

Prognosis

* In contrast to pancreatic cancer, the tumours are slow growing
* Mean survival is 14 months, but may be up to 5 years

6.6 Clinical dilemmas

Postcholecystectomy symptoms and biliary dyskinesia

Recurrent symptoms occur in 15% patients who have an elective cholecystectomy. Most are attributed to ill-defined motility disorders (irritable bowel syndrome or biliary dyskinesia), but there are several important causes.

Causes

* Retained common bile duct stone
* Duodenal or gastric ulcer
* Chronic pancreatitis
* Renal tract disease (including pelviureteric junction obstruction)
* Irritable bowel syndrome
* Biliary dyskinesia (sphincter of Oddi dysfunction, or postcholecystectomy syndrome)

Biliary dyskinesia

* Biliary dyskinesia or sphincter of Oddi dysfunction describes recurrent

colicky pain, fat intolerance, often with diarrhoea and dyspepsia, without a retained stone or other cause

• Three types have been described by Geenan and Hogan: I (biliary pain, twofold elevation of ALP and AST on two occasions, dilated common bile duct and delayed biliary drainage at ERCP), II (biliary pain and one or two of the objective criteria of biliary obstruction) and III (biliary pain and none of the criteria of biliary obstruction). This influences treatment (below)

• Endoscopic manometry of the sphincter of Oddi shows increased baseline pressure (> 40 mmHg) in about 60%, but even without manometry, the classification helps management (see below)

Management

Careful history
To identify differences from precholecystectomy symptoms and associated features of other diseases.

Initial investigation
• Blood tests for ALP, γ-GT (elevated in retained stones) and full blood count
• Urine for blood, protein, bilirubin and urobilinogen
• Abdominal ultrasound (the common bile duct is usually slightly dilated after cholecystectomy, 7–9 mm)
• If these tests are normal, irritable bowel syndrome is the likely diagnosis

Subsequent investigations and treatment
Indicated if severe symptoms persist, or if initial investigations are abnormal:
• Upper gastrointestinal endoscopy
• ERCP—to exclude a retained stone or chronic pancreatitis. ERCP is more often complicated by pancreatitis (5–10%) than normal and should only be performed when there is objective evidence of obstruction
• Sphincterotomy is indicated for retained calculi, or Geenan–Hogan type I or II biliary dyskinesia. In prospective studies, long-term symptomatic relief occurs in 60–70%, but in < 10% with type III obstruction
• A long cystic duct remnant is not an indication for surgery
• Antispasmodics (mebeverine 135 mg three times daily) are sometimes helpful, together with tricyclic antidepressants (such as Motival 1–3 tablets daily) and reassurance that the symptoms do not represent anything serious. The many alternatives (aluminium-containing antacids, cholestyramine, treatment for non-ulcer dyspepsia (p. 90), other antidepressants, laxatives, exclusion diet) indicate how difficult it can be to treat effectively

7 Small Intestine

7.1) Diarrhoea

Food, fluid and intestinal secretions amount to 7 L/day. Normally 5 L is absorbed by the small intestine and 1.5–2 L by the colon. The residual 100–200 mL (or 100–200 g when solid) is excreted as faeces. Consequently a 10% decrease in fluid absorbed by the colon will double the stool volume. There is, however, considerable reserve colonic absorptive capacity which compensates for increased ileal effluent volume in osmotic or secretory conditions (Table 7.2, p. 238), until that capacity is exceeded, when diarrhoea develops.

Diarrhoea means increased stool water. Stool volume of > 200 mL/day (weight > 200 g/day) is a practical definition and usually results in an increased stool frequency. Patients may describe increased stool frequency alone, a single loose motion or even rectal discharge as diarrhoea. A careful history is essential and stool weight should be measured on a 24-h basis when the cause of diarrhoea is not apparent.

Causes

Common causes of recurrent or persistent diarrhoea are shown in Table 7.1. Classification into osmotic, secretory, motility and combined types (Table 7.2) helps when planning later investigations (Fig. 7.1, p. 241), but diagnosis initially depends on excluding colonic causes and identifying common conditions.

Table 7.1 Causes of diarrhoea.

Common	Uncommon	Rare
Gastroenteritis	Crohn's disease	Autonomic neuropathy
viral (rota, echo)	Coeliac disease	Tropical sprue
bacterial (*Salmonella*,	Hypogammaglobulinaemia	Ischaemic colitis
Campylobacter spp.)	Bacterial overgrowth	Whipple's disease
parasitic (*G. lamblia*)	Microscopic colitis	Collagenous colitis
toxin (*E. coli*,	Chronic pancreatitis	Addison's disease
Shigella spp.)	Thyrotoxicosis	Hypoparathyroidism
Irritable bowel syndrome	Pseudomembranous colitis	Amyloidosis
Drugs (many, alcohol)	Laxative abuse	Behçet's disease
Colorectal carcinoma	Food allergy	Polyarteritis nodosa
Ulcerative colitis	Ileal/gastric resection	Gastrinoma
Hypolactasia		Mastocytosis
		Carcinoid
		VIPoma
		Medullary thyroid Cancer
		Pellagra
		Zinc deficiency

Table 7.2 Mechanisms of diarrhoea.

Osmotic	Secretory	Motility	Combined
Hypolactasia Drugs (lactulose, magnesium salts)	Toxins *E. coli* *Vibrio cholerae* *Staphylococcus* *aureus* *Clostridium* *perfringens* Peptides VIP	Irritable bowel Drugs (senna, phenolphthalein)	Ulcerative colitis Coeliac disease Malabsorption

- Persistent diarrhoea after acute gastroenteritis may be due to persistent infection (especially *Giardia lamblia*), acquired hypolactasia, hypogammaglobulinaemia, unrecognized disease (coeliac, ulcerative colitis) or postdysenteric irritable bowel syndrome which is the commonest reason
- Common drug-induced causes include antibiotics, magnesium-containing antacids, β-blockers and NSAIDs, as well as alcohol

Osmotic diarrhoea

- Due to malabsorbed osmotically active substances such as carbohydrate and peptides, which retain water in the intestinal lumen. Diarrhoea occurs when the extra ileal effluent exceeds colonic absorptive capacity, and may be intermittent (if the colon compensates for the fluid load), or only present when there is associated colonic disease (such as hypolactasia with Crohn's colitis)
- Characterized by an osmotic gap: measured osmolality is 20% (or 50 mOsm) greater than the osmolality calculated from stool electrolytes (twice the sum of Na + K concentrations) in osmotic diarrhoea
- Laxative abuse with magnesium-containing medicines or lactulose should always be considered

Secretory diarrhoea

- Secretion, stimulated by a toxin (such as cholera toxin) or peptide (such as VIP), is mediated by cyclic nucleotides. 'Travellers' diarrhoea' is usually due to *Escherichia coli* enterotoxin (Table 7.2)
- Characterized by a stool volume > 200 mL during fasting (Fig. 7.2, p. 241)

Combined mechanisms

- Diarrhoea is frequently due to multiple factors

• The diarrhoea of ulcerative colitis, for example, is caused by disordered motility, altered mucosal permeability, prostaglandin or short-chain fatty acid-induced changes in ion transport, decreased capacity of the rectal reservoir and loss of blood or mucus into the lumen

Clinical features

History
• Duration > 3 weeks (or less in the very young, very old, dehydrated or debilitated) needs investigation
• Nocturnal diarrhoea strongly suggests organic pathology
• Morning diarrhoea is a feature of alcohol abuse and irritable bowel syndrome, but may indicate more serious pathology (such as inflammatory bowel disease)
• Weight loss also favours an organic cause and weight loss despite a good appetite is typical of thyrotoxicosis
• Blood (altered or fresh) indicates a colonic cause
• Fat globules in the pan after flushing suggests steatorrhoea
• Recent travel abroad (including USA, Russia or Europe) suggests giardiasis
• Undigested food, odour, abdominal cramps, bloating, flatulence and audible borborygmi are non-specific
• Always ask about drugs, alcohol intake, contacts, family history, arteritis, iritis and skin rashes (erythema nodosum, dermatitis herpetiformis)

Examination
• Look for dehydration, weight loss, skin rashes and abdominal surgical scars. Clubbing sometimes occurs in active Crohn's disease
• Feel for an enlarged thyroid, or an abdominal mass which may indicate colonic carcinoma or Crohn's disease
• Rectal examination, sigmoidoscopy and rectal biopsy are essential

Initial investigations

Appropriate for all patients with recurrent or persistent diarrhoea (> 3 weeks), or for diarrhoea in the very young, very old, dehydrated or debilitated.

Stool sample
• Microscopy for *Giardia lamblia* (other parasites and ova when from abroad), and cysts of *Cryptosporidium* spp. if immunodeficient
• Culture for *Salmonella*, *Shigella*, *Campylobacter*, *Yersinia* spp.

- *Clostridium difficile* toxin assay when antibiotics have been recently taken
- Electron microscopy (for viruses) only in children, or an epidemic

Sigmoidoscopy

- Record the distance reached, stool and mucosal appearance (p. 304)
- Always take a biopsy of any identifiable lesion and a representative area, because 10–20% of patients with Crohn's disease have microscopic changes even when the mucosa looks normal. Microscopic colitis will otherwise be missed, and histology provides an independent record of the sigmoidoscopic findings

Blood tests

- Microcytic anaemia suggests a carcinoma or inflammatory bowel disease
- Macrocytosis may be due to coeliac disease, distal ileal Crohn's disease, or alcohol
- A high ESR indicates active inflammatory bowel disease, carcinoma or occasionally infective causes. If the ESR is normal, the C-reactive protein should be measured, because this can be elevated independently of the ESR. Both Crohn's disease and carcinoma, however, can occur with a normal ESR and C-reactive protein
- Low potassium (< 3.5 mmol/L) occurs in severe diarrhoea. Laxative abuse, colonic villous adenoma or, very rarely, a VIPoma may be the cause
- Albumin, immunoglobulins and thyroid function tests are best checked at the first or second visit, so that they are not overlooked

Imaging the colon

- Always investigate the colon if sustained diarrhoea develops for the first time over the age of 40 years
- Colonoscopy is the best investigation if there is visible blood in the stools, chronic watery diarrhoea (to exclude microscopic colitis), for young patients (to avoid X-ray exposure) and always if inflammatory bowel disease is suspected (to obtain biopsies)
- Local availability of colonoscopy varies and the waiting time for a barium enema in the UK is often shorter. A barium enema is usually preferable if a colonic carcinoma is suspected (to avoid delay), for investigating iron deficiency anaemia (more reliably images the caecum) or if terminal ileal views are needed (some patients with suspected Crohn's disease)
- Flexible sigmoidoscopy (p. 451) can be rapidly performed and is a useful investigation when there is fresh rectal bleeding
- Abdominal CT scan (especially spiral imaging, p. 460) is useful in the frail or elderly (p. 429), because it avoids the need for bowel preparation

- If < 40 years, carcinoma is unlikely. Irritable bowel syndrome is the most likely diagnosis if other tests are normal and infective causes excluded. Review after treatment is often more appropriate than invasive investigation

Subsequent investigations

The following plan is recommended if the results of initial investigations do not establish a diagnosis and symptoms justify invasive investigation (Fig. 7.1).

Difficult diarrhoea

If the cause of diarrhoea remains obscure after outpatient investigation (Fig. 7.1), then admission is usually necessary to distinguish between organic disease and a motility disorder (Fig. 7.2). Diarrhoea due to organic disease has a stool volume > 200 mL/day, which usually does not settle on

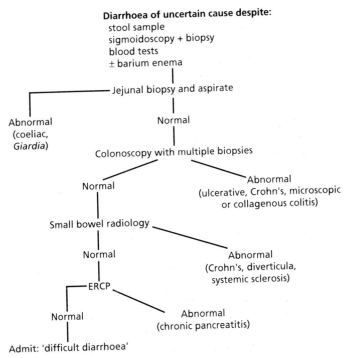

Fig. 7.1 Outpatient investigation of diarrhoea.

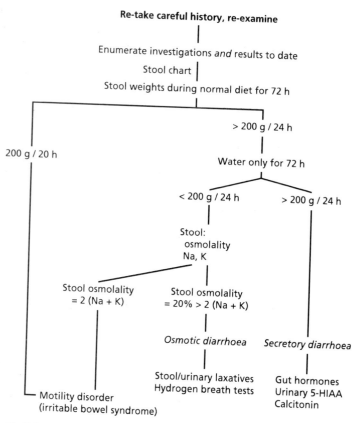

Re-take careful history, re-examine

Enumerate investigations *and* results to date

Stool chart

Stool weights during normal diet for 72 h

200 g / 20 h

> 200 g / 24 h

Water only for 72 h

< 200 g / 24 h   > 200 g / 24 h

Stool: osmolality Na, K

Stool osmolality = 2 (Na + K)

Stool osmolality = 20% > 2 (Na + K)

Osmotic diarrhoea   *Secretory diarrhoea*

Stool/urinary laxatives
Hydrogen breath tests

Gut hormones
Urinary 5-HIAA
Calcitonin

Motility disorder
(irritable bowel syndrome)

Fig. 7.2 Investigation of difficult diarrhoea.

admission. Functional diarrhoea (due to an irritable bowel) often disappears on admission and the stool weight is usually < 200 g/day (volume < 200 mL/day).

General points

- Stool electrolyte assay and osmolality needs to be discussed with the biochemistry laboratory. Don't bother sending solid stool!
- Planned admission for stool weight and frequency measurement on a normal diet for 48–72 h, then (if stool weight exceeds 200 g/24 h) on intravenous fluids for 48–72 h is a simple way of discriminating functional, osmotic and secretory causes of intractable diarrhoea
- Lactulose or glucose breath tests are non-invasive methods of detecting

bacterial overgrowth (p. 462). Breath H_2 normally rises as the lactulose (or any carbohydrate load, including glucose) reaches the colon, but when lactulose is broken down by small intestinal bacteria this rise occurs < 2 h after ingestion

- Lactose breath test is a non-invasive method of detecting lactase deficiency (p. 462). Hypolactasic subjects exhale more H_2 than normal (> 20 p.p.m.) after 2 h. Subjects with normal lactase levels produce little or no H_2
- Xylose absorption is an unreliable screening test for carbohydrate malabsorption. Jejunal biopsy or double sugar tests (p. 464) are preferable
- SeHCAT scans for bile salt malabsorption give less information about the terminal ileum than good small bowel radiology, or reflux of barium during a barium enema
- Peroral pneumocologram (discuss with radiologists) give the best views of the caecum and terminal ileum
- Stool should be examined for laxatives (addition of sodium hydroxide turns the stool red in the presence of phenolphthalein), and the urine for anthracene derivatives or senna alkaloids, if the diagnosis is obscure. Examination of the patient's bedside locker ('lockerotomy') is acceptable if laxative abuse is strongly suspected and there is no alternative

Management

- The cause of diarrhoea should be identified and treated if possible
- Oral rehydration solution (sodium chloride 3.5 g, sodium citrate 2.9 g, potassium chloride 1.5 g and glucose 20 g in 1 L (World Health Organization formula), or Dioralyte is indicated for severe diarrhoea in the young or elderly
- Codeine phosphate 30–60 mg/day is the first choice when stool frequency needs to be controlled
- Loperamide 4 mg, then 2 mg after each loose stool can be used for acute gastroenteritis or motility disorders. Although drugs are best avoided if possible, there is no convincing evidence that clearance of intestinal pathogens is delayed. It should not be used in children, because fatal paralytic ileus has been reported
- Amitriptyline 10–25 mg at night, or Motival 1–3 tablets daily, are sometimes effective for motility disorders, because of anticholinergic effects
- Antibiotics are only indicated for a few infections (*Giardia lamblia*, *Yersinia enterocolitica*, severe shigellosis, or bacterial overgrowth; p. 258). Excretion of *Salmonella* spp. is prolonged by inappropriate antibiotics and increases the risk of a carrier state

Travellers' diarrhoea

Enterotoxigenic *Escherichia coli* cause most acute, self-limiting episodes of diarrhoea in travellers (Table 7.3). *Cryptosporidium* spp. and *Cyclospora* spp. are other causes

- Incubation is 1–5 days
- Sudden onset of severe diarrhoea with abdominal pain is only serious in the young, debilitated or elderly
- Resolution within 48–96 h is usual; < 5% persist for more than 3 weeks and then need investigation to exclude underlying disease
- Symptomatic treatment (p. 243) is indicated and drugs avoided if possible. If the patient's job is affected and rapid control of symptoms needed, a single dose of ciprofloxacin 750 mg is usually effective
- Preventive advice includes avoiding salads, uncooked vegetables, shellfish, ice cream and unsterilized water (including ice) in uncertain

Table 7.3 Differential diagnosis of diarrhoea after foreign travel.

Travellers' diarrhoea (enterotoxigenic *E. coli*)
*G. lambia**
Infective diarrhoea
  Salmonella spp.
  Shigella spp.†
  Campylobacter spp.†
  Cyclospora spp.
  Y. enterocolitica
  E. coli 0157†
  rotavirus
Postinfective irritable bowel syndrome
Postinfective hypolactasia* (when drinking milk)
Latent disease revealed by infection*
  ulcerative colitis†
  coeliac disease
  Crohn's disease
  ileocaecal tuberculosis
Other infections
  Strongyloides stercoralis†
  hepatitis A, B or E (community acquired non-A, non-B)
  acute falciparum malaria
  Cryptosporidium spp.
  amoebic dysentery† (*Entamoeba histolytica*)
  fasciolopsiasis,* capillariasis*
  schistosomiasis,† enterobiasis,† trichuriasis†
Tropical sprue*

*Usually chronic diarrhoea.
†Often bloody diarrhoea.

areas. Antibiotics are not recommended, although sulphonamide combinations (cotrimoxazole 2 tablets twice daily) provide partial protection. Sulphonamides can produce sensitivity to sunlight
- Persistent diarrhoea may be due to postdysenteric irritable bowel syndrome, persistent infection (consider *Cyclospora* spp., *Giardia lamblia*), hypolactasia or unmasked latent disease (Fig. 7.3), and is investigated in the same way as for other causes (p. 239; Fig. 7.1, p. 241)
- For severe symptoms in the absence of adequate microbiological facilities, empirical treatment with ciprofloxacin followed by cotrimoxazole (2 tablets twice daily for 1–2 weeks) in the case of *Cyclospora* infection, then metronidazole 800 mg three times daily for 3 days in case of *G. lamblia* is reasonable

7.2 Malabsorption

Defective luminal digestion, mucosal disease, or structural disorders are the mechanisms of malabsorption. Fat, carbohydrate, protein, vitamin or mineral malabsorption may predominate, but combined deficiency is usual except in metabolic defects.

Causes

- Knowledge of the mechanism is more useful for deciding about investigations than for classifying causes (Table 7.4). More than one mechanism commonly operates, mucosal disease may be associated with defective digestion and sometimes with structural change as well

Table 7.4 Causes of malabsorption.

Common	Uncommon	Rare
Coeliac disease	Pancreatic cancer	Small bowel lymphoma
Chronic pancreatitis	Parasites (*G. lamblia*)	Lymphangiectasia
Crohn's disease	Bacterial overgrowth	Whipple's disease
Postinfective	Drugs	Thyrotoxicosis
Biliary obstruction	Short bowel	Zollinger–Ellison
Cirrhosis	Resection	Metabolic defects
	gastric	Mesenteric ischaemia
	terminal ileal	Mastocytosis
	pancreatic	Amyloidosis
		HIV enteropathy
		α-chain disease
		Tropical sprue
		Starvation

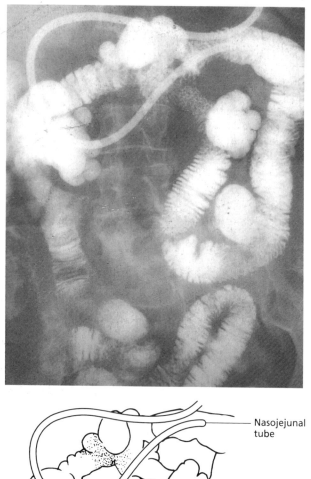

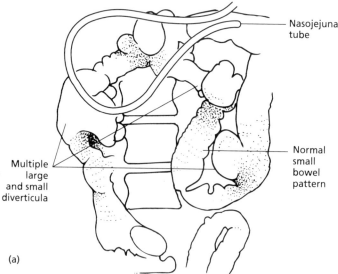

Nasojejunal tube

Multiple large and small diverticula

Normal small bowel pattern

(a)

Fig. 7.3 Small bowel radiology and malabsorption. (a) Small bowel enema showing multiple jejunal diverticula, causing malabsorption due to bacterial overgrowth. (*Continued* on p. 247)

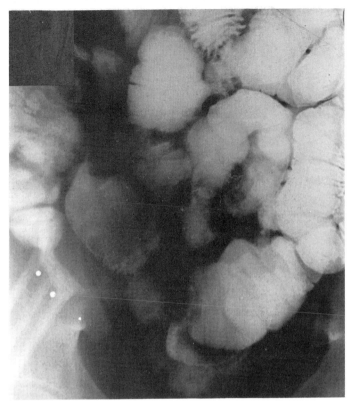

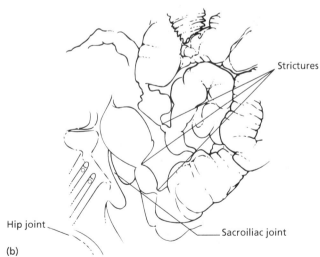

Strictures

Hip joint

Sacroiliac joint

(b)

Fig. 7.3 (*continued*) (b) Small bowel study in a patient with malabsorption due to extensive Crohn's disease, causing multiple strictures.

- Hypoalbuminaemia and vitamin K or D deficiency in cirrhosis may be due to liver disease as well as malabsorption
- Crohn's disease causes malabsorption from distal ileal disease (vitamin B_{12} and bile salts), mucosal disease, disaccharidase deficiency, enteroenteric fistulae, bacterial overgrowth, or a short bowel (p. 262)
- Other causes are discussed below

Clinical features

Diarrhoea

- Steatorrhoea is due to defective digestion of fat, resulting in malabsorption. Pancreatic exocrine insufficiency (p. 135) is the usual cause and severe steatorrhoea is rare in mucosal or structural disease. It is characterized by pale, bulky, malodorous motions, with oily globules in the pan after flushing
- Stool bulk is increased more than frequency, unlike the diarrhoea of colonic disease
- Malabsorption occasionally occurs without diarrhoea. Intestinal causes (coeliac disease, bacterial overgrowth) are then likely

Weight loss

Weight loss occurs whatever the cause of malabsorption, but may be minimal during malabsorption of specific nutrients (such as B_{12} malabsorption from bacterial overgrowth).

General symptoms

Lassitude, anorexia, abdominal bloating, discomfort and borborygmi may be inappropriately dismissed as an irritable bowel.

Specific features (Tables 12.2–12.4, pp. 401–403)

- Hypoalbuminaemia causes dependent oedema or, rarely, ascites when severe
- Hypocalcaemia or hypomagnesaemia cause paraesthesiae and tetany if severe
- Vitamin deficiencies can cause cheilitis (riboflavin), glossitis (B_{12}), bruising (K), bone pain or myopathy (D), night blindness or xerophthalmia (A), dermatitis (niacin), neuropathy or psychological disturbance (thiamine or E)
- Mineral deficiencies can cause paraesthesiae or tetany (calcium), muscle weakness (calcium, magnesium), skin rashes, anaemia or leucopenia (zinc, copper). Deficiencies are rare and often multiple

Investigations

Once malabsorption has been documented, the site and severity must be established.

Documentation

- The combination of diarrhoea, documented weight loss and abnormal blood tests (full blood count, INR, calcium, haematinics or albumin) are sufficient in most patients to document malabsorption prior to further investigation
- Full blood count, folate and B_{12} estimation (anaemia and folate deficiency are common in mucosal disease and B_{12} deficiency in terminal ileal disease or bacterial overgrowth)
- Prothrombin time or ratio (INR), may indicate vitamin K deficiency and is necessary before invasive tests such as jejunal biopsy
- Albumin, calcium and alkaline phosphatase (hypoalbuminaemia indicates severe malabsorption and osteomalacia causes hypocalcaemia or an elevated ALP). Serum magnesium should be measured if symptoms of hypocalcaemia respond slowly to treatment, since it may be low (< 0.7 mmol/L)
- Stool sample for fat globules which are rarely present except in malabsorption, is a qualitative method of documenting malabsorption, but false-negative results are common
- 3–5-day faecal fat estimation is rarely helpful and is not diagnostically discriminating. If malabsorption cannot be documented in other ways, it can be measured (> 5 g/day (13 mmol/day) is abnormal on a normal diet), although not popular with the laboratory. Careful explanation to the patient is necessary to ensure a proper collection. Results are more accurate if expressed as a percentage of intake over a 5-day collection (> 7% of fat intake (> 7 g on a 100 g fat diet) is abnormal)
- The xylose test to assess carbohydrate absorption has a 25% false-negative rate and is not recommended (p. 463). Enteric protein loss can be documented by assessing faecal radioactivity after intravenous ^{131}I-albumin injection. It is rarely necessary and is best done at a specialist referral centre

Identify the site

- Jejunal biopsy is the definitive investigation for mucosal lesions and small bowel radiology for structural causes. Defective luminal digestion may be confirmed by lactose breath test or mucosal enzyme assay
- Distal duodenal biopsies (D3, beyond the papilla) at endoscopy are usually satisfactory for detecting villous atrophy, but normal villi may

appear flattened over duodenal glands. Jejunal biopsy using a peroral paediatric colonoscope, Crosby capsule, steerable Meditech catheter or multiple Quinton biopsy instrument (p. 449), is indicated if endoscopic biopsies are not definitive. Causes of villous atrophy are shown in Table 7.5

• Aspiration of jejunal juice for *G. lamblia* and culture is advisable in any patient who has a jejunal biopsy. Swallowing a piece of string (whilst retaining the end!) and examination for parasites is not used in Britain, because jejunal biopsy is always necessary as well

• Small bowel radiology will usually identify distal ileal disease, diverticula, strictures, systemic sclerosis or tumours. Small bowel enema demonstrates the mucosal pattern better than a barium meal and follow-through (p. 458). Flocculation, thickened folds and slight dialatation are all non-specific

• Lactose breath test is the most convenient non-invasive way of establishing hypolactasia, but it is usually simpler to document symptoms before and after stopping milk and milk products (p. 418) for a week. Enzyme assay is usually impracticable and unnecessary

• Ultrasound and then ERCP to detect chronic pancreatitis is indicated once mucosal and structural causes of malabsorption have been excluded

Assess severity

• Document weight and height (body mass index; Appendix 3, p. 489) and laboratory evidence of malabsorption

• Other methods of nutritional assessment are rarely necessary in clinical practice (p. 401)

Table 7.5 Other causes of villous atrophy.

G. lamblia
Acute infectious enteritis
viral
bacterial
Hypogammaglobulinaemia
Bacterial overgrowth
Tropical sprue
Cows' milk sensitivity*
Soya protein sensitivity*
Lymphoma
Whipple's disease
NSAIDs
Radiation
HIV enteropathy
Starvation

*Children only.

Coeliac disease

Coeliac disease (gluten-sensitive enteropathy) is defined as small intestinal villous atrophy (Fig. 7.4) which resolves when gluten is withdrawn from the diet. Gluten is a group of proteins derived from wheat, barley and rye but not oats, rice or maize; α-gliadin is the toxic moiety. The most plausible mechanism is that α-gliadin, which has high affinity for a peptidase called tissue transglutaminase and reticulin in the lamina propria, unmasks epitopes on this peptidase which trigger the production of reticulin/endomysial autoantibodies in susceptible individuals. Specific HLA class II molecules on antigen-presenting cells then present this modified tissue transglutaminase to activate the autoreactive T-cell population. Mucosal inflammation, with consequent villous atrophy, then continues until the environmental trigger α-gliadin is removed.

Distinguishing features
- Coeliac disease may present at any age, but is now most commonly diagnosed as chronic or recurrent iron-deficiency anaemia in adults, rather than failure to thrive in infancy, or growth retardation in childhood
- Symptoms of malabsorption may be provoked by infection, pregnancy or surgery
- Non-specific symptoms (lethargy, bloating, flatulence, abdominal discomfort) may be present for many years and attributable to an irritable bowel. The combination of such symptoms with iron-deficiency anaemia should always raise the possibility of coeliac disease
- Diarrhoea may be absent or intermittent. Constipation may coexist with coeliac disease
- Aphthous ulcers are common, but clubbing is rare. Hyposplenism (Howell–Jolly bodies, target cells) may be detected on the blood film
- Recurrent or refractory iron-deficiency anaemia may be the only feature
- Isolated nutritional deficiencies (megaloblastic anaemia, myopathy and bone pain) may occur, especially in the elderly
- Examination is often normal (even well nourished), or reveal signs of nutritional deficiencies (p. 401) through to severe malabsorption

Associated disorders
- Dermatitis herpetiformis (intensely itchy vesicular papules on the elbows or buttocks)—up to 96% have villous atrophy and even those without villous atrophy respond to gluten withdrawal
- Autoimmune disease—diabetes, thyrotoxicosis, Addison's disease

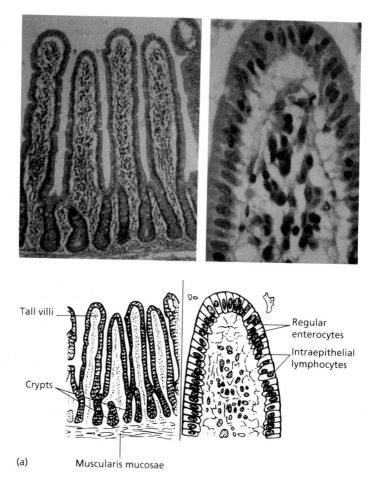

(a)

Tall villi

Regular enterocytes

Intraepithelial lymphocytes

Crypts

Muscularis mucosae

Fig. 7.4 Histological features of coeliac disease. (a) Histological appearance of normal jejunal mucosa. Tall villi (left, ×~70). The villus height: crypt depth ratio is at least 3:1. Tip of a villus showing a few intraepithelial lymphocytes (right, ×~320). Haematoxylin and eosin stain.

- Arthritis—rheumatoid or seronegative arthritis are unusual associations
- Pericarditis, spinocerebellar degeneration, pancreatic insufficiency and liver disorders are very rare associations

Diagnosis in adults

- There is no alternative to distal duodenal biopsy and a second biopsy to document resolution of villous atrophy, after 3–6 months on a gluten-free diet. Clinical recovery after gluten withdrawal may be coincidental, if

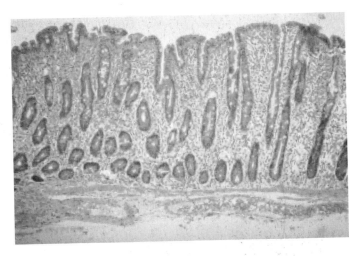

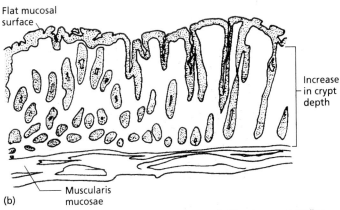

Flat mucosal surface

Increase in crypt depth

Muscularis mucosae

(b)

(b) Sub-total villous atrophy showing total absence of villi and a corresponding increase in depth of the crypts, producing an apparently increased mucosal thickness, but insufficient magnification to see the characteristic increase in intraepithelial lymphocytes. Haematoxylin and eosin stain, ×~70.

villous atrophy is due to a transient cause (such as *G. lamblia,* Table 7.5, p. 250), and the implications of a lifetime gluten-free diet are considerable. Subsequent gluten challenge is unnecessary in adults

• Villous atrophy is occasionally patchy, which can cause diagnostic confusion, especially on distal duodenal biopsies (p. 249)

• Immunoglobulins should be measured, since IgA deficiency (2%) predisposes to intestinal infections and hypogammaglobulinaemia itself can cause villous atrophy, which may respond to globulin infusion

• Antibodies to α-gliadin are non-specific and false negatives (or positives) are common in adults. They cannot be recommended as a screening test to identify or exclude coeliac disease

• Anti-endomysial antibodies (AEA) are more specific, but are also less sensitive and will be negative in patients with IgA deficiency. Only 60% of adults (higher in children) with AEA will have villous atrophy. If positive, such antibodies tend to disappear on gluten withdrawal; however, this is insufficiently reliable to monitor compliance. The main role of AEAs is in diagnostic difficulty in patients with partial villous atrophy; a positive result in these circumstances is consistent with coeliac disease

• A high index of suspicion is justified for children of coeliac patients and other family members with gastrointestinal symptoms (5% risk of coeliac disease), but investigation of family members in the absence of symptoms or anaemia is unjustified

Other causes of villous atrophy

Subtotal villous atrophy is almost always due to coeliac disease in European adults. Partial villous atrophy has other (rare) causes (Table 7.5, p. 250).

Complications

• Malignancy—small intestinal T-cell lymphoma develops in about 5%. Other types of small intestinal lymphoma originate from B cells. Small intestinal adenocarcinoma is also more common. Recrudescence of symptoms, abdominal pain or deterioration despite a gluten-free diet should suggest the diagnosis. Oesophageal and possibly colorectal malignancy is also more common

• Coexistent malignancy should be considered when coeliac disease is diagnosed in the middle-aged or elderly. An elevated C-reactive protein may be the only indicator that there is underlying lymphoma

• A long-term follow-up study in Birmingham (Appendix 2, p. 483) has shown that meticulous adherence to a gluten-free diet reduces the risk of malignant complications

• Ulceration and strictures in the small intestine—rare, but may cause pain, persistent anaemia or bacterial overgrowth. A small bowel enema is diagnostic, but resection may be necessary to exclude lymphoma or multifocal adenocarcinoma

• Osteoporosis is more common in coeliac disease. A good calcium intake is important after diagnosis, with supplements if milk intolerant. Hormone replacement therapy (HRT) is advisable in postmenopausal women, or biphosphonates if HRT cannot be tolerated, or in men with low bone mineral density (p. 437)

Management

- Gluten-free diet (p. 417) for life, with advice from a dietitian. There is now good evidence that this decreases the risk of small intestinal malignancy
- 85% respond, although histological resolution may take 3–12 months. It is advisable to repeat the jejunal biopsy after 3–6 months on a gluten-free diet, but a gluten challenge is not necessary in adults
- Iron and folate supplements are needed if anaemic, until recovery. Specific deficiencies may need treating (hypocalcaemia: effervescent calcium 6–12 tablets daily, but serum calcium must be checked monthly)
- Annual outpatient review is advisable when stable, to confirm adherence to the diet and detect complications. Relapse or poor compliance is most readily detected by anaemia or folate deficiency, followed by repeat jejunal biopsy
- The Coeliac Society (Appendix 1, p. 473) provides useful advice, food lists, recipe books, support and motivation for patients

Poor responders

If there is no clinical or histological improvement after 3 months (less if the patient is unwell), the possibilities are as follows.

Poor compliance

Failure to adhere meticulously to a gluten-free diet. This is also the most common cause of recurrent symptoms after an initial response.

Concomitant

- Hypolactasia (due to mucosal atrophy)
- Infection (G. lamblia, other parasites)
- Endocrine disease (hypothyroidism or Addison's disease—often insidious and not considered)

Untreated nutritional deficiency

- Folate or B_{12} (autoimmune pernicious anaemia is more common in coeliac disease)
- Iron
- Calcium
- Magnesium
- Others deficiencies, less commonly

Other conditions

- Small intestinal lymphoma
- Ulcerative jejunitis

- Hypogammaglobulinaemia
- Reasons unknown
- All, except poor dietary compliance, are unusual

Management of poor responders

- Emphasize the importance of complete gluten exclusion and ask the dietitian to review dietary compliance carefully. Check that contact with the Coeliac Society has been established. Give support, encouragement and motivation
- Exclude dairy products (in case of secondary hypolactasia) and reassess in 4 weeks
- Check that *G. lamblia* has been looked for in jejunal juice, and that hypogammaglobulinaemia or nutritional deficiencies have been corrected. Give a single dose of tinidazole 2 g, even if *G. lamblia* has not been identified
- Check C-reactive protein, perform small bowel radiology and jejunal biopsies using a paediatric colonoscope to exclude lymphoma, Crohn's disease, diverticula or adenocarcinoma
- Start prednisolone 20 mg/day, but only after other causes of a poor response have been rigorously excluded
- Rebiopsy to assess response after 3 months on steroids. Some still do not respond and should be referred to a specialist centre

Prognosis

- Gluten sensitivity persists for life
- Childhood coeliacs often become quiescent as young adults, but symptoms or complications may develop later if the diet is not continued (p. 254)
- Life expectancy is normal on a gluten-free diet

Tropical sprue

Postinfective tropical malabsorption affects adults of any race who have lived in India, Asia or Central America, but is rare in Africa. Tropical sprue is a disease of residents rather than visitors and seems to be increasingly uncommon. It usually follows an acute attack of diarrhoea. The cause of mucosal damage is uncertain although secondary bacterial overgrowth and hypolactasia commonly exacerbate the malabsorption.

Distinguishing features

- Malabsorption in a person who has recently lived in the tropics (rarely in the sub-tropics or several years previously)

- Persisting diarrhoea after an acute attack of gastroenteritis
- Typical features of malabsorption:
  - steatorrhoea
  - weight loss
  - anorexia and lethargy
  - oedema, anaemia, glossitis

Investigation

Diagnosis is established by a consistent history, macrocytic anaemia, partial villous atrophy and response to tetracycline. Other causes of tropical malabsorption should be considered (Table 7.6).

- Macrocytic anaemia is due to folate deficiency, although B_{12} may also be low due to bacterial colonization
- Hypoalbuminaemia is usual and occasionally the AST is elevated
- Jejunal biopsy usually reveals partial villous atrophy (total atrophy is rare), but unlike coeliac disease the changes are more severe in the terminal ileum. Jejunal juice should be examined for *G. lamblia*
- Stools should be examined for parasites
- Small bowel radiology is non-specific, but helps exclude diseases such as tuberculosis. Xylose and Schilling tests are non-specific and unnecessary

Management

- Tetracycline 250 mg four times daily for 4 weeks
- Folic acid 5 mg three times daily for 2 months
- Lactose-free diet (p. 418), for concomitant hypolactasia

Table 7.6 Differential diagnosis of malabsorption from abroad.

G. lamblia
HIV enteropathy
AIDS and associated conditions (p. 393)
Cryptosporidium spp.
Strongyloides stercoralis
Small intestinal tuberculosis
Hypolactasia
Lymphoma (imunoproliferative small intestinal disease)
Visceral leishmaniasis
Clonorchis sinensis cirrhosis
Filariasis
Calcific chronic pancreatitis
Tropical sprue
Idiopathic

Giardiasis

The flagellated protozoan *G. lamblia* is a common cause of diarrhoea and malabsorption, which may be superimposed on coeliac disease, tropical sprue or hypogammaglobulinaemia. Infection may also be asymptomatic.

Distinguishing features
- Incubation is 2–3 weeks
- Transmission is through contaminated water or faecal–oral route
- Travel abroad is not necessary to acquire infection, although it is more prevalent outside Britain, and in male homosexuals
- Persistent diarrhoea after an acute attack of 'gastroenteritis' may continue for months. Frank malabsorption is unusual unless there is an underlying cause such as immunodeficiency
- The diagnosis should always be suspected when a patient first presents with diarrhoea after travelling

Investigations
- Stool examination for cysts or trophozoites detects about 60%
- Jejunal aspiration and biopsy to exclude other causes of persistent diarrhoea or malabsorption (Table 7.1, p. 237; Table 7.4, p. 245), is the most reliable method of diagnosis if no stool cysts are seen
- Measure immunoglobulins if *G. lamblia* is acquired in Britain, or if there is recurrent infection. Family and close contacts should also be checked for symptomatic or asymptomatic carriers
- Treatment (see below) may be given before a jejunal biopsy if stool examination is negative, but only if the patient is going to be followed up and biopsy performed if there is an incomplete response

Management
- Tinidazole 2 g (single dose) is as effective as metronidazole 800 mg three times daily for 3 days
- Mepacrine 100 mg three times daily for 1 week is an alternative for the rate problem of resistant giardiasis. Reinfection or an underlying disease is a more common cause of persistent symptoms after treatment

Bacterial overgrowth

Bacterial contamination of the small intestine results in diarrhoea or typical features of malabsorption. An underlying cause (Table 7.7) is almost always present. Bacterial (anaerobes, *Escherichia coli* and *Klebsiella* spp.)

Table 7.7 Causes of bacterial overgrowth.

Duodenojejunal diverticula
Postsurgical loops ('blind loop')
Obstruction
  Crohn's disease
  tumour
  radiation stricture
  pseudo-obstruction
Fistulae
Hypogammaglobulinaemia
Tropical sprue
Systemic sclerosis
Autonomic neuropathy (diabetes, amyloid)
Anacidity (autoimmune, vagotomy, old age, drugs)

deconjugate bile salts, metabolize B_{12} and carbohydrate, but folate and fat-soluble vitamins are not malabsorbed. Normal jejunal juice contains $< 10^4$ Gram-positive organisms.

Distinguishing features
• Diarrhoea or malabsorption in patients with a structural small intestinal abnormality, or when immunocompromised
• May occur in elderly patients without small intestinal pathology
• Onset of diarrhoea in patients with otherwise stable chronic disease (diabetes, systemic sclerosis, Crohn's disease)
• Malabsorption with a low B_{12} and normal (or elevated) folate

Investigation
• Small bowel radiology is the first investigation when the diagnosis is suspected, to look for jejunal diverticulosis or strictures (Fig. 7.3, p. 246)
• Hydrogen breath test after lactulose is non-invasive. Breath hydrogen > 20 p.p.m. in < 2 h indicates bacterial overgrowth (p. 462). Urinary indican measurements are too unreliable to be useful
• Jejunal aspiration is convenient if a biopsy is being performed to exclude other causes of malabsorption (after normal small bowel radiology), but air insufflation may destroy anaerobes

Management
• Metronidazole 400 mg three times daily for 1 week is often effective
• Tetracycline 250 mg four times daily together with metronidazole 400 mg three times daily for 2 weeks is appropriate if there is no response

- Ciprofloxacin 500 mg twice daily or vancomycin 125 mg four times daily for 1 week are other alternatives, but not first-line therapy
- Replacement vitamin B_{12} (1000 µg intramuscularly for 5 days)
- Recurrent courses when symptoms relapse, or maintenance tetracycline 250 mg daily (not vancomycin, because of potential ototoxicity) are often necessary, because surgical correction of the cause is rarely possible

Disaccharidase deficiency

Hypolactasia

- Hypolactasia is the only common small intestinal enzyme deficiency. Alactasia is rare and presents in neonates
- Usually primary, because the enzyme disappears after weaning in most races except north Europeans
- Secondary causes include any cause of mucosal damage (viral gastroenteritis, coeliac disease, giardiasis, Crohn's disease) and is reversible once the disease is treated. Cows' milk protein intolerance occurs in children (and may cause villous atrophy), but probably not in adults
- The clinical problem is milk intolerance, which may not be recognized by the patient
- Lactose is normally split into galactose and glucose which are rapidly absorbed. Undigested lactose causes an osmotic diarrhoea and excessive flatulence from fermentation. The colon adapts to absorb excess intestinal fluid, so diarrhoea is variable
- Diagnosis is confirmed by a 25 g lactose–hydrogen breath test: a rise of > 20 p.p.m. H_2 2 h after ingestion is abnormal
- Avoiding milk and liquid milk products (yoghurt) is effective (p. 418). Butter and hard cheese contain little lactose, so intake is not restricted

Other deficiencies

- Sucrase–isomaltase deficiency is a rare disorder of childhood
- Trehalase deficiency results in mushroom intolerance

Adverse reactions to food

Terminology

It is important to distinguish between food allergy, sensitivity, intolerance and preference.

- Food allergy is immunological (IgE-mediated type I hypersensitivity) and uncommon

- Food sensitivity best applies to an identifiable non-immunological effect in susceptible individuals, be it pharmacological (tyramine in cheese) or due to enzyme deficiency (hypolactasia)
- Food intolerance applies to reproducible effects of certain foods for undefined reasons (some patients with irritable bowel syndrome, p. 371)
- Food preference or fads are psychological and not a reproducible cause of symptoms on blind testing
- Very few patients who believe food to be the cause of their symptoms have true food allergy. Many apparently have food sensitivity for reasons that cannot be defined scientifically at present. Psychological aversion to certain foods is the most common reason for symptoms

Distinguishing features

- Acute hypersensitivity reactions are usually caused by egg, shellfish, nuts, tomatoes or food additives (commonly tartrazine). Labial or pharyngeal oedema, urticaria, wheeze or anaphylaxis occur rapidly and the relationship is readily recognized by the patient
- Chronic reactions to cows' milk or soya protein are rare in adults, but may cause diarrhoea, vomiting, abdominal pain or steatorrhoea secondary to villous atrophy. The immunological mechanism is uncertain
- Associated atopy (eczema, hay fever, asthma) or drug allergy are clues to the diagnosis of food allergy
- Reproducible food sensitivity or intolerance are recognized by testing with an exclusion diet with the help of a dietitian (p. 421). Lack of reproducibility either means that food is not the cause of symptoms, or indicates a food fad

Investigations

- Document the relationship between exposure to the specific food and symptoms: a food diary (diet on one page, symptoms opposite) is helpful for chronic symptoms
- An exclusion diet of low allergenicity with planned reintroduction of common food allergens (dairy products, egg, fish, nuts, additives and colouring agents) is then appropriate
- Challenge tests, skin tests and radioallergosorbent tests (RAST) are of little value unless done by specialists
- Invasive investigation to exclude other causes of symptoms (small bowel radiology or jejunal biopsy) is only indicated if clinical suspicion of an organic cause is very strong. Partial villous atrophy is almost never due to protein sensitivity in adults

lanagement

- The specific food should be avoided, but subsequent intolerances are common. Foods to which there has been intolerance can often be gradually reintroduced after a few months, for reasons that are obscure
- Mebeverine 135–270 mg three times daily may help abdominal pain, or codeine phosphate 15–30 mg as needed can be prescribed for diarrhoea

Short bowel syndrome

General

- Massive intestinal resection to < 1 m of remaining small intestine may be due to Crohn's disease, mesenteric infarction, trauma or radiation injury. The result is diarrhoea and malnutrition, due to loss of fluid, electrolytes, fat, bile acids, B_{12} or other nutrients. In the acute phase, loss of fluid and electrolytes are most important. Patients with a high jejunostomy lose > 3 L/day, with a sodium loss of at least 90 mmol/L. Adaptation occurs over 2 years. Management of the chronic phase is shown in Table 7.8
- Preservation of the ileocaecal valve, some terminal ileum and some jejunum have the greatest beneficial effect on subsequent symptoms: some patients with 30 cm total (18 cm jejunum, 12 cm terminal ileum) will survive as long as the colon is retained for distal reabsorption of salt and water. Patients with < 100 cm bowel and a stoma will almost all need daily parenteral fluids and electrolyte supplements
- Net absorption of electrolytes from the jejunum only occurs when luminal sodium concentration is 90 mmol/L or more. Since almost all oral fluids contain very little sodium, the more the patient drinks the more intestinal secretion is provoked and the greater the stomal loss. The same is true for hyperosmolar nutritional supplements, including elemental feeds

Symptoms and signs

- Weight loss and high stomal output (> 2000 mL/day) or diarrhoea, despite a good appetite are obvious indications of intestinal failure
- Other causes of ileostomy dysfunction should be considered (p. 316)
- The condition is best anticipated by the surgeon measuring the length of remaining small intestine at intestinal surgery
- Fatigue due to salt depletion, or tetany due to magnesium (less commonly calcium) deficiency may occur
- Chronic vitamin and trace element deficiency can develop insidiously. Unexplained skin rashes or non-specific symptoms (malaise, weakness, paraesthesiae) are very suggestive

Table 7.8 Management of chronic short bowel syndrome.

Problem	Mechanism	Management
Salt and water depletion	Jejunal absorption [Na] > 90 mmol/L	Drink WHO oral rehydration fluid (p. 264) Avoid hypotonic fluids
Diarrhoea or stomal output > 2L/day	Hyperosmolar lumenal contents Gastric secretions (1.5 L/day) Bile salts stimulate colonic secretion Lack of absorptive capacity Rapid transit Secretion > absorption	Avoid elemental/polymeric drinks Proton-pump inhibitor Cholestyramine 4–12 g daily (if colon retained) Small, frequent meals Opioids (loperamide up to 60 mg/day and/or codeine up to 480 mg/day) Octreotide 150–300 µg s.c./day
Malnutrition	Steatorrhoea (calorie wastage) Reduced absorptive capacity Terminal ileal resection	Low-fat diet, but rarely vital Check Mg, folate, Zn, Ca, every 4–12 weeks: give supplements Medium-chain triglyceride diet* Non-total home parenteral feed* B_{12} 1 mg injection every 3 months
Gall stones	Bile acid depletion Octreotide	Cholecystectomy* if symptomatic
Renal stones	Chronic dehydration and chronic salt depletion Hyperoxaluria	Restrict hypotonic fluids. Encourage WHO oral rehydration solution Low-oxalate diet/cholestyramine if colon present, or $CaCO_3$ 7.5 g/day

*When other measures fail.

Therapy

- High sodium fluids in place of ordinary drinks are essential if the residual small intestine is to absorb fluid and electrolytes. Most patients can be encouraged to eat normally. The dietary fat/carbohydrate balance makes no difference to patients without a colon, although patients with a colon absorb more when the diet is high in carbohydrate
- Wrong advice to 'drink plenty of (hypotonic) fluids' and (hyperosmolar) nutritional supplements is commonly given
- The key to management is a modification of the World Health Organization rehydration solution: commercial preparations contain too little (only 60 mmol/L) sodium. The hospital pharmacy can formulate: glucose powder 20 g (110 mmol), sodium chloride 3.5 g (60 mmol) and sodium bicarbonate 2.5 g (30 mmol), made up to 1 L of tap water
- Refrigeration, fruit juice or replacing the bicarbonate by sodium citrate (2.9 g, 30 mmol) may all help palatability
- The patient should drink 750–1000 mL/day of this solution, whilst *restricting* intake of other fluids to 500–750 mL/day

Additional therapy

- A proton-pump inhibitor reduces gastric secretion, which accounts for up to 1500 mL/day
- Octreotide 25–100 µg subcutaneously three times daily also reduces intestinal secretions and high output, but should be reserved for when other measures fail
- Cholestyramine helps patients with a retained colon by chelating bile salts, which otherwise promote chloride secretion
- Very high doses of loperamide (up to 60 mg/day) and/or codeine phosphate (up to 480 mg/day) may also help
- Magnesium deficiency is common. Intravenous magnesium 10–12 mmol/day rapidly restores serum magnesium, followed by oral magnesium 12–24 mmol/day as magnesium glycerophosphate (500 mg twice daily) or heavy magnesium oxide 320 mg two to three times daily as tolerated
- Non-total parenteral nutrition is an important concept if nutrition or electrolyte balance cannot be maintained. Most patients can eat and absorb much, but not all, of their daily requirements. A tunnelled central venous line for administering electrolytes, trace elements (Additrace) and vitamins three or four nights a week is a useful option
- Total home parenteral nutrition may be necessary in a small proportion

Other causes

- Postinfective malabsorption may occur after gastroenteritis from any cause—bacterial, viral, toxin (travellers' diarrhoea) or parasitic (*Giardia lamblia*). Hypolactasia is the usual reason
- Drug-induced causes include:
  - neomycin
  - cholestyramine
  - liquid paraffin and irritant purgative abuse
  - magnesium-based antacids (interfere with iron, antibiotic, antimalarial and sucralfate absorption)
  - alcohol
- Lymphangiectasia may be primary, or secondary to lymphoma, tuberculosis, severe right heart failure or filariasis. Protein leaks into the lumen ('protein-losing enteropathy') and chylous ascites (p. 173) may develop
- Whipple's disease is a rare condition caused by the bacillus *Tropheryma whippelii*. It usually affects middle-aged men, causing malabsorption, arthritis, pleuritic pain, pericarditis or pigmentation, and occasional neuro-logical features. It is diagnosed by jejunal biopsy and cured by tetracycline for a year, although other antibiotics (penicillin or cotrimoxazole) are also effective. Patients are best referred to a specialist centre
- Eosinophilic gastroenteritis is a rare disorder characterized by an intense eosinophilic infiltrate which is mucosal (type 1), submucosal (type 2) or transmural (type 3). There is usually a peripheral eosinophilia, which should suggest the diagnosis once parasitic infections have been excluded. Symptoms are non-specific, with pain, diarrhoea and occasionally frank malabsorption, but type 3 causes ascites with a high eosinophil content. Rapid response to steroids is usual
- Metabolic defects, except hypolactasia, are not acquired by adults. Aminoacidurias (cystinuria, Hartnup disease), chloridorrhoea and acrodermatitis enteropathica (zinc deficiency) occur in children
- HIV enteropathy is characterized by diarrhoea and partial villous atrophy without an identifiable cause (p. 393)
- Starvation causes partial villous atrophy, defective intestinal immunity and possibly calcific pancreatitis. Susceptibility to enteric infection is increased. Impaired digestion of nutrients influences refeeding (calorie intake should be increased gradually, with replacement of vitamins and minerals). Chronic illness and postoperative complications are the commonest cause of starvation in adults in Britain (Section 12.1)
- Small intestinal lymphoma, and immunoproliferative small intestinal disease or α-chain disease is discussed on p. 270

7.3) Diverticulosis

Small intestinal diverticula are asymptomatic, or result in stasis of intestinal contents, bacterial overgrowth and malabsorption (pp. 245, 258). Perforation, inflammation and haemorrhage are much less common than in colonic diverticula.

Duodenal

* A single diverticulum is usually an incidental finding at ERCP or on a barium meal (about 2%), adjacent to or involving the papilla, and associated with gall stones. They make cannulation of the common bile duct more difficult at ERCP
* A diverticulum in the duodenal cap rarely follows ulceration
* Treatment is unnecessary unless complications occur. Surgery is appropriate for perforation, haemorrhage or contamination due to stasis, but these are very unusual

Meckel's diverticulum

2% of the population have this embryological remnant in the terminal ileum, but < 5% cause symptoms.

Haemorrhage
* More common than in other small intestinal diverticula, because 20% have heterotropic gastric or pancreatic tissue which can become inflamed
* Occult gastrointestinal bleeding may occur, especially in the young (p. 24)
* Small bowel enema will show a diverticulum more reliably than a ^{99m}Tc isotope scan, which detects heterotropic gastric mucosa, but still sometimes with difficulty

Diverticulitis and perforation
Cannot be distinguished clinically from appendicitis. Immediate management is similar (p. 268), but the surgeon must look carefully for a Meckel's diverticulum if the appendix is normal.

Other
Bacterial overgrowth, intussusception and herniation (Littré's) are all very unusual.

Small intestinal diverticulosis

- Jejunal diverticula are usually multiple, on the mesenteric margin
- Diarrhoea due to bacterial overgrowth is the commonest presentation (p. 258), but most are asymptomatic
- Small bowel radiology is diagnostic (Fig. 7.3, p. 246)
- Maintenance antibiotics (p. 259), or repeat courses when symptoms recur are indicated once bacterial overgrowth has occurred
- Angiography is necessary for obscure gastrointestinal bleeding in a patient with multiple diverticula, prior to surgery, but such patients are best referred to a specialist centre

7.4 Appendicitis

Appendicitis is usually due to obstruction and invasion by *Escherichia coli* with anaerobes. Crohn's disease, *Yersinia enterocolitica*, tuberculosis, carcinoid tumour, or *Enterobius vermicularis* infestation are other rare causes.

Clinical features

- Occurs at any age, but most commonly diagnosed in the young. Mortality is 25% when age > 70 years
- The pattern of central abdominal pain, shifting to the right iliac fossa, with anorexia and vomiting is most common in adolescents
- Abdominal rigidity may be absent when the appendix is retrocaecal or pelvic, and in obese or elderly patients
- Rectal examination is essential in all cases of abdominal pain
- The pain is higher and more lateral in pregnancy, with a higher incidence of peritonitis
- Subacute obstruction may occur in the elderly
- An appendix mass may be confused with a caecal carcinoma, Crohn's disease, tuberculosis or an ovarian tumour
- Clues to the differential diagnosis (Table 1.4, p. 27) include:
  - recent sore throat (mesenteric adenitis)
  - previous episode (Crohn's disease)
  - anaemia (Crohn's disease, caecal carcinoma)
  - weight loss (Crohn's disease, caecal carcinoma)
  - dyspepsia (cholecystitis, perforated ulcer)
  - arthralgia (*Yersinia enterocolitica*, Crohn's disease)
  - vaginal discharge (salpingitis)
  - mid-menstrual cycle (ruptured follicular cyst)

- frequency (urinary tract infection)
- preserved appetite (non-specific, or gynaecological)
- Asian origin (ileocaecal tuberculosis)

Management

- Abdominal ultrasound is often helpful in excluding other diagnoses (see above) and should always be performed in women
- Metronidazole 1 g suppository, oral clear fluids and observation for 8 h is reasonable if peritonism is absent and the diagnosis uncertain
- Surgery is needed for acute abdominal pain with peritonism
- Metronidazole 1 g suppository should be given 1 h before and 8 h after operation
- A normal appendix is found in up to 30%. Mesenteric adenitis, *Y. enterocolitica* ileitis, Crohn's disease, Meckel's diverticulitis, tubo-ovarian and non-specific causes (p. 41) should then be considered

Conservative management

- Indicated for an appendix mass, or when the risk of operation is too great—such as in a ship at sea
- Intravenous fluids, metronidazole 500 mg, ampicillin 500 mg and gentamicin 80 mg are given 8 hourly
- 30 mL water can be allowed every hour
- Careful charts of pulse and temperature, as well as regular examination determine progress
- Surgery must be performed if peritonitis develops

Appendix mass and abscess

- A tender right iliac fossa mass may be palpable after 5 days of untreated appendicitis. Pain and pyrexia resolve with bed rest
- Interval appendicectomy is indicated after 3 months. Small bowel radiology to exclude Crohn's disease is necessary before operation, if the history is atypical in any way
- An appendix abscess is distinguished by a swinging pyrexia and point tenderness on rectal examination. Ultrasound will identify the site and surgical drainage is indicated forthwith

'Grumbling appendix'

- Recurrent right iliac fossa pain has often been attributed to a 'grumbling appendix'. The diagnosis is doubtful

• Repeated attacks of appendicitis may occur, but the patient is well in between.

• Chronic pain with evidence of organic disease (weight loss, elevated ESR) is usually due to Crohn's disease at any age, caecal carcinoma in the elderly or, rarely, lymphoma or tuberculosis

• Pain without signs or abnormal investigations is likely to be due to the irritable bowel syndrome (p. 367), but a small bowel enema is still warranted if pain persists, to exclude more unusual causes

7.5 Small intestinal tumours

Polyps

Single

Isolated small intestinal polyps are rare and suggest malignancy (Table 7.9), although they may be benign. Secondaries from melanoma or lung should be considered. Symptoms are unusual, but bleeding or intussusception can occur. Surgical resection is indicated to establish the nature of a polyp if one is detected by small bowel radiology, but localization at operation is difficult without peroperative endoscopy.

Polyposis

Multiple polyps are more common (Table 7.9) than single polyps. They are usually lymphoid (nodular lymphoid hyperplasia, in the ileum or rectum of children, or associated with hypogammaglobulinaemia), non-neoplastic hamartomas (Peutz–Jeghers syndrome, associated with buccal or labial pigmentation and intussusception, p. 45) and rarely adenomatous (Cronkhite–Canada syndrome, associated with alopecia and nail dystrophy, p. 333).

Associated features are usually sufficient for diagnosis, although jejunal biopsy or laparotomy may be necessary to exclude lymphoma.

Table 7.9 Causes of small intestinal polyps.

Single	Multiple
Adenocarcinoma	Nodular lymphoid hyperplasia
Carcinoid	Peutz–Jeghers syndrome (hamartomas)
Secondary deposit	Lymphomatous polyposis
Benign adenoma	Multifocal adenocarcinoma
Lipoma	Endometriosis
Leiomyoma	Cronkhite–Canada syndrome (adenomas)

Lymphoma

Intestinal lymphoma is rare, but after the stomach (p. 113) is the most common extranodal origin of lymphoma. Mediterranean lymphoma (immunoproliferative small intestinal disease, or α-heavy chain disease) is discussed below.

Features

• Present with obstruction (70%), haemorrhage (50%) or perforation
• Associated with coeliac disease (5–10% coeliacs, usually > 50 years and following dietary non-compliance, p. 255). These are T-cell lymphomas, as opposed to the more usual B-cell lymphomas
• Weight loss, non-specific symptoms or failure to respond to gluten withdrawal in coeliac disease are characteristic. A mass may be palpable

Management

• Diagnosis is established by small bowel radiology (Fig. 7.5), followed by laparotomy. Lesions may be annular, ulcerating, multiple or occasionally diffuse, or missed by contrast radiology. Lymphoma may occur anywhere in the bowel
• Staging (Table 3.4, p. 113) is performed by thoracoabdominal CT scan, bone marrow and frozen-section biopsies at laparotomy
• Resection of annular lesions is often possible, but lymphoma in coeliac disease has a bad prognosis
• Postoperative chemotherapy is usually indicated and should be discussed with an oncologist
• Annual follow-up after treatment should include abdominal examination for a mass, blood count, ESR and small bowel radiology if intestinal symptoms recur

Immunoproliferative small intestinal disease

• Immunoproliferative small intestinal disease is common in the Middle East (especially Iraq), but important to recognize in Europe because the early stage can be cured by antibiotics
• Mediterranean lymphoma or α-heavy chain disease are synonyms. Only 70% excrete α-chains in the urine and immunoproliferative small intestinal disease has been recorded in indigenous Europeans
• Hypogammaglobulinaemia is commonly associated and nodular lymphoid hyperplasia in adults may be premalignant

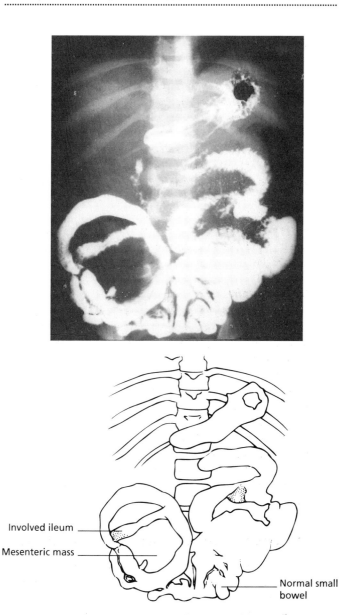

Fig. 7.5 Radiological features of small intestinal lymphoma. Small bowel lymphoma in a patient with coeliac disease giving rise to a large mesenteric mass in the right iliac fossa. This is displacing and compressing several ileal loops which show effacement of the fold pattern and nodular irregularity, indicating mucosal invasion.

- Lymphomatous polyposis, which is definitely malignant, is distinguished from immunoproliferative small intestinal disease histologically by normal intestinal mucosa between areas of lymphoid infiltration
- Diarrhoea, malabsorption, finger clubbing and weight loss in a young Middle Eastern adult are characteristic. Urine for α-chains, small bowel radiology and jejunal biopsy establish the diagnosis. Tetracycline 500 mg four times daily for 6 months is effective before extraintestinal spread occurs, but prognosis is poor after dissemination

Carcinoma

- Small intestinal carcinoma is rare and usually of unknown cause
- It is occasionally associated with coeliac disease, familial adenomatous polyposis (Gardner's syndrome) or Cronkhite–Canada syndrome (p. 269)
- Obstruction or chronic blood loss are the usual presenting features. Other causes of a small intestinal stricture are shown in Table 7.10
- Laparotomy is necessary, after small bowel radiology (Fig. 7.3, p. 247), for histological diagnosis and resection. Duodenal carcinomas are treated by pancreaticoduodenectomy (Whipple's procedure)

Table 7.10 Causes of small intestinal strictures.

Crohn's disease
Adenocarcinoma
Lymphoma
Tuberculosis
Vasculitis
Secondary deposit
NSAIDs
Radiation
Surgical anastomosis
Y. enterocolitica

8 Inflammatory Bowel Disease

8.1 Crohn's disease

Crohn's disease is characterized by chronic transmural granulomatous inflammation, with a tendency to form fistulae or strictures. It predominantly affects the ileocaecal region, but may affect any part of the gastrointestinal tract, often in discontinuity. The cause remains unknown.

General information

A few facts are helpful when explaining the disease to the patient:

- First recognized in 1932, but described earlier (1913, Dalziel)
- Affects 70–100 per 100 000 population, but studies from primary care on hospital-diagnosed cases report a higher prevalence (156/100 000)
- Five to seven new cases per 100 000 per year in northern Europe, USA and Australia, but appears uncommon in other areas of the world
- Incidence has doubled since 1950, and increased until 1990, but appears stable in northern Europe. It does not differ markedly between race, sex or social class in Britain, although more common among Jews in the USA
- Presents at any age, but usually 15–40 years. The site of disease and pattern of onset are unrelated to age
- 15% have a relative with Crohn's disease or ulcerative colitis; children of an affected parent have an 80–90% chance of *not* being affected. Affected parents are older at diagnosis (may indicate genetic anticipation) and pattern of disease within families is similar. Twins (8 of 18 monozygotic pairs) often have Crohn's disease together
- Immunogenetics of sibling pairs show highly significant allele sharing on chromosomes 7 and 12. If susceptibility gene(s) can be identified, the cause and pattern of disease may be predicted. Chromosome 12 is the site for genes synthesizing inflammatory mediators and modulators
- Four times more common in smokers than non-smokers; stopping smoking reduces risk of relapse. Probably not associated with oral contraceptive use
- Infective agents (measles, *Listeria* spp., *Saccharomyces* spp., *Mycobacterium paratuberculosis*) mucins and altered cell-mediated immunity, diet (high refined sugar) and anti-inflammatory drugs are postulated causes, but none explain disease discontinuity. Microvascular changes are probably secondary to inflammation
- At least half the patients have periods of remission lasting 5 years

Clinical features

It is clinically useful to classify Crohn's disease according to the site, extent and pattern of disease (Table 8.1), since this influences medical management, likelihood of surgery and prognosis. The site of disease influences the presentation. Exacerbations of existing disease produce similar features that may be due to active inflammation, infection or other complication. Although one pattern of disease tends to predominate in an individual, patterns are not mutually exclusive.

All sites and patterns

• Three symptoms occur in most patients: diarrhoea, abdominal pain and weight loss

• Acute abdominal pain may be confused initially with appendicitis or yersinial ileitis (Table 1.4, p. 27), but a careful history usually detects previous episodes that have not been recognized

• Fever, malaise, anorexia and lassitude are usual in active disease

• Weight loss alone, without diarrhoea or pain, may be the presenting feature in extensive inflammatory small bowel disease and may be confused with anorexia nervosa in adolescents

Small bowel disease

• Aphthous ulcers are common with active disease, but true oropharyngeal Crohn's ulcers are rare

• Duodenal ulcers that are postbulbar, difficult to heal or associated with a high ESR may be due to Crohn's disease, although they are exceptionally rare

• Colicky abdominal pain without systemic illness or local tenderness suggests a fibrotic stricture

• Abdominal pain may also be due to biliary colic or renal calculi

• Malnutrition is usually due to anorexia

Table 8.1 Site, extent and pattern of Crohn's disease.

Site	Extent	Pattern
Ileocolic (33%)	Localized (< 100 cm)	Fibrostenotic
Colonic (30%)	Extensive (> 100 cm)	Inflammatory
Small bowel (29%)		Fistulating
Other (8%)		

- Malabsorption is rare except in extensive small intestinal disease, or after resection
- An abdominal mass is frequently palpable in small intestinal disease, often in the right iliac fossa, but can be anywhere

Colonic disease (Crohn's colitis)

- Severe diarrhoea is more common than in small intestinal disease
- The rectum is usually spared, although perianal disease is common and can be very difficult to treat (p. 295)
- Extraintestinal manifestations (Table 8.2, p. 278) are more common than in small intestinal disease
- Rectal bleeding is uncommon compared to ulcerative colitis, but profuse haemorrhage is a very rare complication. Bleeding may indicate a colonic carcinoma in chronic Crohn's colitis, but this is rare
- Toxic dilatation is also much less common than in ulcerative colitis, but may be the presenting feature (p. 46)

Perianal disease

- Associated with ileocolonic disease, less common in isolated small bowel disease
- Recurrent abscesses, fistulae and violaceous fleshy skin tags, with or without ulceration, are characteristic. Appearance is often disproportionately severe compared to symptoms: pain and systemic illness are infrequent except with an abscess
- Anal or rectal stenosis may cause constipation and spurious diarrhoea

Extent of disease

- Extensive (> 100 cm) colonic or small bowel disease is associated with more profound weight loss and poor nutrition
- > 100 cm distal ileum must be diseased or resected before B_{12} malabsorption occurs
- Localized disease tends to follow a fibrostenotic or fistulating course, rather than inflammatory pattern

Pattern of disease

- Fibrostenotic disease is commonly ileocaecal or small bowel, causing localized strictures and obstructive symptoms
- Inflammatory disease is more commonly colonic, causing profuse diarrhoea, pronounced weight loss and marked elevation in inflammatory markers (C-reactive protein, ESR)

Table 8.2 Extraintestinal manifestations of Crohn's disease.

	Common (5–20%)	Unusual (< 5%)

Related to activity	Aphthous ulcers
	Erythema nodosum
	Finger clubbing
	Ocular
	   conjunctivitis
	   episcleritis
	   iritis
	Arthritis (large joint)
	Osteoporosis
		Pyoderma gangrenosum

Unrelated to activity	Gall stones
	Sacroiliitis
	Arthralgia (small joint)
	Nutritional deficiency
		Liver disease
		   fatty
		   primary sclerosing cholangitis
		Ankylosing spondylitis
		Renal
		   stones
		   ureteric stricture
		   right hydronephrosis
		   nephropathy (oxalate) amyloid
		Osteomalacia
		Sweet's syndrome
		Systemic amyloidosis

- Fistulating disease especially occurs in perineal Crohn's causing enterocutaneous fistulae, or pelvic and abdominal abscesses when there is small bowel or colonic disease

Extraintestinal manifestations

Occur in about 15%, but up to 30% in colonic disease. Some are markers of active disease and respond to treatment, others are unrelated to disease activity (Table 8.2). Differences from ulcerative colitis are discussed in Table 8.9 (p. 302).

- Sacroiliitis is unrelated to HLA-B27, unlike ankylosing spondylitis
- Fatty liver and abnormal liver function tests are common in sick patients and non-specific
- Renal calculi are more commonly due to chronic dehydration and salt depletion than hyperoxaluria
- Nutritional deficiencies may account for obscure symptoms (p. 402), including weakness (vitamin D, potassium, magnesium), lassitude (iron, B_{12}, folate), rashes (niacin, zinc) or altered taste (zinc), but only occur in very extensive disease or after major resection

Investigations

Diagnosis depends on clinical *and* radiological *and* endoscopic *and* histological features. There is no specific diagnostic test. All patients should be completely investigated to establish the site, extent and pattern of disease, even if the diagnosis is confirmed on a single test (e.g. finding granulomas on rectal biopsy).

Establishing the diagnosis

Sigmoidoscopy and rectal biopsy
Necessary even when the mucosa is macroscopically normal (up to 20% have microscopic granulomas).

Small bowel radiology (p. 458)
Performed first if diarrhoea, pain and weight loss are the presenting features. Colonoscopy should subsequently be arranged to exclude Crohn's colitis (Fig. 8.1, Table 8.3).

Colonoscopy
Colonoscopy is preferable to a barium enema if there is diarrhoea or visible rectal bleeding, since aphthoid ulcers are more readily detected and multiple biopsies can be taken. A barium enema may be more readily available and can obtain views of the terminal ileum, which may be helpful if pain predominates. Complete small bowel radiology is then advisable, even if the terminal ileum has been demonstrated by reflux of barium, to exclude more proximal disease.

Blood tests
- Anaemia is common, usually due to iron deficiency rather than B_{12} or folate deficiency

Table 8.3 Summary of radiological features of Crohn's disease.

General	Structural	Mucosal
Rectal sparing	Strictures	Aphthoid ulcers
Discontinuity	Fistula	Rose-thorn ulcers
('skip lesions')	Asymmetrical disease	Linear ulcers
	Dilatation	Thickened valvulae
	Pseudodiverticula	Cobblestoning
	Caecal distortion	Pseudopolyps
	Mass effect	

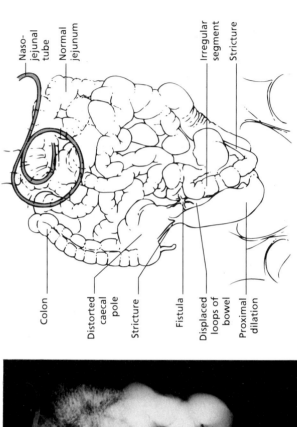

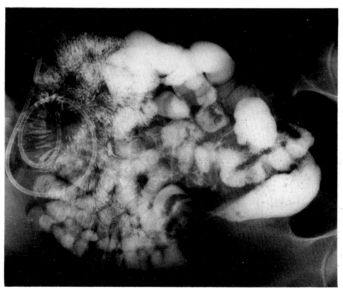

(a)

Fig. 8.1 Radiological appearance of Crohn's disease. (a) Small bowel enema in distal ileal Crohn's disease, showing dilatation of the ilium proximal to a stricture, displaced loops of bowel due to a mass, a distorted caecum and a fistula. (*Continued* on p. 281)

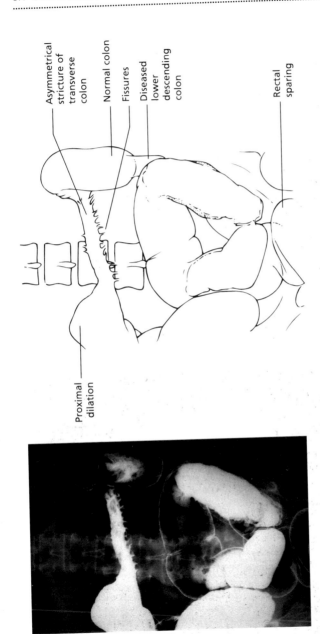

Asymmetrical stricture of transverse colon

Normal colon

Fissures

Diseased lower descending colon

Rectal sparing

Proximal dilation

(b)

Fig. 8.1 (*continued*) (b) Barium enema illustrating colonic Crohn's disease.

- C-reactive protein is the most sensitive inflammatory marker, but an elevated ESR or platelet count and a low albumin in a patient with recurrent abdominal pain and weight loss is usually due to Crohn's disease
- Antibodies to *Yersinia enterocolitica* are indicated when terminal ileal disease is diagnosed at laparotomy for suspected appendicitis

Stool

- Examination for pathogens and *Clostridium difficile* toxin assay if diarrhoea is severe
- Laparotomy is occasionally necessary to distinguish Crohn's disease from other causes of a small bowel stricture (Table 7.10, p. 272), including malignancy. Resection will also be therapeutic

Assessing activity

Once the diagnosis has been made it is necessary to establish whether symptoms are due to active disease or complications. Assessment of disease activity is often difficult, because symptoms such as diarrhoea or abdominal pain may be due to conditions other than active disease (Table 8.6, p. 290). A combination of clinical, blood and imaging tests is needed, as no one test is sufficient.

Clinical

- Anorexia, malaise, fever, tachycardia and weight loss indicate active disease
- Severe disease may be present without all these features and superimposed infection can mimic any of them

Blood tests

Low serum albumin or anaemia, a high ESR, C-reactive protein, plasma viscosity or platelet count all indicate active disease.

Radiology

Ulcers (aphthous, rose-thorn or linear), fistulae or disease at a new site found on small or large bowel radiology suggest activity.

Endoscopy and other techniques

- Visible ulcers or histological evidence of acute inflammation on biopsies are specific indicators of activity, although these do not correlate well with symptoms and the site of active disease (small intestine) may be inaccessible

- Ultrasound of the abdomen is valuable in experienced hands. It can demonstrate thickened bowel loops, an inflammatory mass or an abscess
- [111]I-labelled leucocyte scanning helps differentiate active disease from a fibrotic stricture and may locate an abscess, but may not be available locally
- Crohn's disease activity index, the Bradshaw or Dutch activity (Van Hees) index, are useful for coordinating clinical trials, but of less value for assessing individual patients

Investigation of recurrent symptoms

Recurrent symptoms may have to be investigated as above, to detect active disease or disease at a new site, but the reasons for reinvestigation must be clearly formulated. They should be relevant to subsequent therapeutic strategies, rather than to document the current extent of disease for its own sake. Crohn's disease is a chronic condition and therefore patients will have numerous investigations over the years.

Contrast radiology should be limited to symptoms of subacute intestinal obstruction that do not resolve rapidly with treatment, or investigation of complications (fistulae), when surgery may be indicated. Endoscopy is appropriate for colonic or upper gastrointestinal symptoms.

If symptoms do not follow the previous pattern of disease, arrange:

- MSU—for ureteric or renal involvement
- Plain abdominal X-ray—for subacute obstruction or stones
- Ultrasound—for gall stones, nephrolithiasis or hydronephrosis
- Lactulose hydrogen breath test—for bacterial overgrowth (p. 462)

Differential diagnosis

As much care must be taken to avoid inappropriately labelling a patient as having Crohn's disease, as not to overlook the diagnosis in the first place. Features are diverse and the clinical alternatives are many, but only a few cause real difficulty (Table 8.4). Do not forget that other disease can also develop after a diagnosis of Crohn's disease has been made.

Weight loss as the sole symptom

- May be inappropriately attributed to anorexia nervosa in an adolescent. Anaemia, a high ESR or platelet count strongly suggest Crohn's disease
- In older patients, gastrointestinal malignancy (pancreas, gastric carcinoma or lymphoma) must be considered. Gastroscopy and ultrasound are indicated before small bowel radiology
- Diabetes can cause weight loss and recurrent perianal sepsis

Table 8.4 Differential diagnosis of Crohn's disease: site of disease.

Site	Condition	Differentiating features
Duodenal	Tuberculosis	Biopsy persistent ulcers, chest X-ray
	Sarcoidosis	Chest X-ray, serum ACE, Kveim test
	Zollinger–Ellison syndrome	Diarrhoea common. Serum gastrin
Jejunoileal	Appendicitis, mass or abscess	Abrupt onset. No anaemia
	Laparotomy	
	Tuberculosis	Asian/African patients, Mantoux test
		Laparotomy
	Lymphoma	Smooth stricture(s). Laparotomy
	Adenocarcinoma	Single or multiple strictures (p. 272)
	Other tumours	Ovarian, carcinoid, metastases
	Y. enterocolitica	Acute ileitis. Yersinial antibodies
	Behçet's disease	Aphthous ileal and orogenital ulcers
	Coeliac disease	Ulcerative jejunitis may occur (p. 254)
	NSAID stricture	Ingestion of slow-release NSAID, with no systemic illness
Colonic	Ulcerative colitis	Table 8.12, p. 307
	Indeterminate colitis	p. 319
	Ischaemic colitis	Table 9.5, p. 352
	Carcinoma	Shouldered stricture(s). Biopsy
	Infective colitis	Stool samples, biopsy
	Amoebic colitis	Hot stool, biopsy (p. 388)
	Schistosomiasis	Japan/Middle Eastern patients
		Cyst excretion, biopsy
	Radiation	History of pelvic malignancy, biopsy
	Solitary rectal ulcer	Constipation, anterior position, biopsy, no systemic illness (p. 332)

ACE, angiotensin-converting enzyme.

Abdominal pain

- Symptoms resembling the irritable bowel syndrome (p. 369) with weight loss or anaemia are indications for further investigation
- Gall stones or renal calculi may coexist with Crohn's disease

Diarrhoea

- Ulcerative colitis, indeterminate colitis (p. 319), pseudomembranous, infective or ischaemic colitis (Table 9.5, p. 352) are usually distinguished by biopsy and stool culture, which must be repeated in cases of doubt
- Isolated diarrhoea that remains undiagnosed after colonic investigation is an indication for small bowel radiology, then jejunal biopsy and aspirate (Fig. 7.1, p. 241)

Right iliac fossa mass
- Caecal carcinoma is more common than Crohn's in the elderly
- Appendix abscess or ileocaecal tuberculosis occur at any age.
Tuberculosis, amoeboma or actinomycosis should be considered in Asian, African or South American patients. Ultrasound and serology help, but laparotomy may be necessary. The surgeon needs as much information as possible before operating

Rectal and perianal ulceration
Carcinoma, lymphogranuloma venereum, syphilis, Behçet's disease, HIV infection, herpes simplex, cytomegalovirus or tuberculosis are less common causes than Crohn's disease. Biopsy and serology are usually diagnostic.

Disease at other sites
Radiology resolves most of the dilemmas, but other conditions occasionally mimic the radiological appearances of Crohn's disease (Table 8.3, p. 279).

Management principles

General
- A confident and consistent approach, attention to nutrition, medical treatment of active disease and surgical management of complications are the principles of management
- Close liaison between medical and surgical teams is essential for optimal management of functional and structural problems
- Crohn's disease is only treated if there are symptoms: treat the patient, not the X-ray

Approach
- Explain that although the cause is unknown, inflammation and infection can be treated effectively. General information (p. 275) is often helpful for the patient
- Availability to deal with recurrent problems is reassuring. The patient should have a telephone number to call, either the medical secretary for an appointment or an experienced nurse
- Patients should be seen and followed up by an experienced gastro-enterologist, who can avoid unnecessary investigations and provide continuity
- Cautious optimism is advisable
- Patients often benefit from contact with the National Association for Colitis and Crohn's (NACC, Appendix 1, p. 477). Useful information leaflets are also available from the British Digestive Foundation (Appendix 1, p. 472)

Nutrition

Most patients can eat anything. Patients should avoid foods that upset them and try to eat a balanced diet. A special diet is occasionally needed (Table 8.5). Many patients find that avoiding vegetables and other foods high in fibre mitigate abdominal pain during an acute episode, especially if there is small intestinal disease.

• Good nutrition is especially important in children and adolescents, to ensure adequate growth

• A liquid elemental diet is beneficial in active disease, but polymeric feeds are as effective and more palatable. Neither are as effective as steroids, but offer an alternative treatment for active disease, especially for extensive small bowel disease, or if consequences of steroids and surgery are best avoided (children, multiple operations). About 60% respond to 6 weeks elemental or polymeric feeding. An experienced dietitian is essential to maintain compliance

• Adequate nutritional supplementation (as sip-feeds, nocturnal nasogastric tube feeding or parenteral nutrition) improves growth velocity in children

• Liquid polymeric diet helps maintain remission in children

• Parenteral feeding is only indicated when there is gut failure, due to obstruction, high output fistulae or massive resection

• There is no evidence that decreasing sugar intake alters the pattern of disease, although a high sugar intake has been implicated in the aetiology (p. 275)

Table 8.5 Indications for special diets in Crohn's disease.

Situation	Diet
Small intestinal stricture	Low-residue diet (p. 419)
Persistent diarrhoea without active disease	Try a lactose-free diet (p. 418), but see also Table 8.7 (p. 296)
Malnourishment	
during active disease	Enteral supplements (p. 408)
perioperatively	Parenteral nutrition, central or peripheral (p. 410)
jejunoileostomy	Diorylate for excess fluid loss (p. 262)
short (< 100 cm) bowel	Enteral or parenteral nutrition (p. 262)
Steatorrhoea	Low-fat diet (p. 49)
Active disease unresponsive to steroids	Elemental diet (p. 286), but see also p. 298 or polymeric diet for 6 weeks
Specific deficiencies	Iron, folate, B_{12}, fat-soluble vitamins, calcium, zinc p. 422

Medical management

Severity can be difficult to assess. All symptoms should be taken seriously. The differentiation between severe and mild attacks is not as clear as in ulcerative colitis (p. 301).

Basic investigations for any acute episode include a full blood count, ESR or C-reactive protein, albumin, electrolytes and stool sample for pathogens, including *Cl. difficile* toxin. A plain abdominal X-ray is also indicated in severe attacks to look for large or small bowel dilation and contrast radiology is advisable before surgical intervention.

Severe attacks
- Patients look ill, with severe symptoms, vomiting, fever > 38°C, tachycardia > 90 b.p.m., or laboratory evidence (albumin < 35 g/dL, high ESR, leucocytosis) of inflammation or infection. These features are indications for admission to hospital
- Intravenous fluids and replacement of electrolytes (especially K) are important. The patient may be dehydrated
- Intravenous hydrocortisone 100 mg four times daily should be started
- Metronidazole 400–500 mg three times daily, orally if possible, can be useful, because there is often associated infection which may be impossible to distinguish from inflammation. It may also have a specific effect
- Blood transfusion may be needed to bring the haemoglobin up to 10 g/dL
- Fluids are allowed by mouth, but no food. It is uncertain whether avoiding food is of specific value, but patients are often anorexic and symptoms may be exacerbated by food
- Intravenous hydrocortisone and fluids are best continued for 5 days, then feeding restarted, with oral prednisolone 40 mg/day
- Response should be monitored by symptoms (bowel frequency, pain, anorexia), examination (abdominal tenderness, fever, tachycardia) and blood tests (alternate daily full blood count, C-reactive protein, albumin, electrolytes)
- Deterioration during intravenous treatment suggests a complication, or disease that is not going to respond to medical treatment, and is usually an indication for surgery (p. 290). Deterioration once feeding is restarted has similar implications
- Further investigations can be arranged when the patient is stable
- Once appetite returns and abdominal tenderness resolves, the patient can be discharged home, with an outpatient appointment for 2–4 weeks time. The weight on discharge should be recorded

- Prednisolone is decreased to 20 mg/day over 2 weeks, then continued at 20 mg for a month, before decreasing by 5 mg/day every 1–2 weeks. More rapid reduction can provoke early relapse, but the aim must always be to stop steroids during remission. Some patients are very sensitive to minor changes in steroid dosage and the minimum dose needed to control symptoms in these patients should be established
- Alternatives to steroids and maintenance therapy are discussed below

Mild attacks

- Patients are symptomatic and uncomfortable, often with abdominal tenderness and an elevated ESR or C-reactive protein. Vomiting, fever or a low albumin usually indicate a severe attack (p. 287)
- Outpatient treatment is reasonable
- Prescribe prednisolone 40 mg daily for a week, then 30 mg daily for a week, then 20 mg/day for 1 month. A low-residue diet is advisable if colicky pain is prominent
- Prednisolone can then be decreased slowly if symptoms have resolved, by 5 mg/day every 1–2 weeks
- Response should be regularly assessed in outpatients (every 2–4 weeks). Symptoms, examination and blood tests (full blood count, C-reactive protein, albumin) are the guide. It is usually unwise to stop steroids until all have returned to normal

Maintenance therapy

- Until recently, maintenance therapy was rarely indicated. Prophylaxis with mesalazine (released in the small bowel) after surgery or a relapse should now be routine unless it cannot be tolerated
- High doses of salicylates (mesalazine ≥ 2 g/day) appear to halve the risk of relapse in controlled trials, especially when started within 3 months of surgery (Pentasa 1 g twice daily is convenient because 500 mg tablets are available in the UK; Asacol 800 mg three times daily is an alternative). Lower doses do not work
- Azathioprine 1.5–2.5 mg/kg/day also halves the risk of relapse and is indicated in the group of patients in whom complete steroid withdrawal is difficult (p. 297). Treatment should continue for 4–5 years if tolerated

Alternatives to steroids

- Surgery is usually indicated for steroid-resistant disease, including stricturoplasty for small bowel strictures, split ileostomy for colonic or perianal Crohn's disease and resection when necessary (p. 290)

- Mesalazine 4000 mg/day is effective for active ileocaecal or colonic Crohn's disease, but not as effective as steroids
- Budesonide-CIR is a steroid with low systemic bioavailability and minimal systemic side-effects for treatment of ileocaecal or ascending colonic Crohn's disease. A dose of 9 mg daily for 6 weeks, then 6 mg daily for 4 weeks is comparable to prednisolone. Continued treatment may reduce relapse
- Azathioprine (1.5–2.5 mg/kg/day) is indicated as a steroid-sparing agent for patients with side-effects from steroids, or for those who relapse rapidly when steroids are reduced. It is ineffective alone for active disease and takes about a month to have an effect
- An elemental or liquid polymeric diet for 6 weeks (p. 286) can be used alone or as an adjunct to steroids for extensive small intestinal, perianal or steroid-resistant disease. Palatability is poor and needs expert dietetic support to be tolerated
- Metronidazole 400 mg three times daily is indicated with steroids for perianal disease, or when infection coexists with active disease (see below)
- Methotrexate 15–25 mg once weekly is sometimes effective for active, steroid-resistant disease when surgery needs to be avoided, but should not be used outside specialist centres
- Antitumour necrosis factor antibody (either a human CDP571, or chimeric cA2 antibody) and interleukin-10 infusion have been shown to improve symptoms and macroscopic inflammation after a single infusion in about 70% with steroid-resistant disease, but are not widely available and should be considered as 'one-off' rescue therapy
- Cyclosporin has not been shown to work in controlled trials

Outpatient review in Crohn's disease

Routine follow-up of patients (every 3–6 months) aims to detect early recurrence or complications and to monitor long-term therapy.

Documentation

Needed for each patient and most helpfully recorded on a special card at the front of the notes:

- Date of onset of symptoms
- Site and extent of disease
- Presence or absence of positive histology
- Date of last small bowel/colonic examination
- Chronology of operations and complications

At each review
- Ask about present symptoms and extraintestinal manifestations
- Consider causes of diarrhoea or abdominal pain other than active Crohn's disease (Table 8.6)
- Record weight and abdominal signs
- Check full blood count and liver function every 6 months, even if asymptomatic, to detect sub-clinical nutritional deficiency or other complications such as sclerosing cholangitis. Full blood count every 4–8 weeks is necessary during azathioprine therapy
- Explain the importance of early review if symptoms recur

Indications for surgery

70–80% of patients have an operation at some stage. The decision to operate depends on the degree of disability caused by the symptoms.

Major indications
- Symptomatic disease despite medical therapy
- Intestinal obstruction (sub-acute or acute) from strictures
- Local complications:
  - fistulae
  - abscess
  - perforation

Principles
- Limited resection of the most diseased area by an experienced surgeon
- Avoid bypass surgery: recurrence is common. End-to-end anastomosis is always preferable
- Staged procedures for sick patients with colonic disease (e.g. ileostomy, then resection of the diseased area, then restoration of continuity) are now

Table 8.6 Causes of abdominal pain in Crohn's disease.

Inflammatory markers present	Inflammatory markers absent
Active Crohn's	Stricture
small intestinal	small intestinal
colonic	colonic
Abscess	Biliary colic
Pyelonephritis	Renal colic
Cholecystitis	Adhesions
Drug-induced pancreatitis	Steroid-induced peptic ulcers
(azathioprine, mesalazine, steroids)	Other disease—ovarian, pelvic

performed less commonly because of better supportive care, including parenteral nutrition

- Perioperative corticosteroids may reduce postoperative relapse, including after elective procedures during remission. Give intravenous hydrocortisone 100 mg twice daily whilst nil by mouth, then prednisolone 20 mg/day decreasing by 5 mg/week
- Postoperative salicylates (Pentasa 1 g twice daily or Asacol 800 mg three times daily) halve the risk of relapse and should be started before the patient leaves hospital. Whether azathioprine usefully reduces postoperative relapse is being investigated

Special situations

- Stricturoplasty is preferable for small intestinal strictures, since it avoids resection and anastomosis and minimizes loss of bowel
- Limited resection (rather than a right hemicolectomy) is appropriate for ascending colonic or terminal ileal disease
- Localized transverse or distal colonic disease with a stricture or fistula may first be resected, but the relapse rate is fairly high and more extensive disease that needs surgery is best treated by proctocolectomy, which has a lower relapse rate
- Ileorectal anastomosis may avoid a permanent ileostomy if the rectum is spared, but the relapse rate is higher than with a proctocolectomy. Ileoanal pouch formation is considered absolutely contraindicated by most surgeons because of the risk of postoperative sepsis or fistulae, but success in some patients has been reported
- Split ileostomy and hydrocortisone 100 mg in 100 mL instilled into the distal limb daily may heal resistant colonic or perianal disease. Continuity can be restored after 18 months and a permanent ileostomy avoided in about half of patients
- Local surgery should be avoided for perianal fistulae, ulcers, skin tags or haemorrhoids, because symptoms are usually few and recurrence common

Complications

Small intestinal obstruction

Diagnostic investigations
Plain abdominal X-ray, markers of activity and cautious small bowel radiology.

- Usually due to active disease, but may be caused by bolus obstruction at a fibrotic stricture

- Chronic symptoms with few signs of active disease suggests a fibrotic stricture
- Radiographic intestinal diameter correlates poorly with symptoms

Toxic dilatation (p. 46)

Diagnostic investigations
Temperature > 38°C, colonic diameter > 6.0 cm on plain X-ray) Fig. 1.5, p. 47; repeated daily), stool culture for pathogens and *Cl. difficile* toxin and blood cultures.
- Much less common than in ulcerative colitis

Abdominal, pelvic or ischiorectal abscess

Diagnostic investigations
Temperature chart, white cell count, ultrasound and culture of pus after aspiration. Magnetic resonance imaging (MRI) (Fig. 8.2, p. 293) effectively demonstrates the location and any fistulous connections of pelvic abscesses, but may not be locally available.
[111]In-labelled leucocyte scanning is sometimes helpful if an abscess is suspected and cannot be detected by other methods
- Surgery is necessary to drain the abscess before antibiotics can be effective (intravenous cefotaxime 1 g and metronidazole 500 mg three times daily until apyrexial, then oral equivalent for 1 week). Steroids are also indicated (oral for ischiorectal, intravenous for abdominal abscesses) to suppress active Crohn's disease

Fistulae
Diagnostic investigations
Contrast radiology, preferably when disease is quiescent, MRI is best for perianal fistulae if available, but surgical examination under anaesthetic by an experienced surgeon is the traditional alternative.
- Perianal fistulae produce a discharge and may interfere with anal sphincter function (faecal soiling) or produce a stricture (palpable on rectal examination). Treatment is only indicated for symptoms (p. 297). MRI defines the complexity of fistulous tracks in relation to the levator muscles
- Vesicocolic or vaginal fistulae (causing pneumaturia or faecal vaginal discharge) usually connect with the terminal ileum. Small bowel radiology is indicated before surgery. Rectovaginal fistulae can heal spontaneously
- Enterocutaneous fistulae follow surgery. Antibiotics, steroids and nutritional support allow a minority to heal spontaneously, but surgical

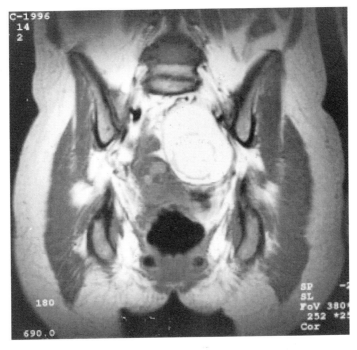

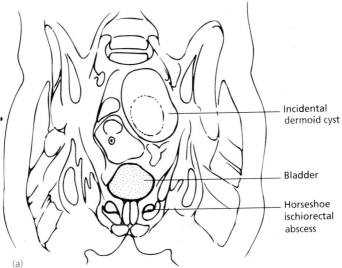

Incidental dermoid cyst

Bladder

Horseshoe ischiorectal abscess

(a)

Fig. 8.2 (a) **Pelvic MRI showing coronal section.** (*Continued* on p. 294)

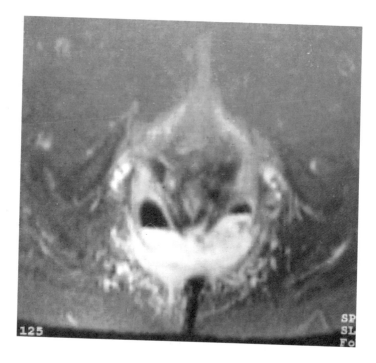

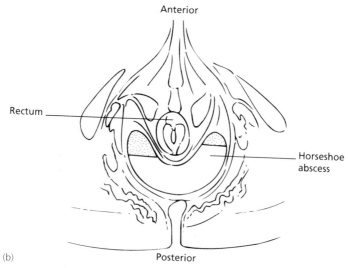

Fig. 8.2 (*continued*) (b) Pelvic MRI showing enlarged sagittal section of horseshoe abscess in (a).

resection of the fistulous track and connecting bowel is usually needed. The anatomy must be clearly defined by sinograms, small and large bowel radiology before surgery
- Enterocolic or enteroenteric fistulae cause profound weight loss, often, but not always, with diarrhoea. Steroids (prednisolone 40 mg/day), metronidazole (400 mg three times daily) and an elemental diet or parenteral nutrition should be tried for a month or more, before considering surgery

Short bowel syndrome
- Cumulative resection to < 100–200 cm leads to short bowel syndrome, especially if there is persistent small intestinal disease or if the colon has been removed
- Surgeons should measure the length of bowel from the ligament of Treitz at the time of laparotomy for resection in any patient with Crohn's disease
- Management is discussed on p. 262

Perforation

Diagnostic investigations
Plain abdominal and erect chest X-rays.
- Rarely presents acutely because an abscess cavity often forms, although features may be suppressed by steroids
- Surgery is indicated if perforation is detected

Massive rectal bleeding

Diagnostic investigations
Clinical evidence, full blood count, prothrombin time.
- Rare in colonic disease (1%) and very rare in terminal ileal disease
- Transfusion alone is almost always sufficient. Colonoscopy is indicated after the bleeding stops
- Surgery for persistent bleeding (> 8 unit transfusion) may be preceded by angiography if the distribution of colonic disease is unknown

Carcinoma

Diagnostic investigations
Colonoscopy, biopsy.
- Occurs in < 5% of patients with colonic disease, related to the extent and duration (> 10 years) of Crohn's colitis. Diagnosis is often too late for a curative colectomy

- New symptoms, such as rectal bleeding without signs of active disease, are an indication for colonoscopy
- The risk of small intestinal carcinoma is increased, but remains very rare (2/373 patients followed for > 10 years)

Extraintestinal complications

See Table 8.2, p. 278.

Management problems

Recurrent symptoms are not always due to active disease. When inflammation or infection are present the ESR, C-reactive protein and platelet count are usually elevated and the albumin low ('inflammatory markers').

Persistent abdominal pain (Table 8.6, p. 290)

- Urine examination is always necessary, to look for haematuria (calculi), proteinuria (infection or inflammation) and for culture
- A plain abdominal film may show fluid levels, dilated bowel, loops separated by a mass or calcified calculi
- Ultrasound of a mass, to look for an abscess cavity, inflammatory mass, thickened bowel loops or calculi is advisable before repeat small bowel radiology, because it is less invasive. Intestinal gas may, however, obscure views

Persistent diarrhoea (Table 8.7)

- Active Crohn's colitis may be extensive or an enteroenteric fistula unsuspected. Imaging should be reviewed and colonoscopy or small bowel enema arranged if necessary
- Small bowel bacterial overgrowth is diagnosed by a lactulose hydrogen breath test (p. 462), except after ileocolonic resection or enteroenteric

Table 8.7 Causes of persistent diarrhoea in Crohn's disease.

Inflammatory markers present	Inflammatory markers absent
Active Crohn's disease	Small intestinal bacterial overgrowth
	Hypolactasia
	Bile-salt malabsorption after ileal resection
	Short bowel after resection
	Irritable bowel syndrome
	Other disease (coeliac, chronic pancreatitis)

fistula, when jejunal aspiration is more reliable. It is treated with tetracycline 250 mg four times daily and metronidazole 400 mg three times daily for 2 weeks (p. 258). Recurrent courses every few months may be necessary

- Avoiding milk helps patients with hypolactasia
- Diarrhoea due to distal ileal disease or resection responds to cholestyramine 4 g one to three times a day
- Symptomatic control with codeine phosphate (up to 90 mg/day) or loperamide (up to 12 mg/day) is appropriate if other measures fail

Rapid relapse upon steroid withdrawal

Patients who relapse when steroids are reduced below 10 mg, or within 6 weeks of complete withdrawal whilst taking maintenance mesalazine ≥ 2 g/day (p. 288), are best treated by:

- Prednisolone 30 mg daily to induce remission again, with azathioprine 2–2.5 mg/kg/day (usually 100–150 mg/day)
- Decrease prednisolone to 20 mg/day upon remission, then by 5 mg every 2–4 weeks. It is occasionally not possible either to withdraw steroids or to control symptoms completely, and a compromise may have to be struck between symptom control and steroid dosage. Budesonide-CIR 3–9 mg daily is appropriate in place of prednisolone for ileal or ascending colonic disease if steroids cannot be withdrawn and surgery considered for persistent symptoms
- Continue azathioprine after steroids are withdrawn for up to 5 years. A full blood count every 1–2 months, or during any acute infection, is advisable to detect the rare complication of agranulocytosis (< 3%). Concomitant treatment with allopurinol or co-trimoxazole should be avoided because toxicity is enhanced
- Mesalazine ≥ 2 g/day should be continued as maintenance therapy

Perianal disease

- Treatment is only necessary for symptoms, which are frequently mild compared to the often horrific appearance
- Resolution is often independent of disease activity elsewhere
- Metronidazole 400 mg three times daily and topical steroid suppositories twice daily are indicated for symptomatic disease, with sulphasalazine or mesalazine 2 g daily for associated ileocolonic disease
- Spreading fistulation is an indication for oral steroids (prednisolone 30 mg daily) with metronidazole 400 mg three times daily. Azathioprine is often useful as a steroid-sparing agent, but otherwise offers no specific advantage
- An elemental diet sometimes helps

- Surgery is indicated for drainage of an abscess (acute local pain and tenderness). Complicated fistulae that fail to respond to intensive medical treatment usually respond well to defunctioning of the colon or rectum (split ileostomy or colostomy), but are best treated at a specialist centre
- Pads are helpful for discharging sinuses

Ileostomy dysfunction
See p. 316.

Crohn's disease in pregnancy (see also p. 428)

- Advise patients to avoid conception until disease is inactive. There is then little risk to the pregnancy or the course of Crohn's disease
- Active disease during pregnancy is often relatively resistant to treatment, but sometimes remits spontaneously. Steroids and salicylates are used in the normal way (p. 287), because the risks of active disease are greater than any drug side-effects. Immunosuppression with azathioprine can be continued if essential for maternal health (such as remission in refractory disease or recurrent relapse only achieved with azathioprine)
- Delivery by caesarean section is advisable if there is active perianal disease or previous anorectal surgery for fistulae

Crohn's disease in adolescence

- Retardation of growth and puberty, as well as loss of schooling, are additional problems, although the course of disease and treatment principles are the same as in adults
- Nutritional assessment and support are essential. Height and weight must be recorded on a centile chart at each visit. Falling below centile lines for height or weight is an indication for blood tests to assess activity and nutritional status (full blood count, folate, B$_{12}$, iron studies, calcium). Nutritional supplements (enteric sip feeds, p. 408) are usually tolerated, but if not, continuous or nocturnal enteral feeding are alternatives
- Active disease may be treated as in adults, with prednisolone (starting at 1 mg/kg daily). However, many paediatric gastroenterologists use nutritional therapy in place of steroids as first line therapy. Once symptoms are relieved, steroids may be prescribed as a double dose on alternate days, to decrease adverse effects on growth. Rapid control of disease activity with adequate steroids, whilst providing nutritional supplements, also minimizes the adverse effects of steroids. Surgical resection of the most diseased area should be considered if the response is slow

Prognosis

It is currently impossible to predict the course of Crohn's disease in an individual patient. Relapses tend to follow the previous pattern of disease (fibrostenotic, fistulating, inflammatory). Up to 80% concordance of disease distribution or pattern has been reported in family members affected by Crohn's. Most patients have a good prognosis, although morbidity may be considerable for short periods.

Risk of relapse
- Crohn's disease cannot be cured
- A year after diagnosis, about 50% have no symptoms, 25% have low activity and 25% high disease activity in any given year
- Working capacity is normal in 75%. After 5–10 years, 15% are not working due to the disease
- Patients with jejunoileal disease relapse more commonly than those with Crohn's colitis

Need for surgery
- 60% of patients have an intestinal resection within 10 years of the onset of symptoms and 80% after 20 years
- Half the operations are emergencies
- After 15 years a third have had no operation, a third have had a single operation and a third have had two or more operations
- The need for surgery is more common (80% at 5 years) in those presenting with ileocaecal disease compared to those with Crohn's colitis or disease at other locations (40%)
- About 10% with colonic disease have a permanent ileostomy after 10 years

Recurrence after surgery
- 30% relapse within 5 years and 50% within 10 years, but only half of these need further surgery
- Recurrence is less common in colonic disease and the elderly, but more common in children

Mortality
- In population-based studies, overall mortality is no different from that of the general population
- Patients with extensive (> 100 cm) small intestinal disease, proximal (gastroduodenal or jejunal) disease, or those aged 20–29 years at diagnosis,

however, have a higher mortality in the first 5 years after diagnosis (relative risk three- to sixfold)

8.2) Ulcerative colitis

Ulcerative colitis is an inflammatory disorder of the colonic mucosa characterized by relapses and remissions. The cause remains unknown.

General information

A few facts are helpful when explaining the disease to patients:

• Affects 90–170 per 100 000 population (twice as common as Crohn's), but studies from primary care on hospital-diagnosed cases report a higher prevalence (up to 268 per 100 000). These higher prevalence figures need to be confirmed

• Seven to 22 new cases per 100 000 per year, with no apparent increase in incidence recently. Sex and social class are not associated, although it is uncommon outside Western societies. Asian immigrants have a much higher incidence than those in the sub-continent

• Most patients present aged 15–30 years, with a second peak at age 55–70 years, although no age is exempt. Proctitis is more common than total colitis, especially in the elderly

• 15% have a member of the family with ulcerative colitis or Crohn's. Ulcerative colitis in monozygotic twins affects both twins about half the time, but concordance in twins with Crohn's disease is more common

• The genotype may be related to the pattern of disease (HLA-DR1*103 is five to 11 times more common in patients who have a colectomy than those who do not)

• Twice as common in non-smokers

• Seasonal variation occurs, with presentation in the winter (1.48-fold increased risk in December) being twice as common as in early summer (0.76-fold risk in May, relative to annual mean)

• Appendicectomy is uncommon (3%) compared to controls (16%) or patients with Crohn's (34%)

• The cause is unknown, but deficient immunoregulation, non-steroidal anti-inflammatory drugs (72% in 6 months prior to diagnosis, compared to 7% controls), cell-wall deficient bacteria and diet (low fibre, milk) have been implicated. Stress may exacerbate existing symptoms, but not cause the disease

• The pattern is usually intermittent. Chronic continuous symptoms with varying severity are less common. Single attacks with no recurrence are rare, and probably not true ulcerative colitis but caused by infection

Clinical features

General

- Bloody diarrhoea is the hallmark, usually with mucus
- Onset is usually gradual but can be abrupt, and there may sometimes be a previous history of episodic diarrhoea. Infection may trigger an abrupt onset or toxic dilatation
- Bowel frequency is broadly related to the severity of disease
- Crampy abdominal discomfort is common, but severe persistent pain suggests a complication or different diagnosis
- Systemic features (anorexia, malaise, fever) are common during an acute attack, except in ulcerative proctitis
- Signs (tachycardia, fever, abdominal tenderness or distension) are important when assessing severity (Table 8.8)
- Other features that help distinguish severe attacks are systemic upset (anorexia, malaise, weight loss), tender colon (but often notable by its absence), leucocytosis and hypoalbuminaemia
- Steroids can mask clinical features of severity
- Young patients with severe disease may appear misleadingly well

Table 8.8 Assessing the severity of ulcerative colitis.

Feature	Mild	Moderate	Severe
Motions/day	< 4	4–6	> 6
Rectal bleeding	Small	Moderate	Large amounts
Temperature	Apyrexial	Intermediate	> 37.8°C on 2 days out of 4
Pulse rate	Normal	Intermediate	> 90 b.p.m.
Haemoglobin	> 11 g/dL	Intermediate	< 10.5 g/dL
ESR	< 20 mm/h	Intermediate	> 30 mm/h

Extraintestinal manifestations

- 10–20% are affected, especially those with pancolitis
- Similar to those in Crohn's disease (Table 8.2, p. 278), with some important exceptions (Table 8.9, p. 302)

Investigations

The aim is to confirm the diagnosis, assess the severity and extent of disease, and to detect complications.

Table 8.9 Distinctions between extraintestinal manifestation of ulcerative colitis and Crohn's disease.

Extraintestinal feature	Comment
PSC (p. 229)	Affects 2–3% 80% with PSC have UC, 70% are male Less common in Crohn's disease
Cholangiocarcinoma	Usually complicates PSC, but very rare in Crohn's disease
Skin lesions	Consider drug-induced lesions, such as sulphasalazine, especially in UC
Large joint arthritis	Possibly becoming less common in UC due to maintenance sulphasalazine
All extraintestinal manifestations	Relieved by proctocolectomy in UC, except ankylosing spondylitis and hepatobiliary disease, but not in Crohn's disease

PSC, primary sclerosing cholangitis; UC, ulcerative cholitis.

Establish the diagnosis

Sigmoidoscopy and biopsy
- Diffuse mucosal changes in the rectum are invariable during active disease
- Infective colitis and occasionally Crohn's disease or ischaemia can look similar
- Characteristic microscopic features are a chronic inflammatory infiltrate, glandular distortion, goblet-cell depletion and crypt abscesses

Colonoscopy
- Always preferable to a barium enema as the initial investigation of bloody diarrhoea, because it provides better mucosal definition and allows biopsies to be taken
- In the acute stages a flexible sigmoidoscopy 30–60 min after a phosphate enema is more appropriate than full colonoscopy, which can be dangerous (perforation)

Air contrast barium enema
- Only appropriate if colonoscopy is unavailable or not possible
- Shows symmetrical and confluent changes (Fig. 8.3, p. 303, Table 8.10, p. 304)
- Establishes the extent of disease after an acute attack

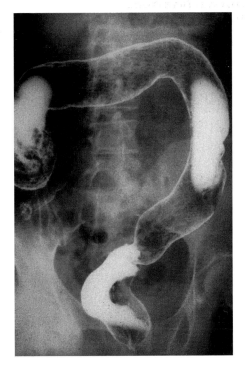

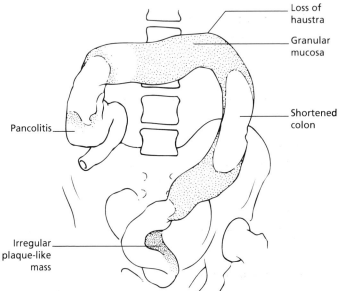

Loss of haustra

Granular mucosa

Shortened colon

Pancolitis

Irregular plaque-like mass

Fig. 8.3 Radiological features of ulcerative colitis. Barium enema radiograph showing carcinoma in long-standing ulcerative colitis, presenting as an infiltrative plaque.

Table 8.10 Summary of radiological features of ulcerative colitis (approximate order of severity).

Acute	Chronic
Normal (proctitis)	Increased retrorectal space
Granular mucosa	Granular mucosa
Absent faecal shadows*	Loss of haustra
Punctate ulcers	Tubular colon
Collar-stud ulcers	Pseudopolyps
Mucosal islands*	Backwash ileitis (pancolitis)
Toxic dilatation (> 6.0 cm)*	Carcinoma

*Visible on plain abdominal X-ray.

- Should not be performed during severe disease unless major doubt exists about the diagnosis. An unprepared, single contrast 'instant enema' is only appropriate if immediate management will be altered, but is not good for estimating the true extent of disease

Stool examination

Always necessary to exclude pathogens (*Esherichia coli* 0157, *Shigella* spp., *Campylobacter* spp., *Clostridium difficile* toxin, *Salmonella* spp., *Entamoeba histolytica* after foreign travel, or CMV in immunocompromised).

Establish the severity

- Clinical criteria (Table 8.8, p. 301)
- Sigmoidoscopy (Table 8.11), but mucosal changes may have been ameliorated by rectal steroids
- Blood tests
  - anaemia (Hb < 10.5 g/dL) and an ESR > 30 mm/h indicate severe disease. If the ESR is normal, a C-reactive protein > 10 mg/L has the same significance
  - leucocytosis, hypoalbuminaemia (< 35 g/L) and hypokalaemia are also common in severe disease

Table 8.11 Sigmoidoscopic appearances in ulcerative colitis.

Mild	Moderate	Severe
Diffuse erythema	Granular mucosa	Intense inflammation
Loss of vascular pattern	Petechial haemorrhages	Purulent exudate
Contact bleeding	Spontaneous bleeding	Discrete ulcers

Establish the extent of disease

- In a population-based study of 1161 patients, distribution of disease at diagnosis was proctitis (48%), distal or left-sided (33%) or total (19%)
- Proctitis means that the upper limit of inflammation can be seen on rigid sigmoidoscopy (usually < 15 cm from anal verge)
- Distribution of faecal shadows on a plain abdominal X-ray during an acute attack is a useful guide to the extent of disease: faecal shadows are absent from bowel with active mucosal inflammation. It can be misleading, however, in those with proximal constipation
- Colonoscopy and serial biopsy is the best way of establishing the extent. Biopsies frequently show microscopic inflammation proximal to the limit of macroscopic inflammation, but the implications of microscopic changes are not clear. Prognostic factors (for carcinoma, or risk from a severe attack) are based on the extent of macroscopic disease
- Barium enema (see above) documents the extent of macroscopic disease
- The risk of proximal extension of distal disease is conventionally estimated at 15%, but in one retrospective study of 145 patients was 16% at 5 years and 31% 10 years after diagnosis

Investigation of relapse

- Sigmoidoscopy and biopsy are necessary to assess the severity (Table 8.11, p. 304), in association with the clinical features
- Stool for culture and *Clostridium difficile* toxin assay must be taken
- Full blood count, ESR or C-reactive protein, electrolytes and albumin should be measured. The C-reactive protein may be elevated when the ESR is normal and has the same significance as a high ESR
- A plain abdominal X-ray is necessary in severe disease to look for signs of toxic dilatation or mucosal islands (Fig. 1.6, p. 48). When a moderate relapse is slow to settle, proximal constipation may be visible (p. 315)
- Repeat colonoscopy is unnecessary unless the extent of the disease is thought to have changed (such as after a severe attack in a patient with previous proctitis)

Outpatient follow-up in remission

- Duration and extent of disease should always be documented, preferably on a summary card at the front of the notes
- Sigmoidoscopy is only necessary if a relapse occurs
- Rectal biopsy is recommended at every sigmoidoscopy, because it provides an independent record of the macroscopic appearances, consolidates the diagnosis and, rarely, detects dysplasia
- Surveillance colonoscopy and multiple biopsy may be indicated for total

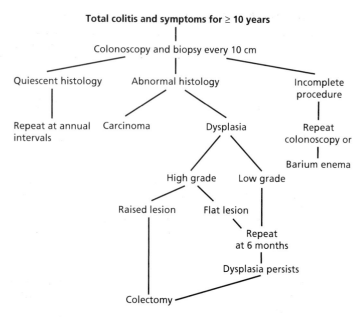

Fig. 8.4 Surveillance colonoscopy in ulcerative colitis.

colitis after symptoms for 8–10 years (discussed in Fig. 8.4). It is not necessary for left-sided disease

• Annual full blood count and liver function tests are recommended. Macrocytosis can be due to sulphasalazine or azathioprine therapy, but other causes (alcohol, B_{12} or folate deficiency, myxoedema or haemolysis) should not be overlooked

• A mildly elevated AST is an indication for complete abstinence from alcohol for 4–8 weeks before repeating the test. Drug-induced liver damage should be considered (p. 160) and if the AST continues to rise, all drugs should be stopped if possible. A liver biopsy is indicated if > twofold elevation persists for 3 months

• Persistently (> 3 months), or > threefold elevation in ALP, are indications for ultrasound to exclude gall stones, before ERCP to look for primary sclerosing cholangitis

Differential diagnosis

There are many causes of bloody diarrhoea, but only a few cause diffuse rectal changes visible on sigmoidoscopy. The main problems are differentiating ulcerative colitis from infective or Crohn's colitis (Table 8.12).

Table 8.12 Differentiation of ulcerative from Crohn's colitis.

	Ulcerative colitis	Crohn's colitis
Clinical		
Bloody diarrhoea	90–100%	50%
Abdominal mass	Very rare	Common
Perianal disease	Very uncommon	30–50%
Sigmoidoscopy		
Rectal sparing	Never	50%
Histology		
Distribution	Mucosal	Transmural
Cellular infiltrate	Polymorphs	Lymphocytes
Crypts	Distorted	Normal
Goblet cell depletion	Common when active	Absent
Granuloma	Absent	Diagnostic
Radiology		
Distribution	Continuous	Discontinuous
Symmetry	Symmetrical	Asymmetrical
Mucosa	Shallow ulcers	Deep ulcers
Strictures	Very rare	Common
Fistulae	Never	Common

Infective colitis

- Identification of *Escherichia coli* 0157, *Campylobacter* spp., *Clostridium difficile*, *Salmonella* spp., *Shigella* spp. or *Entamoeba histolytica* in the stool do not exclude ulcerative colitis
- Infective colitis causes macroscopic and microscopic inflammation, but unlike ulcerative colitis, does not usually distort microscopic glandular architecture
- Repeat sigmoidoscopy and biopsy after the acute episode has settled is always advisable if doubt exists. The patient can be reassured if the second biopsy is normal, but follow-up is necessary if inflammation persists
- Colitis (caused by CMV, herpes simplex or other opportunistic pathogens) can be a feature of AIDS (p. 396)

Crohn's colitis

A definitive diagnosis is not initially possible in 10–15% (see indeterminate colitis, p. 319) and some turn out on long-term follow-up to have Crohn's colitis. This is one reason for repeat rectal biopsies (p. 444).

In distinguishing ulcerative from Crohn's colitis, the clinical *and* endoscopic *and* histological *and* radiological features should all be considered, rather than depending on a single investigation such as rectal biopsy or barium enema for diagnosis.

Other possibilities

• Ischaemic colitis—clinical features can be identical. Rectal sparing, 'thumb-printing' on plain abdominal X-ray and a flexible sigmoidoscopy establish the diagnosis (Fig. 9.6, p. 354)

• Radiation colitis—history of pelvic or abdominal node irradiation, with mucosal telangiectasia

• Microscopic colitis—no bleeding and macroscopically normal mucosa (p. 320)

• Pseudomembranous colitis (p. 321)

• Diverticular-associated colitis, polyps and colorectal carcinoma are readily distinguished as the cause of bloody diarrhoea, by colonoscopy

• Irritable bowel syndrome may coexist with ulcerative colitis (p. 374)

Management

The principles of management are:
• Prompt treatment of acute attacks
• Maintenance therapy to reduce the relapse rate
• Selection of patients for colectomy
• Detection of colorectal carcinoma
• Patient education is essential to ensure early presentation during relapse

Treatment of an acute attack involving any site other than proctitis depends on the severity (Table 8.13, below). Proctitis is a special case because proximal progression is uncommon (< 10%). The term 'fulminant attack' is best avoided, because treatment is no different from that for a severe attack.

Table 8.13 Treatment of active ulcerative colitis after topical steroid or 5-ASA enema for up to 2 weeks.

Drug	Mild	Moderate	Severe
Prednisolone	20 mg/day 1 month 15 mg/day 1 week 10 mg/day 1 week 5 mg/day 1 week	40 mg/day 1 week 30 mg/day 1 week then as for mild attacks	Admit for i.v. steroids; telephone gastroenterologist
Enemas	Colifoam/Asafoam once or twice daily whilst bleeding		
Salicylates	Continue unchanged		

Mild attacks

General
- Prompt and decisive treatment brings rapid relief to the patient and reduces the risk of complications, so oral steroids are recommended, although they may initially appear unnecessary for mild symptoms
- Whilst it is reasonable to give a trial of local treatment (steroid or 5-aminosalicylic foam enemas) alone in the very early stages (bleeding for < 2 weeks), far too many patients are expected to suffer continuing symptoms from inadequate treatment with oral salicylates and liquid enemas for prolonged periods. Such treatment may be better than placebo, but is not nearly as effective as the combination of oral and topical steroids
- The role of newer salicylates such as balsalazide remains to be determined. Whilst more effective than mesalazine in one of five trials, some aspects of the trials (inclusion of patients with severe colitis, or concomitant treatment with oral steroids) remain unusual

Recommended treatment
- 2 week trial of topical treatment (above)
- Oral prednisolone 20 mg daily for 1 month, then reduce by 5 mg/week
- Steroid retention enemas twice daily (foam enemas are usually better tolerated and retained than liquid enemas)
- Continue maintenance therapy unchanged (sulphasalazine 1 g twice daily, mesalazine or olsalazine for intolerance)
- Failure to improve after 2 weeks is an indication for treatment as a moderate attack. Deterioration is an indication for admission

Moderate attacks
- Prednisolone 40 mg daily for 1 week, then 30 mg/day for 1 week, then 20 mg/day for 1 month, before decreasing by 5 mg/day
- Steroid enemas morning and night
- Sulphasalazine 1 g twice daily (mesalazine or olsalazine for intolerance). A higher dose (up to 4 g/day) is slightly more effective, but cannot usually be tolerated
- Admission is not essential unless symptoms fail to improve within 2 weeks, although for some patients (especially the elderly), bed rest and enemas in hospital are more comfortable

Severe attacks
- Immediate admission is necessary when clinical features of a severe attack are present (Table 8.8, p. 301). Surgical colleagues should be informed.

A severe attack may occur without colonic dilatation ('toxic dilatation') although this may subsequently develop

- A plain abdominal X-ray and blood tests are taken on the way to the ward. Daily abdominal X-rays are appropriate until fever, abdominal tenderness and tachycardia resolve, to detect mucosal islands, dilatation (Fig. 1.6, p. 48) or perforation

- Intravenous hydrocortisone 100 mg four times daily is given for 5 days

- Rectal steroids should also be given twice daily. Hydrocortisone 100 mg in 100 mL 0.9% saline, dripped into the rectum through a soft catheter via an intravenous giving set, is often more comfortable for the patient than commercial enemas

- Stool frequency and appearance should be carefully documented by nursing staff, as well as pulse and temperature every 6 h, because these provide the objective measurements for clinical decisions

- Sips of fluid only by mouth; although the benefit of withdrawing food has not been proven, patients are usually anorexic and the response to reintroduction may help decide whether colectomy is indicated in difficult cases (p. 311). Parenteral nutrition is needed for malnourished patients or those who come to colectomy. Peripheral intravenous feeds (p. 311) are a useful temporary measure

- Intravenous fluids are needed to correct dehydration and maintain serum K at 4.0–4.5 mmol/L

- Blood transfusion is advisable if Hb < 10 g/dL. Serum should be grouped and saved for possible surgery

- Daily (or twice daily in very sick patients) re-examination is essential, looking for a rise in pulse or temperature, increasing abdominal girth or tenderness

- After 3 days treatment the simple prognostic factors (stool frequency and C-reactive protein) should be assessed (p. 311)

- Daily full blood count, C-reactive protein and electrolytes should be checked until it is clear that the patient is responding to treatment

- Failure to respond after 5 days, or deterioration at any stage, is an indication for colectomy. Delay increases the mortality

- 50% are in remission after 5 days, and 25% deteriorate and have a colectomy. Another group (25%) improve but continue to need careful observation. Relapse on reintroducing food and changing to oral steroids usually means that colectomy is required

- For those who improve, oral prednisolone 40 mg/day can be started after 5 days and decreased after 1 week to 30 mg/day for a week, then to 20 mg/day for a month. It can then be decreased by 5 mg/week unless relapse occurs (p. 297)

- Sulphasalazine is poorly tolerated in severely ill patients and should be stopped. It can be reintroduced with oral steroids
- Antibiotics, including metronidazole or ciprofloxacin, offer no benefit
- Cyclosporin (4 mg/kg/day intravenously, then 5 mg/kg/day orally) may be effective in avoiding surgery when severe colitis fails to respond to intravenous steroids. Experience in the UK is not as favourable as reported from the USA and there is a risk of morbidity (and mortality) from further delaying surgery, opportunistic infections, seizures, or renal impairment. It should only be used in specialist centres and its main role is in treatment of a severe first attack or in refractory distal disease whilst the patient comes to terms with the prospect of surgery. Most patients relapse again after cyclosporin is withdrawn

Indications for emergency surgery
- Toxic dilatation (p. 46)
- Perforation
- Massive haemorrhage
- Failure of a severe attack to respond to intravenous steroids within 5 days. The decision and timing can be difficult, and should be made jointly by a senior physician and surgeon. Whilst some prefer to continue steroids for longer periods, the operative morbidity (and mortality) increases if surgery is inappropriately delayed
- A prospective study has provided a simple clinical guide to the need for surgery in severe colitis without colonic dilatation: after 3 days' intravenous treatment if the stool frequency is > 8/day, or if the frequency is 3–8/day together with a C-reactive protein > 45 mg/L, then there is an 85% chance that colectomy will be needed on that admission
- Mucosal islands on a plain abdominal X-ray, a sustained fever > 38°C and stool frequency > 8/day after 24 h treatment, predict a high probability that colectomy will be needed
- Patients with a severe attack who make an incomplete response to intravenous steroids after 5 days, but then deteriorate when food is reintroduced usually need surgery. In a prospective study, 40% incomplete responders (stool frequency > 3/day, or visible blood in the stools 1 week after starting intensive treatment) came to colectomy within a few months of admission and 60% continued to need immunosuppressive therapy

Proctitis
- Local steroids and oral salicylates are often sufficient, but proctitis can be very refractory, even to oral steroids

- Steroid retention enemas morning and night, then only at night when bleeding stops until 1 week after bowel frequency returns to normal
- Mesalazine enemas are more effective than steroid enemas, but also more expensive and should be reserved for those who do not respond to steroid enemas alone
- Patients usually find foam enemas or suppositories easier to retain than fluid enemas. It is a matter for personal choice, although suppositories may be useful for very localized disease
- Sulphasalazine 1 g twice daily (mesalazine or olsalazine for intolerance)
- Failure to control symptoms within 2 weeks is an indication for prednisolone 20 mg daily, reducing by 5 mg/week after a month.
- Refractory proctitis is discussed on p. 315

Maintenance treatment

- All 5-ASA compounds (sulphasalazine, mesalazine, olsalazine) reduce the relapse rate by about fourfold, from 80 to 20% at 1 year
- Maintenance treatment should be continued for life, because the benefit is sustained
- Sulphasalazine 1 g twice daily is usually the drug of first choice, because it is cheap (25% of the cost of other salicylates) and well established. Higher doses (up to 4 g/day) are more effective and may be tried if relapse occurs whilst taking a lower dose, but are poorly tolerated. Enteric-coated sulphasalazine may help
- Nausea or abdominal discomfort occur in 10–20% taking sulphasalazine 2 g/day, but more specific side-effects (rash, haemolysis) are rare. Reversible oligospermia is frequent, so potential fathers should be started on olsalazine or mesalazine
- Mesalazine (400–500 mg three times daily) or olsalazine (500 mg twice daily), are indicated for sulphasalazine intolerance
- Higher doses of olsalazine (2 g/day) are more effective at maintaining remission in proctitis for 1 year after a relapse. Diarrhoea can be provoked by olsalazine, but is ameliorated by taking tablets with food
- Trials have shown that azo compounds such as olsalazine 1 g/day are more effective than mesalazine (Asacol) 1.2 g/day in patients with distal disease
- Salicylates have a local action on colonic epithelium. Azo-bonded (sulphasalazine, olsalazine, balsalazide) and slow-release (Pentasa) compounds lead to lower serum concentrations of mesalazine, which is potentially nephrotoxic, than pH-dependent release compounds (Asacol, Salofalk)
- Steroids have no effect on relapse rate and should be stopped once remission occurs

• Patients often benefit from contact with the NACC, even if symptoms are mild (Appendix 1, p. 477). A booklet on ulcerative colitis is also available from the British Digestive Foundation amongst others (Appendix 1, p. 472)

Detection of colonic carcinoma

Risk
• The risk of cancer increases with the extent and duration of disease. It may be unrelated to age of onset, although there is anecdotal evidence that it is more common when disease starts in childhood, who often have a pancolitis
• It is more prevalent in patients whose symptoms run a chronic continuous course and those lost to specialist follow-up
• An active medical and surgical approach to treatment as outlined above also found no increase in the risk of colorectal cancer among 1161 patients with ulcerative colitis treated in Copenhagen

Surveillance
• Whether surveillance colonoscopy is cost-effective or even effective at all is hotly debated. Once symptomatic and interval cancers that present between planned colonoscopies are excluded, a huge number of colonoscopies have to be performed to detect the occasional case of dysplasia or early cancer. Colonoscopy also carries a small but definable mortality and probably has to be performed annually with serial biopsies every 10 cm to be effective. However, many patients with pancolitis like the reassurance that surveillance colonoscopy affords
• Until more data are available the decision about surveillance is probably best discussed with individual patients after discussing the pros and cons and current evaluation of risk, taking into account the patient's own preference
• Colitis distal to the splenic flexure does not justify surveillance
• There is some evidence that maintenance sulphasalazine decreases the risk of cancer in ulcerative colitis
• If a surveillance programme is part of the unit's policy, a register and recall system for patients with total colitis is essential
• Some advise that all patients with symptoms of ulcerative colitis for 8–10 years should have a colonoscopy to reassess extent of disease and then to follow up those with pancolitis in a surveillance programme (Fig. 8.4, p. 306). The best surveillance programme has not been established
• The alternative is promptly to investigate by colonoscopy any new or persistent symptoms in patients with a pancolitis

Indications for surgery

Colectomy is the only cure for ulcerative colitis, although it does not affect some of the extraintestinal manifestations (Table 8.9, p. 302). Colectomy with a temporary ileostomy and later ileoanal pouch construction is now the operation of choice, but proctocolectomy and permanent ileostomy retains a definite place.

Indications for elective surgery

Disease is usually extensive, but colectomy is occasionally needed for distal colitis. The patient should talk to an ileostomist of the same gender and similar age before surgery.

- Continuous symptoms (often with general ill health and anaemia) despite treatment
- Frequent relapses unresponsive to medical treatment that materially affect the patient's life
- High-grade dysplasia, or frank malignancy

Indications for emergency surgery (p. 311)

Type of operation

- Colectomy and later formation of an ileoanal pouch ('restorative proctocolectomy', J, W or S pouches) is popular because there is no permanent ileostomy. Good results (continence and five or fewer bowel actions/day) are obtained in 80–90% in experienced hands, but some need revision to a permanent ileostomy
- Proctocolectomy with a permanent ileostomy remains the standard procedure for older patients or those with poor continence during acute attacks. Mortality is < 2%, but ileostomy dysfunction occurs in about 15% (Table 8.14, p. 316)
- For emergency surgery in patients who may subsequently have an ileoanal pouch, then sub-total colectomy is appropriate, leaving the rectal remnant in place. Otherwise a one-stage proctocolectomy is safer than sub-total colectomy and ileostomy for emergencies, in experienced hands
- Segmental resection or ileorectal anastomosis cannot be justified in ulcerative colitis, as disease starts distally or will continue in the colonic remnant

Complications

Toxic dilatation

Clinical features of severe disease with mucosal islands and a colonic diameter of > 6.0 cm on plain X-ray are diagnostic (Fig. 1.6, p. 48).

Perforation
- Diagnosed by free gas on plain X-ray, usually complicating toxic dilatation when surgery has been delayed too long, or colonoscopy during a severe attack
- Common signs (pain and peritonism) are often few and masked by steroids
- Colectomy after fluid, blood and electrolyte replacement is vital

Massive haemorrhage
- Diagnosis is not difficult except at presentation, when the mucosal pattern may be obscured by blood
- Coagulation should be checked and corrected with FFP if the INR is > 1.5 (prothrombin time > 22 s)
- As the underlying disease is likely to recur, colectomy is usually indicated if bleeding has not stopped after transfusing 4 units

Carcinoma
See p. 312.

Management problems

Refractory distal colitis or proctitis
- Distal colitis is resistant to treatment in about 25%, but surgery is better avoided for limited disease. The therapeutic options below also apply to patients who relapse rapidly after a course of steroids, or who appear to be dependent on steroids
- Take a plain X-ray and relieve proximal constipation if visible by sodium picosulphate and magnesium citrate (Picolax) 1 sachet orally, or lactulose 30–60 mL/day
- Start mesalazine enemas at night, in addition to steroid enemas in the morning. Foam enemas are best tolerated, but some patients still find them difficult to retain
- Restart prednisolone 40 mg/day, as for a moderate attack (Table 8.13, p. 308), together with azathioprine 2–2.5 mg/kg/day. A full blood count should be performed every 1–2 months, or if unwell, to detect the unusual complications of agranulocytosis or aplasia. Azathioprine should be continued if tolerated after steroids are withdrawn for up to 5 years
- Avoiding milk relieves diarrhoea in a minority, but does not affect disease activity
- Anecdotal treatment options with lignocaine 2% gel (10–30 mL twice daily), arsenic suppositories (Acetarsol 250 mg twice daily), bismuth or

butyrate enemas have either not been subjected to or not substantiated by controlled trials
- Admission for intensive treatment before considering colectomy may be needed if there is still no response, but patients are best referred to a specialist centre

Pregnancy
- Pregnancy has no consistent effect on colitis
- Maintenance therapy should almost always be continued, because long experience with salicylates has not revealed any adverse effect on the baby and the risk of relapse is more serious than that of treatment
- Relapse during pregnancy is treated in the standard way

Chronic continuous symptoms
Usually an indication for colectomy if the disease is extensive.

Stomas and pouches (Table 8.14)

Ileostomists and patients with pouches produce 500 mL effluent/day, which is largely fluid and high in sodium. Urine volume is decreased to compensate. Ileal adaptation develops over 12 months and volume decreases. Nutrient absorption is normal except when there is coexistent small intestinal disease or terminal ileal resection.

Ileostomy dysfunction
- Ileostomy dysfunction means an overactive ileostomy with an increase in effluent
- Loss of fluid and electrolytes causes lassitude, postural hypotension and dehydration

Table 8.14 Complications of ileostomies.

Early	Late
Ischaemia	Dysfunction (fluid loss > 1000 mL/day)
Wound infection	Small bowel obstruction
Small bowel obstruction	Parastomal herniation
Delayed perineal healing	Stenosis
	Retraction
	Local dermatitis
	Psychosexual/social
	Gall stones
	Renal calculi

- Partial obstruction (parastomal hernia, adhesions), prestomal ileitis, recurrent disease (in Crohn's), or infection may be the cause, but often no reason is apparent
- Culture of effluent, plain abdominal X-ray and serum electrolytes are necessary. Small bowel radiology, if there is abdominal pain, and urinary and ileal effluent electrolytes guide replacement in severe cases
- Admission and intravenous fluids are indicated if there is clinical evidence of dehydration or postural hypotension
- Loperamide, up to 12 mg/day, decreases moderately increased fluid loss
- Oral electrolyte solutions (p. 243) are indicated for chronic losses. The amount depends on electrolyte loss, but is often 2000–3000 mL/day

Partial ('subacute') small bowel obstruction

- Adhesions, twisted ileal loops, stenosis, recurrent Crohn's disease or parastomal herniation may be the cause
- Examination with a fibreoptic sigmoidoscope is advisable, but is often limited even in normal ileostomies
- Most settle spontaneously with intravenous fluids, nasogastric suction if there is vomiting and intramuscular pethidine 50–100 mg for pain

Stenosis or retraction

- Digital examination of the ileostomy spout will detect stenosis and is advisable at outpatient visits during the first 6 months and if obstruction or bleeding occurs
- Retraction of the spout causes maceration of the skin and difficulties with bag adhesion. Surgical revision is usually necessary

Practical problems

- A specialist nurse (stomatherapist) is invaluable before elective procedures to help plan the site or relieve anxiety and to assist with management after a stoma has been formed
- A badly sited stoma is rapidly recognized by the patient. Revision may be necessary if the stoma substantially interferes with daily activities (including sitting, if at an abdominal crease)
- Odour may be reduced by odour-proof bags or dietary changes (eggs, onions and beans are common culprits)
- Local dermatitis may be due to an allergy to the adhesive, or leaking effluent. Changing the type of appliance and an effective seal are the solutions
- Psychosocial difficulties may be helped through patient support groups

(the Ileostomy Association, NACC, Appendix 1, p. 471), although patients without problems benefit as well

Ileoanal pouches

Indications
• After proctocolectomy for ulcerative colitis or familial adenomatous polyposis and occasionally for other patients with cancer
• Crohn's disease is usually considered an absolute contraindication, but indeterminate colitis is acceptable
• Relative contraindications include faecal incontinence during acute attacks, age > 65 years, rectal cancer, during emergency colectomy for severe ulcerative colitis (delay procedure until recovery)

Complications
• All the problems of ileostomists may occur with ileoanal pouches.
• Pouchitis occurs in 10–20%, causing diarrhoea (occasionally bloody), urgency and an inflamed pouch mucosa. It probably does not occur in pouches for familial adenomatous polyposis. Infection must be excluded and the diagnosis confirmed by pouchoscopy (rigid sigmoidoscope) *and* biopsy. Metronidazole 400 mg three times daily, ciprofloxacin 500 mg twice daily, Colifoam enemas twice daily, or catheter emptying of the pouch should be tried, in that order. Attacks are often isolated
• Other causes of pouch dysfunction include too small a pouch, incomplete emptying, anastomotic stenosis, cuffitis, or parapouch sepsis. A pouchogram (isotope or contrast imaging) to assess design and function and MRI can aid diagnosis
• Local patient groups (such as the Kangaroo Club, or Plymouth Possums) provide help and support

Prognosis

• The pattern of relapse and remission 1 year after diagnosis tends to continue for any individual. 90% have intermittent activity and 50% are in remission at any one time. 20% will relapse every year and 10% have continuous symptoms
• Prolonged remission on maintenance therapy occurs, with 50–60% remaining in remission for more than 2 years, but < 5% are symptom free for 15 years
• Proximal extension in proctitis is rare (< 10%), but occurs in 15–35% with distal or left-sided disease

• The colectomy rate varies with the local approach to refractory disease. Following the approach above, the cumulative colectomy rate in 1161 patients was 24% at 10 years and 32% 25 years after diagnosis
• Distribution of disease affects the likelihood of colectomy. In the study of 1161 patients, 9% with distal, 19% with substantial and 35% with total colitis had a colectomy within 5 years of diagnosis. Thereafter the colectomy rate was 1% per year, whatever the extent
• There appears to be a substantial difference in mortality during a severe attack between those managed in specialist centres (< 1%, including operative mortality) and those managed elsewhere (5%)
• Mortality is otherwise similar to that of the general population
• Up to 12–15% with pancolitis for 20 years develop colonic carcinoma, but some population-based studies have not shown any increased risk (p. 312). The risk of carcinoma in colitis distal to the splenic flexure is no higher than in the general population

Other types of colitis

General information

If a definitive diagnosis of the type of colitis cannot be made after clinical, endoscopic, histological and radiological examination, this should be stated in the notes. This is an indication for regular follow-up, repeated sigmoidoscopy and biopsy, until a diagnosis is established.

Differentiation between postinfective, ulcerative and diffuse Crohn's colitis is the usual problem (Table 8.12, p. 307). Small bowel radiology is essential if doubt about the diagnosis persists, because typical lesions of Crohn's disease may be asymptomatic.

Indeterminate colitis

Features
• Features of both ulcerative colitis and Crohn's colitis (such as non-bloody diarrhoea with diffuse inflammation on colonoscopy, or bloody diarrhoea with relative rectal sparing and histology suggesting ulcerative colitis, or clinical and endoscopic features of ulcerative colitis, but histology showing sub-mucosal inflammation)
• Distinction between ulcerative colitis and Crohn's colitis is not possible in 10–15%
• Incidence may be two per 100 000 and prevalence 27 per 100 000 (giving

a total prevalence of inflammatory bowel disease of up to 450 per 100 000 in one study in primary care, or just less than one in 200 population)

Treatment
- As for ulcerative colitis
- Careful histological examination of colectomy specimens by an experienced gastrointestinal pathologist prior to ileoanal pouch surgery is necessary in cases of diagnostic doubt. Patients with indeterminate colitis appear to do as well with ileoanal pouch surgery as those with ulcerative colitis, although there is some evidence that a substantial proportion subsequently turn out to have Crohn's colitis

Microscopic colitis

Features
- Watery diarrhoea
- Often female, aged > 60 years, but can occur in much younger patients
- Macroscopically normal mucosa on sigmoidoscopy and colonoscopy
- Multiple biopsies show microscopic inflammation and lymphocytic infiltration (the term 'lymphocytic colitis' is also used)
- Other causes of diarrhoea (Table 7.1, p. 237), including coeliac disease, should be excluded

Treatment
- No treatment has been definitely established, but it is probably best to start with salicylates (e.g. sulphasalazine 2 g/day). About half respond
- Prednisolone 20 mg daily until diarrhoea stops, then decreased slowly (5 mg/month) if there is no response to sulphasalazine
- Metronidazole 400 mg three times daily, or cholestryamine help a proportion, but these are empirical
- Long-term results remain unknown

Collagenous colitis

Features
- A rare disorder, causing persistent watery diarrhoea
- Characterized by a sub-epithelial band of collagen on colonic biopsies
- Possibly associated with microscopic colitis, but unrelated to connective tissue diseases

Treatment

Treatment with steroids or salicylates is empirical.

Diversion colitis

Inflammation in the defunctioned loop of a colostomy, causing a mucous discharge, usually responds to topical steroid enemas. Thought to be due to epithelial short chain fatty acid deficiency and sodium butyrate enemas may be effective, although these are not commercially available.

Pseudomembranous colitis

Features

- Caused by *Clostridium difficile*, usually after prolonged or multiple antibiotics, especially ampicillin, clindamycin or lincomycin
- *Cl. difficile* causes about 4% of acute gastroenteritis in adults and cases in hospitals are increasing exponentially
- Pseudomembranous colitis only represents the severe end of the spectrum
- Diagnosed by sigmoidoscopy (punctate, adherent yellow–white plaques on an inflamed rectal mucosa) and detecting *Cl. difficile* toxin in stool. Histology may be diagnostic if a plaque ('summit lesion') is included in the biopsy, but may be difficult to distinguish from ulcerative colitis or ischaemic colitis (Table 9.6, p. 335). Either condition may coexist

Treatment

- Oral metronidazole 400 mg three times daily for 1 week in the first instance
- Relapse may occur (up to 30%) and should be treated with vancomycin 125–250 mg four times daily for a week or longer (sometimes several weeks, decreasing the dose gradually)
- Both antibiotics and steroids (p. 309) are advisable if doubt exists about the diagnosis of pseudomembranous or acute ulcerative colitis, followed by colonoscopy once symptoms resolve
- Recurrent infection despite metronidazole and vancomycin is rare and patients are best referred to a specialist centre

Ischaemic colitis

See p. 352.

9 Large Intestine

Constipation

Constipation means the passage of hard faeces infrequently, often with straining and discomfort. Patient reporting of constipation depends on early training, preoccupation with the bowel and expectations (p. 327). Some make exacting demands. Most people have five or more bowel evacuations each week, but frequency is of less concern than inability to defaecate at will, or the effort in evacuating hard stools. Only the rectum is normally evacuated during defaecation. It is harder for normal people to evacuate a 2 cm solid sphere than a 50 mL compressible balloon—consistent with the experience of constipated patients passing 'rabbit-droppings'.

Causes

- Diet or faulty bowel habit cause the vast majority, but less common, treatable causes should not be overlooked (Table 9.1)
- Dietary causes are common in the elderly or depressed, although tricyclic antidepressants and pseudo-obstruction are additional causes in these groups
- Faecal impaction in the elderly or mentally impaired may cause spurious diarrhoea, urinary retention or exacerbate neurological irritability
- Chronic stimulant laxative use causes cathartic megacolon, hypokalaemia or melanosis coli
- Idiopathic slow transit constipation is discussed on p. 329
- Neurological disorders may cause constipation due to inactivity or failure

Table 9.1 Causes of constipation.

Common	Uncommon	Rare
Diet	Anorectal disease	Metabolic/endocrine
inadequate fibre	fissure	hypothyroidism
Motility disorders	stricture	hypercalcaemia
irritable bowel	mucosal prolapse	hypokalaemia
Age	Drugs	porphyria
Pregnancy	opiates	lead poisoning
Immobility	aluminium antacids	hypopituitarism
	anticholinergics	Idiopathic slow transit
	iron	Neurological disorders
	cathartic colon	cerebral disease
	Intestinal obstruction	spinal cord lesions
	carcinoma	aganglionosis
	pseudo-obstruction	autonomic neuropathy
	Anorexia nervosa	myopathy

of rectal sensation and rectal reflexes. Constipation is a key feature of spinal cord lesions (such as transection, transverse myelitis or cauda equina tumours). Drugs often contribute to constipation in Parkinson's or cerebrovascular disease

• Aganglionosis (due to Hirschprung's or Chagas' disease) very rarely presents in adults, with constipation and megacolon

Investigation

General
• The history must determine the frequency, nature and consistency of stool, so as to establish whether the patient really is constipated. Also ask about duration, diet and drugs
• Rectal examination is essential
• Investigation of the colon is only indicated if there has been a recent change in bowel habit (< 6 months), especially if age > 40 years, or if there are associated features (rectal bleeding, weight loss)

Initial investigations
• Blood tests—a full blood count, electrolytes, calcium and thyroid function tests will identify most organic and treatable causes
• Proctosigmoidoscopy is always indicated if dietary measures fail, in patients > 40 years, or if there are additional symptoms (rectal bleeding, weight loss). Anorectal disorders, or melanosis due to chronic use of anthraquinone laxatives (such as senna) may be detected
• Barium enema is only indicated to exclude an organic lesion, if the change in bowel habit is recent in a patient age > 40 years

Special investigations
• Testing perineal sensation with an orange stick is essential in severe constipation when considering spinal cord pathology. Further careful clinical examination by asking the patient to strain may reveal perineal descent (p. 331) or mucosal prolapse
• MRI is the most sensitive test to exclude a cauda equina lesion
• Transit studies are useful to document slow intestinal transit when the bowel frequency is less than once a week. Fybogel three sachets/day is given for 2 weeks (to eliminate dietary causes of slow transit), then 20 oral radio-opaque markers are taken at once. Plain abdominal X-rays at 2 and 5 days normally show > 75% excretion of markers by day 5 (Fig. 9.1, p. 330)
• Anorectal manometry (p. 467) is rarely indicated in adults, unless there is faecal incontinence, a defaecation disorder (p. 331) is suspected, or if there

is megacolon or megarectum (to identify aganglionosis, when the rectosphincteric reflex is absent)
• Defaecography at a specialist centre may demonstrate anterior mucosal prolapse or a rectocoele

Management

Constipation due to colonic, anorectal or systemic disease must be identified and treated appropriately. The patient's idea of a normal bowel habit should be discussed. A reasonable aim is a soft motion every 1–2 days. The call to stool should not be ignored.

Diet
• Increased fibre intake is the key, but is not always well tolerated. There is no universal dose, but it must be accompanied by adequate fluids (about 1500 mL/day), which the elderly are sometimes reluctant to increase
• 100% wholemeal bread, leguminous vegetable (peas, beans and lentils) and fruit are simple dietary changes (p. 416)
• A tablespoon of bran (added to breakfast cereal, yoghurt or soup) may be necessary, but it should be of the coarse-milled variety
• Flatulence or abdominal distension may be increased on a high-fibre diet, and the elderly may develop faecal soiling if the softer stool cannot be controlled. A gradual increase in fibre intake is wise
• Constipation due to colonic strictures or spinal cord lesions may be exacerbated by increased dietary fibre

Laxatives
• Laxatives are indicated to alleviate painful defaecation, when straining will exacerbate a condition (such as a hernia), for drug-induced constipation, before surgery or colonic examination. There are four groups of laxatives and 60 preparations, but bran and an osmotic laxative, with only an occasional stimulant, work for most. The diagnosis should be reassessed if two sorts of laxative are ineffective. The ultimate sanction for simple constipation is magnesium sulphate. Any laxative is dangerous in obstruction.

Bulk-forming laxatives
• For dietary constipation and painful anorectal conditions, with extra fluid
• Isphagula husk (Fybogel), or sterculia (Normacol) are more palatable than coarse bran (1–2 tbs/day), but more expensive

Osmotic laxatives

• Indicated when bulk-forming laxatives are ineffective, for proximal constipation in ulcerative colitis or hepatic encephalopathy

• The dose of lactulose (30–100 mL/day) is easier to regulate according to effect, but more expensive, than magnesium sulphate (10–20 mL of crystals in water 2 hourly, until effective)

• Sodium picosulphate with magnesium citrate (Picolax 1–2 sachets) works for intractable constipation (p. 329), but has some stimulant action. Smaller doses (Laxoberal 5–20 mL daily, available over the counter in the UK) can be given regularly to prevent recurrence

• Polyethylene glycol (PEG-3350, Movicol) 1 or more sachets daily helps chronic constipation; it has no role in hepatic encephalopathy. It is also effective for faecal impaction (p. 329)

Stimulant laxatives

• For opiate-induced constipation, bowel clearance, neurological disorders or temporary use in stubborn constipation

• Colic may be exacerbated and long-term use should be avoided (p. 325)

• Bisacodyl suppositories (1–2) act within an hour, senna tablets (2–4 at night) act the following morning

• Codanthrusate (1–3 capsules, or 5–15 mL at night) should be given to patients on long-term morphine to prevent constipation

Faecal softeners

• Arachis oil enema, or glycerine suppositories are useful and a disposable enema (such as Relaxit) is good for stubborn cases

• Liquid paraffin can cause granulomas or lipoid pneumonia, and is not recommended

General advice on constipation

Re-education is an important part of improving bowel habit:

• Do not ignore the call to stool
• Develop a regular time for defaecation each day
• Avoid excessive straining—this makes defaecation disorders worse
• Avoid prolonged sitting
• Aim for a soft, easily passed motion every day or two

Intractable constipation

• Many patients with chronic constipation have tried 'all the laxatives'
• First make a record of the dose and type of all that have been tried

- Then work from first principles: retake the history, repeat a careful clinical examination including proctosigmoidoscopy, check that the calcium, thyroid function and other appropriate tests have been performed, before discussing a constipation strategy with the patient
- The best strategy is usually to clear the bowels out with Picolax, followed by a regular osmotic laxative in effective (often large) doses to prevent 'silting up' again. Polyethylene glycol (Movicol 1–3 sachets daily) is an alternative. An appropriate diet with plenty of fluid is important, but excessive fibre can be counterproductive
- Avoid using two laxatives with the same mode of action and increase the dose of any laxative to a maximum, before changing the type

Faecal impaction and soiling

Faecal impaction is distressing for the patient and may cause stercoral ulceration. Patients usually have neurological disease, or are elderly with multisystem disease. A history of long-standing constipation is followed by anismus, spurious diarrhoea or general irritability in the neurologically subtunded. Diagnosis is made by rectal examination revealing a hard mass of stool.

- Polyethylene glycol (Movicol, 8 sachets in 1 L drunk over 6 h) is frequently effective and well tolerated
- Regular osmotic laxatives (p. 328) or stimulant laxatives in neurological constipation are necessary to prevent recurrence
- In faecal soiling, regular enemas (Micralax or Relaxit, three times weekly) will keep the rectum empty and prevent soiling
- Faecal soiling in younger patients is often a feature of psychological distress, which should be explored. It may be a feature of sexual abuse. Biofeedback to relearn early recognition signals of the call to stool may help, along with appropriate psychological support

Slow transit constipation

- Young women (exceptionally men), occasionally present with gross constipation (bowel frequency once or twice a fortnight), abdominal discomfort and painful defaecation, but are otherwise in good health. No cause can be found and the diagnosis is confirmed by transit studies (Fig. 9.1). Barium enema is usually unnecessary, but rarely shows faecal loading in a dilated colon—idiopathic megacolon (p. 331)
- The diagnosis is important and should be distinguished from constipation-predominant irritable bowel syndrome, because life-long use

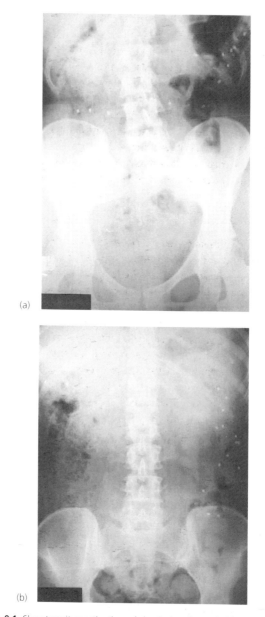

(a)

(b)

Fig. 9.1 Slow transit constipation: abdominal radiograph (a) 3 and (b) 5 days after ingesting 20 radio-opaque markers, all of which remain visible, indicating prolonged transit. From Travis S.T. *Shared Care Gastroenterology*, by permission of Isis Medical Media Ltd.

of osmotic laxatives is needed, often in large doses. This should be emphasized to the general practitioner

- The bowel should initially be cleared with Picolax (1–3 sachets), then osmotic laxatives in sufficient doses (lactulose 50–150 mL daily, Laxoberal 10–20 mL daily or Movicol 1–3 sachets daily). The patient should adjust the dose according to the stool consistency. Stimulant laxatives may be needed at times of crisis (no defaecation for > 7 days), but regular use should be avoided, because of the risk of cathartic colon in the long term. Bulking agents may make abdominal discomfort worse
- Cisapride or erythromycin (as a motilin agonist) are rarely beneficial. Colectomy and ileorectal anastomosis are the last resort for disabling symptoms

Megacolon

Megacolon or megarectum in adults is usually idiopathic. A long history of constipation is usual, although it may be intermittent and interspersed with episodes of faecal impaction with spurious diarrhoea. A barium enema is diagnostic. Aganglionosis must be excluded by anorectal manometry (p. 467). Full-thickness rectal biopsy and silver stain to show the myenteric plexus is only justified if manometry shows inhibition of sphincteric relaxation.

- Idiopathic megacolon is treated in the same way as slow transit constipation, but referral to a specialist centre is necessary for manometry and makes subsequent management easier. Laxatives must be continued for life, to avoid episodes of faecal impaction, and this should be made clear to the patient and the general practitioner

Defaecation disorders

Obstructed defaecation causes a sensation of incomplete evacuation (tenesmus). A local cause (tumour, rectal ulcer, mucosal prolapse) must be excluded by rectal examination, proctoscopy and sigmoidoscopy. The patient must strain during proctoscopy for mucosal prolapse to be seen. The descending perineum syndrome, with or without mucosal prolapse and ulceration, should be considered. Tenesmus is likely to be a feature of the irritable bowel syndrome (p. 367) if a cause is not visible on rectal examination and proctosigmoidoscopy.

Descending perineum syndrome

Women are most commonly affected, sometimes as a sequel to pudendal nerve damage during childbirth. Marked perineal descent during excessive straining at stool causes a sensation of incomplete evacuation and further straining. This results in rectal mucosal prolapse, ulceration and bleeding. Incontinence may develop. Diagnosis is made by careful inspection of the perineum during straining, which can be measured at a specialist centre; > 2 cm descent is abnormal.

Solitary rectal ulcer

This presents with rectal bleeding and a sensation of incomplete evacuation and must be distinguished from proctitis or Crohn's disease. Patients are often male. Constipation with excessive straining at stool is thought to cause mucosal prolapse with anterior rectal inflammation. Sigmoidoscopy shows a patch of erythema, a single, or sometimes several ulcers; biopsies are diagnostic and are essential to exclude Crohn's disease, carcinoma or other causes of rectal ulcers (p. 285). Histopathology shows the muscularis characteristically interdigitating into the mucosa, with some fibrosis. Solitary rectal ulcers are sometimes caused by insertion of a finger or foreign body, in a desperate attempt to initiate defaecation by severely constipated patients.

Management of defaecation disorders

Treatment of constipation, advice to avoid straining at stool and excluding serious disease are the principles of management. Local steroids may relieve bleeding from mucosal ulceration, but are otherwise unhelpful since the condition is not primarily inflammatory. Barium enema, follow-up and repeat biopsies are indicated if rectal biopsies are equivocal, to exclude Crohn's disease and other pathology. Pronounced rectal mucosal prolapse may be treated surgically, but this is best done by an experienced colorectal surgeon.

Should symptoms persist, referral to a specialist centre is advised, for anorectal studies (p. 467), pelvic nerve conduction studies and defaeco-graphy, before surgery in selected cases. Anal dilatation for constipation in inappropriate cases (such as descending perineum syndrome with a lax anal sphincter) can provoke faecal incontinence, which is a disaster.

9.2 Colonic polyps

Adenomatous polyps precede colorectal cancer, which can be prevented by the early recognition and treatment of polyps. Not all polyps are premalignant.

Classification

Polyps are mucosal projections into the lumen and may be sessile or pedunculated. There are four types, which cannot be reliably distinguished macroscopically, so polypectomy and histology are always indicated.

Metaplastic

- Commonest type (75% of those in the rectum of adults > 40 years, often multiple, usually sessile, shiny and < 5 mm in diameter)
- No malignant potential

Adenomas

- Also common (50% of colonic polyps in patients > 55 years)
- A third of older Western patients have one or two colonic adenomas, but only 2–3% develop colorectal cancer
- Malignant potential in an individual is related to size (> 10 mm), histology (villous > tubulovillous > tubular, or presence of dysplasia), and number of polyps (> 5)
- 25% are multiple
- Villous adenomas tend to recur locally after removal

Inflammatory

- Pseudopolyps after severe colitis of any cause
- May have a sessile or cylindrical appearance
- Not neoplastic

Hamartomatous

- Juvenile polyps are developmental malformations, often large, pedunculated and vascular, but usually solitary. Very rarely there are multiple (> 5) polyps—juvenile polyposis
- Peutz–Jeghers syndrome of buccal pigmentation and multiple small intestinal hamartomas, also affects the colon in over 50% (p. 269)
- No apparent malignant potential, but occasional foci of dysplasia in solitary polyps increase the risk of small or large bowel cancer in Peutz–Jeghers syndrome (about half of patients aged 50 years) and juvenile polyposis
- Cronkhite–Canada syndrome is a rare disorder affecting middle-aged adults, causing diffuse gastrointestinal polyposis (adenomas), malabsorption due to protein-losing enteropathy, nail dystrophy and hyperpigmentation. It is not inherited. Antibiotics may help diarrhoea due to bacterial overgrowth, but there is no specific treatment

Other

- Nodular lymphoid hyperplasia in the rectum or terminal ileum is a normal variant in young people and recognized histologically, although radiological features may resemble Crohn's disease or polyposis (p. 269)
- Pneumatosis coli (p. 337) can be mistaken for multiple polyps or Crohn's disease by the uninitiated

- Lipomas, leiomyomas or neurofibromas occasionally occur in the colon, but are of no significance

Clinical features

Most colonic polyps are asymptomatic and detected on barium enema or endoscopy for unrelated gastrointestinal symptoms. Some present with rectal bleeding at any age, but diarrhoea (sometimes with profuse mucus and hypokalaemia) is a rare presentation of a villous adenoma.

Management

- Polyps identified on sigmoidoscopy or a barium enema are an indication for total colonoscopy and polypectomy; small polyps other than those detected radiologically may be present
- Polyps recur in 30–40% of patients, so surveillance is appropriate
- The time interval from a small polyp to malignancy is measured in years and may be more than a decade. Explanation of the polyp–cancer sequence is important and should reassure patients, who might otherwise think that every examination can be expected to reveal a cancer
- Optimum timing for surveillance remains a matter for debate. The American Gastroenterological Association have produced guidelines for polyp surveillance (1997, Appendix 2, p. 484), but factors driving health care differ between USA and other countries. Figure 9.2 presents a reasonable guide
- All polyps must be examined histologically and the pathologist should say whether polypectomy has been complete
- A good way of permanently marking the site of suspicious or partially removed polyps, for follow-up or surgical identification, is by 'tattooing', with 1 mL intramucosal Indian ink
- Complications of polypectomy include immediate or delayed (up to 2 weeks) bleeding. Perforation is rare
- The main problem of colonoscopic surveillance is administrative. Endoscopy units should have a system for checking on defaults and general practitioners have an important role in ensuring patients do not 'slip through the net'. A related role of the general practitioner is to communicate any major change in the patient's medical condition that makes further colonoscopy inappropriate (such as major cardiorespiratory or cerebrovascular disease)

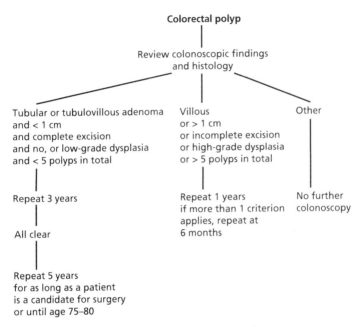

Fig. 9.2 Surveillance programme for patients with polyps.

Familial adenomatous polyposis

Multiple (> 100) colonic polyps invariably progress to colorectal cancer in this autosomal dominant condition, unless colectomy is performed. Sporadic cases occur. Polyps may occur in childhood, but the increased cancer risk starts in teenagers. Gastric cancer and small intestinal adenocarcinoma are also more common and Gardner's syndrome (colonic polyposis and osteomas) is a variant. Other rare associations are tumours of the central nervous system in adolescence (Turcot's syndrome), congenital hypertrophy of the retinal pigment epithelium (CHRPE), thyroid (papillary carcinoma), adrenal or large intra-abdominal desmoid tumours.

The incidence is about 1:10 000 live births. It is caused by one of several mutations in the APC (tumour suppressor) gene on the q21–22 region of chromosome 5.

Management

Early diagnosis is the key to management, usually achieved by meticulous screening of family members of an index case. Colorectal cancer in the relative of an index case is a treatment failure.

• Proctocolectomy should be performed once the diagnosis is made. The operation of choice is a total colectomy and ileoanal anastomosis, but some

patients will still opt for an ileorectal anastomosis (assuming the rectum is clear of polyps), or a proctocolectomy and permanent ileostomy
• The details of all patients should be sent to the FAP Registry (St Mark's Hospital, Northwick Park, Harrow, Middlesex)
• Ophthalmological examination to detect congenital hypertrophy of the retinal pigment epithelium (see above), causing multiple areas of pigmentation in the peripheral retina is appropriate, because this can aid screening of relatives if present
• Long-term follow-up is essential, not only to manage pouch function and perform sigmoidoscopy in patients with an ileorectal anastomosis but also to detect other complications. Chronic abdominal pain may be caused by desmoid tumours, diagnosed by CT scan. Ampullary carcinoma is more common and screening by biennial endoscopy or endoscopic ultrasound, if available, is advocated by specialist centres. Pouchitis (p. 318) is extremely rare in ileoanal pouches for familial adenomatous polyposis, unlike ulcerative colitis

Screening relatives
• All first-degree and probably all second-degree relatives should currently have screening for familial adenomatous polyposis
• Screening by fibreoptic sigmoidoscopy or colonoscopy is appropriate after age 15 years, but some advocate starting in adolescence (11–14 years)
• Flexible sigmoidoscopy every 2 years until polyps are detected (indicating the need for colectomy) or until age 40 is currently advisable
• Genetic markers are not currently used, because of the number of mutations and risk of false-negative results. However, prenatal diagnosis by using gene probes to detect deletions in chromosome 5 is possible. Genetic counselling of index cases and relatives is essential

Prognosis
Although colectomy prevents colorectal cancer, mortality is still more than twice the general population owing to the development of desmoid tumours, duodenal or ampullary carcinoma.

Hereditary non-polyposis colorectal cancer (Lynch syndrome)

Rare families have a high incidence of colorectal cancer without polyposis (although preceded by adenomas), especially at a young age (< 45 years) and in the proximal colon. The inheritance is dominant, due to a mutation in the DNA mismatch repair gene on the long arm of chromosome 2.

- Carcinoma of the caecum or ascending colon at a young age (< 45 years) should raise the suspicion of hereditary non-polyposis colorectal cancer
- Family members may be at risk from other primary tumours (breast, ovary, endometrium). Only a thorough family history identifies those at risk
- First-degree relatives should have colonoscopic screening every 5 years and annual pelvic ultrasound after age 25 years. Genetic counselling is essential and referral to a specialist centre may be advisable (Appendix 1, p. 476)
- Screening for colorectal cancer is also recommended if a first-degree relative (parent, sibling or child) has developed colorectal cancer aged < 45 years, or if two first-degree relatives have had colorectal carcinoma at any age (Table 9.2, p. 342)

Pneumatosis coli (pneumatosis cystoides intestinalis)

A rare condition with gas-filled sub-mucosal cysts that look like polyps at colonoscopy, but which collapse on needle aspiration. A plain X-ray or barium enema show multiple radiolucencies along the wall of the bowel, or throughout the abdomen if the small intestine is involved. It may be misdiagnosed as multiple polyps, Crohn's disease, lymphoma or carcinoma if the diagnosis is not recognized at colonoscopy or barium enema. Histology of colonic biopsies is diagnostic. Sub-mucosal spaces and associated giant cells are characteristic.

- There may be no symptoms, but diarrhoea with bleeding, mucus or abdominal pain are common. No cause can usually be found, although it may be associated with emphysema
- Treatment is only necessary for symptoms. 70% inspired oxygen through an oxygen mask and rebreathing apparatus for 5 days usually gives relief for long periods. The improvement in colonoscopic appearance is dramatic. Oxygen should be used with care if the patient has emphysema. Metronidazole has been advocated, but is rarely helpful. Hyperbaric therapy also has its advocates, but is very rarely necessary if atmospheric oxygen is properly administered. Persistent symptoms are often due to coexistent irritable bowel

9.3 Colorectal cancer

Adenocarcinoma of the colon is the commonest malignancy in Britain after lung cancer (lifetime incidence 2–3%, about 20 000 deaths per year in the UK). It is potentially curable and preventable.

Causes

The polyp–dysplasia–cancer sequence is now generally accepted. Adenocarcinomas almost always arise from pre-existing adenomatous polyps except in ulcerative or Crohn's colitis. The proposed sequence from normal mucosa through hyperplastic to adenoma then carcinoma is accompanied by serial mutations, first in the APC gene, then in the *ras* oncogene, followed by inactivation of the p53 tumour suppressor gene, resulting in loss of control of epithelial growth and repair mechanisms. Other mutations are certainly involved.

- Genetic—sporadic colorectal cancer is considered a polygenic disorder susceptible to environmental influences. Although only 1% have familial adenomatous polyposis, acquired mutations in the APC gene occur in up to 80% of all colorectal cancers and at least 50% have mutations in a well-defined position in the *ras* oncogene

- Environmental—lack of dietary fibre causing slow transit and excessive fat with increased exposure to toxic bacterial products of digestion, may explain the prevalence in Western communities. Colonic cancer is rare in the Far East and Africa, but the incidence is increasing. How dietary factors influence gene mutations is not understood

- Chronic inflammation (ulcerative or Crohn's colitis, pp. 295, 312) increases the risk

- Suggested associations with Barrett's oesophagus, cholecystectomy, coffee drinking or cholesterol are unproven

Clinical features

- Features vary with the site of the tumour. Most colorectal cancers are left-sided, but a third are proximal to the splenic flexure. Cancers associated with pancolitis are evenly distributed

- Bleeding—less than half have visible rectal bleeding. Fresh blood on the outside of faeces does not exclude a tumour, which may coexist with haemorrhoids. Negative occult blood tests do *not* exclude a colorectal cancer

- Change in bowel habit—more common in distal tumours. Tenesmus is common in rectal cancer. Any patient with change in bowel habit over the age of 40 years should be referred for investigation

- Abdominal pain is non-specific. It may be due to spasm, partial obstruction in distal lesions or local invasion in caecal tumours

- Anorexia, weight loss or an abdominal mass (especially caecal) are late features, but do not always indicate incurable disease

- Emergency presentation with obstruction (15%, usually at the splenic flexure), perforation (< 5%) or other reason (anaemia, jaundice) occurs in 30%
- Iron-deficiency anaemia in middle-aged men or postmenopausal women suggests a caecal neoplasm until proven otherwise (Section 9.7, p. 359)
- Colorectal cancer is an unusual cause of a persistent pyrexia, and is rarely the cause of pyogenic liver abscesses

Investigations

Patients with rectal bleeding, change in bowel habit or iron-deficiency anaemia (especially in postmenopausal women) must always be investigated for colonic cancer. Once the diagnosis is established, operability must be assessed.

Initial investigations

Rigid sigmoidoscopy

- Any patient with rectal bleeding
- The whole colon should then be examined by barium enema or colonoscopy, preferably preoperatively, but if necessary postoperatively, because tumours may be multiple in about 3%. The terms 'synchronous' (more than one tumour at one time) and 'metachronous' (a second tumour after resection of the first) for multiple tumours are sometimes used

Blood tests

- Anaemia may be the only feature of caecal tumours. ESR is often normal
- Raised ALP may be due to hepatic or bony metastases. Elevated γ-GT or AST indicates hepatic origin

Air contrast barium enema

- Usual initial colonic investigation for patients with an altered bowel habit (single contrast examinations are obsolete) radiological features of cancer are strictures with shouldering ('apple core'), or irregular filling defect in the bowel wall (Fig. 9.3)
- Colonoscopy is necessary if a barium enema is normal or views were poor in a patient with persistent rectal bleeding

Colonoscopy

- Appropriate initial colonic investigation for patients with rectal bleeding, polyp(s) seen on sigmoidoscopy, or those with a strong family history of colorectal cancer

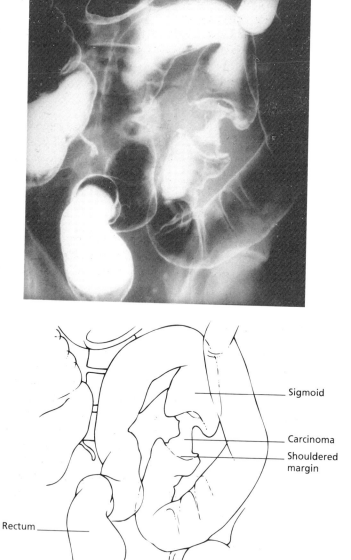

Sigmoid

Carcinoma

Shouldered
margin

Rectum

Fig. 9.3 Colorectal cancer. Barium enema showing a typical annular carcinoma in the mid-sigmoid.

- Detects polyps or cancer that has been missed at barium enema in 20–30% with rectal bleeding
- Provides a histological diagnosis which is desirable before surgery, but not essential if the radiological appearances are typical

Subsequent investigations

Ultrasound
- To exclude hepatic metastases in all patients with abnormal liver function tests
- Intracavitary rectal ultrasound is valuable for assessing tumour stage in rectal cancer, but is not widely available

Chest X-ray and other tests
- Look for lung metastases
- Other preoperative tests include ECG and blood crossmatch, depending on the age of the patient. However, blood transfusion may best be avoided before surgery as some studies (none are prospective) suggest a poorer outcome

Management

Early diagnosis and treatment improves prognosis (p. 343), so a high index of suspicion and early referral for definitive treatment is the key to management. Management depends on the site and extent of the tumour, although surgery is almost always necessary to prevent obstruction or relieve bleeding. Palliative laser therapy is occasionally used if surgery is contraindicated, but may not be available locally. The site and prospect of a possible colostomy should be discussed with the patient. Good bowel preparation and prophylactic antibiotics are needed before elective colorectal surgery. Antibiotics (intravenous metronidazole 500 mg and cefotaxime 1 g three times daily, although regimes vary) should be started on induction and continued for 24 h.

Rectal cancer
- Experienced colorectal surgeons produce the best results in terms of survival and local recurrence, making a strong case for sub-specialization in surgery
- Preoperative radiotherapy over 3–6 weeks reduces local recurrence and improves outcome

- Anterior resection (rectal and mesorectal excision with stapled anastomosis and no colostomy) is now possible even for rectal tumours to within a few centimetres of the anal margin. Abdominoperineal resection is still necessary for low rectal tumours
- Small tumours < 10 cm from the anus can often be removed by local excision in the elderly

Transverse/distal colon cancer
- Transverse or left hemicolectomy is indicated
- Emergency operations for obstruction need two or three stages (decompression, resection and anastomosis). A defunctioning colostomy decompresses the bowel, relieves symptoms and can be closed later

Caecal/ascending colon cancer
Right hemicolectomy is appropriate during elective or emergency surgery.

Adjuvant therapy
- Chemotherapy with 5-fluorouracil for infiltrating tumours (Dukes' B or C; Table 9.3, p. 343) improves survival. Colorectal surgeons should work closely with an oncology colleague and arrange direct referral. Different treatment regimens and delivery systems are under evaluation
- Radiotherapy is useful for rectal tumours (see above) and for subsequent palliation of metastatic disease

Surveillance
- Surveillance colonoscopy after surgical removal of the primary tumour is recommended, except for those with advanced disease (Dukes' C) at the time of surgery. Surveillance as for polyps (Fig. 9.2, p. 335) is appropriate
- A detailed family history to detect relatives at risk of cancer is essential (Table 9.2)

Table 9.2 Family history and risk of colorectal cancer.

Family history	Risk
None	1 : 50 (2%)
One first-degree relative age > 45 years	1 : 17 (6%)
One first- and one second-degree relative (any age)	1 : 12 (8%)
One first-degree relative age < 45 years	1 : 10 (10%)
Two first-degree relatives (any age)	1 : 12 (17%)
Hereditary non-polyposis colorectal cancer or familial adenomatous polyposis	1 : 2 (50%)

• Carcinoembryonic antigen measurements are often used as an adjunct to surveillance, but are potentially unreliable, because they fail to rise in a third with recurrent tumour

• An aggressive approach to detection and treatment of recurrence is justified in young patients. Resection of isolated hepatic metastases should be considered at a specialist centre, because survival may be improved. Ultrasound surveillance, probably every 6–12 months, is needed for detection of metastases

Recurrent or inoperable disease

• Symptoms of obstruction or recurrent rectal bleeding must be relieved even when a cure is not possible, because the quality of life (and death) is so poor with no intervention

• Local ethanol injection or laser photocoagulation may alleviate bleeding, but palliative surgery is needed to relieve incipient obstruction. Self-expanding metal stents are under evaluation for ameliorating obstruction in recurrent rectal or distal cancers

Screening for colorectal cancer

Screening aims to detect cancer at a treatable stage. The target groups and method of screening remain controversial, but there is good evidence that screening for colorectal cancer in the general population over the age of 50 would be at least as cost-effective as mammography screening for breast cancer.

General population

Screening asymptomatic individuals at standard risk of colorectal cancer aims to detect polyps that are premalignant, or cancer at a curable stage (Table 9.3). The present options are faecal occult blood testing or flexible sigmoidoscopy.

Table 9.3 Prognosis in colorectal cancer.

Stage	Description	5-year survival (%)
Dukes' A	Tumour limited to the bowel wall	95–100
Dukes' B	Tumour penetrating the wall, but no lymph nodes	65–75
Dukes' C	Lymph node involvement	30–40
'D'	Distant metastases	< 1

Faecal occult blood testing

- Four double-blind trials from Nottingham, Sweden, Denmark and Minnesota have shown that annual occult blood testing more than doubles the detection of curable (Dukes' A) cancers compared to controls. The Nottingham, Danish and Minnesota studies have also shown a reduction in mortality

- The problems are a low take-up rate (54–75%), poor sensitivity (20–50% of cancers are missed through false negatives), poor specificity (many unnecessary colonoscopies for false positives), bias towards motivated patients (potentially at higher risk) and possible detection of less aggressive tumours earlier (lead-time bias)

- Careful technique (three stool samples after no red meat in the diet for 3 days, repeated if positive before proceeding to colonoscopy), with rehydration of the specimen, is necessary

- The advantages of low cost, simplicity and demonstrable efficacy, however, make it appropriate to recommend for patients who remain concerned about their risk of cancer in spite of being at average or only slightly increased risk (Table 9.2, p. 342). General introduction should not occur until resources are available for colonoscopic examination

Flexible sigmoidoscopy

Flexible sigmoidoscopy every 5 years from the age of 50 is now recommended in the USA, but a single examination at age 55–60 years may be as effective. This would identify most polyp-formers and allow more intensive surveillance. Three randomized trials are in progress.

Other techniques

- Faecal analysis for tumour DNA is being developed, but the problem is to reduce 'background noise' in whole faecal samples when trying to detect *ras* mutations

- Full colonoscopic screening at the age of 55–60 years has its advocates

High-risk groups

Screening by colonoscopy every 3 years is widely accepted for high-risk groups such as patients with polyps, relatives with familial adenomatous polyposis, hereditary non-polyposis colorectal cancer (p. 336), or other strong family history of cancer (Table 9.2, p. 342), extensive ulcerative colitis (p. 312) or after resection of colorectal cancer. These represent a minority of all patients with colorectal cancer. Faecal occult blood screening in these high-risk groups is not worthwhile, because it has a low negative predictive value.

- If the family history suggests a risk of 10% or greater, colonoscopic screening should be offered, from the age of 20–25 years (younger in dominantly inherited syndromes)
- Screening patients with ulcerative colitis is only appropriate for pancolitis > 10 years duration, but remains controversial (p. 312)

Prognosis

Histopathological criteria of spread and differentiation are the most useful guide. Adaptations of Dukes' classification are most widely used (Table 9.3, p. 343).

- Well-differentiated tumours have a better prognosis than poorly differentiated tumours at any stage
- Older patients have a higher operative mortality. Young patients may have more aggressive tumours, but this is disputed
- Women have a better prognosis than men
- Duration of symptoms is inversely related to prognosis, except in obstruction, when survival is halved, or perforation, when 5-year survival is < 10%

9.4 Colonic diverticular disease

Colonic diverticula are present in 50% aged > 50 years in Europe, but most are asymptomatic. The term 'diverticular disease' is in common usage, but is hardly appropriate for describing the presence of uncomplicated diverticula. 'Colonic diverticulosis' avoids the connotations of the word 'disease', which may worry patients unnecessarily. Symptomatic diverticulosis may become complicated by inflammation or abscess (diverticulitis).

Asymptomatic diverticulosis

Diverticula are an incidental finding on barium enema when there are no abdominal symptoms (a patient being investigated for iron-deficiency anaemia, for instance), or when symptoms that are present are uncharacteristic.

Symptomatic diverticulosis

Symptoms

Colonic symptoms in the elderly are likely to be due to irritable bowel syndrome and coexistent diverticulosis, but colorectal cancer must always be considered. It remains debatable whether uncomplicated diverticula can

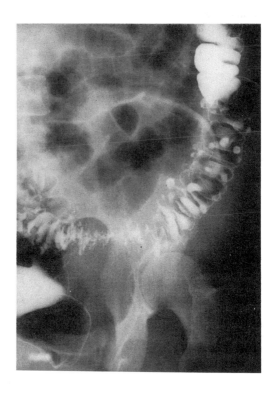

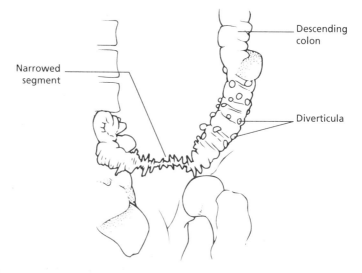

Fig. 9.4 Radiological appearance of colonic diverticulosis. Barium enema radiograph showing a narrowed segment in the sigmoid colon due to diverticulosis: thickened muscle is compressing the necks of the diverticula and the redundant mucosa is restricting the lumen.

cause any symptoms, since it is far more probable that diverticula are simply a peripheral feature of an underlying motility disorder. Muscle hypertrophy is striking in pathological specimens, but less visible on barium enema except in extreme cases (Fig. 9.4, p. 346).

Common symptoms

- Colicky left iliac fossa pain relieved by defaecation, lasting for weeks or months. Pain is sometimes central or in the right iliac fossa, and persistent
- Constipation (which is thought to promote formation of diverticula), with pellety stools, often covered in mucus
- Bloating and flatulence
- Dyspepsia is common, but likely to be due to coexisting gastro-oesophageal reflux or gall stones
- Rectal bleeding, recently altered bowel habit, right-sided or upper abdominal pain, diarrhoea or tenesmus must not be attributed to diverticulosis without investigation

Diagnosis

- Characteristic symptoms, normal blood tests (full blood count, ESR) and diverticula on barium enema (Fig. 9.4) are sufficient for diagnosis
- Rigid sigmoidoscopy should always be performed before a barium enema, because the rectum can be more closely examined. A biopsy should always be taken, because histology may show disease (Crohn's microscopic colitis) even when the rectal mucosa looks normal
- Colonoscopy is only indicated when a barium enema shows distortion of the bowel wall in association with diverticula (Fig. 9.4), but should be performed by an experienced colonoscopist because of the risk of perforation. Carcinoma, Crohn's disease, ischaemia or a pericolic abscess from diverticulitis may be impossible to distinguish radiologically from muscle hypertrophy or stricture

Management

- Increasing dietary fibre (p. 416) relieves pain if constipation is present, but existing diverticula do not regress
- Antispasmodic agents (dicyclomine 10–20 mg, mebeverine 135–270 mg, or 2 peppermint oil capsules three times daily) may help pain
- Stimulant laxatives should be avoided for treating constipation because these may increase colonic pressure and provoke pain. Osmotic laxatives (p. 328) are preferable

Complicated diverticulosis

Diverticulosis may be complicated by inflammation or abscess (diverticulitis), perforation, bleeding or obstruction.

Inflammation

Diverticulitis is recognized by pain, fever, leucocytosis and an elevated ESR. Prior symptoms are often absent. Colonoscopy is contraindicated in the acute stage, but may be done when symptoms settle if diverticulitis cannot be distinguished from a carcinoma or Crohn's disease on the barium enema.

- Pericolic abscess is suggested when a mass is palpable. It may present with obstruction
- Perforation may present with peritonitis, pelvic, paracolic or sub-phrenic abscess. Chronic pyrexia, ill health and weight loss may be the only features in the elderly or debilitated
- Portal pyaemia with liver abscesses is often due to diverticulitis in the elderly, but can also be due to a colorectal cancer or appendicitis
- Fistulae (vesicocolic, ileocolic) are more commonly due to diverticulitis than Crohn's disease in the elderly, but are rare

Management of diverticulitis is usually possible with oral antibiotics (metronidazole 400 mg three times daily and cephradine 500 mg four times daily), but severe cases need admission to hospital. In hospital, blood cultures, intravenous fluids, intravenous antibiotics and analgesia (intramuscular pethidine 50–100 mg every 4 h) are appropriate. A CT scan is indicated if a mass is palpable, to exclude an abscess. Surgery is necessary for abscesses, perforation or fistulae. Subsequent treatment with bulking agents and osmotic laxatives (p. 328) are indicated to treat constipation and reduce recurrence.

Bleeding

Recurrent rectal bleeding is uncommon and usually occurs without other symptoms of diverticulosis.

- Iron-deficiency anaemia is never due to uncomplicated diverticulosis. Carcinoma, ulcerative colitis, Crohn's disease and angiodysplasia must be excluded by colonoscopy, but angiography during active bleeding may be necessary to detect the site of bleeding (p. 24)
- Management is initially conservative (p. 23) unless the patient is on anticoagulants, when FFP is needed. Subsequent anticoagulation then needs a sound reason (such as a prosthetic valve)

Obstruction

Colonic obstruction may be due to inflammation or a fibrotic stricture, but carcinoma in association with diverticulosis is more common.

Indications for surgery

Surgery is only indicated for complications of diverticulosis (Table 9.4). Segmental colectomy for symptomatic diverticulosis is very rarely necessary, and only after medical treatment has been vigorously tried and other causes of symptoms have been excluded. Sigmoid myotomy is now rarely performed.

- Recurrent diverticulitis is unusual, but can be cured by resection and primary anastomosis in between attacks
- Abscesses are best localized by ultrasound and drained percutaneously. Colonic resection is rarely necessary, because perforated diverticula causing an abscess usually seal spontaneously
- Patients with perforated diverticula and peritonitis need adequate rehydration and parenteral antibiotics (metronidazole 500 mg and cefotaxime 1 g three times daily) before emergency laparotomy. Resection of the affected colon and a double-barrelled colostomy is probably best, but when it is not possible to mobilize an inflamed mass of sigmoid colon, resection with closure of the rectal stump and a colostomy (Hartmann's procedure) is then necessary. Attention to nutrition in the postoperative period is vital, because such patients are often frail, elderly and debilitated
- Fistulae are treated by sigmoid colectomy and closure of the bladder or vaginal connection
- Obstruction can be managed conservatively if incomplete (p. 42), but total colonic obstruction needs decompression by a transverse colostomy, with later resection of the stricture

Table 9.4 Indications for surgery in diverticulosis.

Infection
   recurrent diverticulitis
   paracolic or pelvic abscess
   peritonitis
Perforation
Fistulae
   colovesical
   colovaginal
   ileocolic
Obstruction
Major haemorrhage

Prognosis

Treating symptomatic diverticulosis with increased dietary fibre appears to reduce the complication rate to around 5%.

9.5) Intestinal ischaemia

Intestinal ischaemia includes small intestinal ischaemia, but this is rare compared to ischaemic colitis. Vascular disease may be acute or chronic, but does not always involve arterial occlusion. Focal ischaemia (due to vasculitis) or venous infarction are rare.

Vascular anatomy

The gut is supplied by the coeliac axis, superior mesenteric artery and inferior mesenteric artery (Fig. 9.5). The stomach and rectum (supplied by the coeliac axis and inferior mesenteric vessels) are well protected by oesophageal and internal iliac anastomoses, respectively. Branches of the superior and inferior mesenteric arteries anastomose through a variable marginal artery, which means that the splenic flexure is at particular risk from ischaemia. Ischaemic colitis is usually microvascular, with no apparent large vessel disease.

Causes

Although there are many causes (Table 9.5, p. 352), intestinal ischaemia is rare and there are only four clinical syndromes: acute, chronic, or focal intestinal ischaemia, which usually affect the small intestine, and ischaemic colitis.

Acute intestinal ischaemia

See p. 38.

Chronic intestinal ischaemia

Chronic small intestinal ischaemia is very rare.

Clinical features
• Abdominal pain 20–60 min after eating ('mesenteric angina') in an elderly patient with other cardiovascular disease

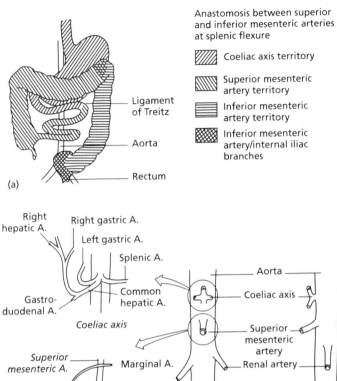

Anastomosis between superior and inferior mesenteric arteries at splenic flexure

▨ Coeliac axis territory

▧ Superior mesenteric artery territory

☰ Inferior mesenteric artery territory

▩ Inferior mesenteric artery/internal iliac branches

Ligament of Treitz

Aorta

Rectum

(a)

Right hepatic A.

Right gastric A.

Left gastric A.

Splenic A.

Gastro-duodenal A.

Common hepatic A.

Aorta

Coeliac axis

Coeliac axis

Superior mesenteric A.

Marginal A.

Superior mesenteric artery

Renal artery

Middle colic A.

Jejunal branches

Ileocolic A.

Ileal branches

Inferior mesenteric artery

Right colic A.

Inferior mesenteric A.

Common iliac artery

Superior rectal A.

Left colic A.

(b)

Sigmoid branches

Anterior view

Lateral view

Fig. 9.5 Mesenteric vascular supply. (a) Vascular territories. (b) Vascular anatomy.

Table 9.5 Causes of intestinal ischaemia.

Common	Uncommon	Rare
Atheroma stenosis thrombosis embolization	Systemic emboli atrial thrombus bacterial endocarditis Non-occlusive infarction cardiac failure septicaemia trauma anaphylaxis	Thrombosis polycythaemia sickle cell oral contraceptive antithrombin III deficiency factor V Leiden mutation protein C deficiency antiphospholipid antibodies microvascular Vasculitis rheumatoid arthritis polyarteritis nodosa systemic lupus Takayasu's disease Behçet's disease Miscellaneous aortic dissection infiltration by tumour iatrogenic (cardiac catheters)

- Weight loss, because the patient becomes afraid to eat
- Audible epigastric bruit, but this is often absent and may be normal in thin adults

Management

The diagnosis should be suspected in an elderly arteriopath when other causes of postprandial pain and weight loss have been excluded. Mesenteric angiography may show a stenosis at the origin of the superior mesenteric artery, but reveals nothing about arterial flow. Doppler ultrasound is potentially useful and non-invasive, but needs a highly skilled radiologist and may not be available.

- Treatment is difficult. Small, frequent meals are advisable
- Anecdotal reports of octreotide (50–100 µg subcutaneously, before meals) are encouraging, but experience is limited
- Angioplasty or arterial reconstructive surgery should be restricted to specialist units

Focal intestinal ischaemia

Trauma, radiation, vasculitis or drugs (enteric-coated potassium, slow-release anti-inflammatory drugs) may cause focal ischaemic damage. These cause a small intestinal stricture that presents as sub-acute obstruction: bleeding or perforation rarely occur. Diagnosis is made by small bowel enema since it may be overlooked on barium follow-through. Management is surgical, to exclude other causes (Table 7.10, p. 272) and to relieve the obstruction.

Strangulated herniae also cause focal ischaemia, but present acutely. The exception is a Richter's hernia (ischaemia of part of the herniated bowel, which subsequently returns to the abdominal cavity), because initial symptoms may resolve temporarily.

Ischaemic colitis

Ischaemic colitis can be acute, chronic or focal, but is classified separately because it is more common and presents differently from small intestinal ischaemia.

Clinical features
• Patients are usually elderly arteriopaths with a history of myocardial infarction, atrial fibrillation, peripheral vascular disease or hypertension. Colonic ischaemia is a recognized complication of aortic aneurysm repair (< 5%)
• Diarrhoea may precede rectal bleeding, or vice versa. The onset of either is usually sudden
• Abdominal pain is usual but not invariable, unlike small intestinal ischaemia
• Toxic dilatation occurs rarely
• Symptoms may occur for days or weeks before presentation, although patients with colonic gangrene present within hours and cannot be distinguished clinically from those with acute small intestinal ischaemia

Diagnosis
• Sigmoidoscopy shows a normal rectal mucosa and blood, or profuse blood-stained mucus, coming from above. The appearances may look like Crohn's disease or ulcerative colitis, with pronounced mucosal oedema, but colonoscopy is not advised because of the risk of perforation
• Limited flexible sigmoidoscopy after a phosphate enema and performed by an experienced colonoscopist is safe and the best diagnostic investigation
• Biopsies show ulceration and a polymorphonuclear infiltrate. Haemosiderin-laden macrophages are characteristic, but uncommon
• A plain abdominal X-ray often shows an abnormal segment, usually at the splenic flexure, with mucosal oedema ('thumbprinting', Fig. 9.6)

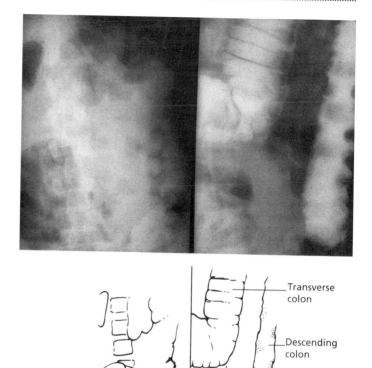

Fig. 9.6 Radiological appearance of ischaemic colitis. Radiographs in acute ischaemic colitis. In the plain film (left) gas outlines smooth indentations of the mucosa in the descending colon: thumbprinting. This is shown on barium enema (right).

- A common dilemma is to distinguish ischaemic colitis from acute Crohn's colitis (Table 9.6). It is normally possible to exclude ulcerative colitis, because the rectum is not inflamed, but occasionally the rectal mucosa can look congested

- An unprepared, single contrast barium enema may help resolve the dilemma, although the radiological features are often visible on a plain abdominal X-ray. Air contrast barium enema in the acute stage may

Table 9.6 Features favouring a diagnosis of ischaemic colitis.

History
Age > 60 years
Vascular disease (angina, hypertension, previous myocardial infarction,
  claudication)
Diabetes
Onset with sudden pain, then bleeding

Signs
No abdominal mass
No perianal or extraintestinal features of Crohn's radiology
Single affected segment
Often localized around the splenic flexure
Thumbprinting (mucosal oedema, distinguished from mucosal islands by
  being larger)
Symmetrical stricture

Endoscopy
Variable appearance, from mild reddening, local ulceration to gangrene

Histology
Minimal changes
Intramucosal haemmorrhage
Fibrosis
Haemosiderin (uncommon)

increase the risk of perforation, and colonoscopy is contraindicated if there
is peritonism. Sometimes diagnosis has to await colonoscopy after an
interval of 3–6 months

Management

- It is often not possible to distinguish colonic gangrene from acute
small intestinal ischaemia as the cause of an abdominal catastrophe, but
resuscitation with intravenous fluids and laparotomy are indicated for both
conditions (p. 38)
- Resolution is the rule for most patients with ischaemic colitis. Intravenous
fluids and transfusion to maintain the haemoglobin at 10 g/dL are indicated,
until bleeding, pain and diarrhoea improve. Deterioration is an indication for
blood cultures, intravenous antibiotics and plain abdominal X-ray: if colonic
dilatation has developed (diameter > 6.0 cm), colectomy is indicated
- Most recover completely and recurrence is surprisingly rare. Follow-up
barium enema is unnecessary if symptoms resolve. About 25% develop a
colonic stricture, which needs resection
- Colonoscopic dilatation of a localized stricture may be an alternative at a
specialist centre, because these patients are often a poor operative risk

9.6 Anorectal conditions

Haemorrhoids

Haemorrhoids are dilatations of the normal rectal submucosal venous plexus, which develop due to straining at stool. They are often associated with redundant mucosa or perianal skin. The traditional classifications into internal or external, first-, second- or third-degree haemorrhoids are better replaced by descriptive terms (such as bleeding, temporarily or permanently prolapsed, thrombosed).

Bleeding
• Bright red blood often spurts round the pan after defaecation, or smears the outside of the stool. This type of bleeding does *not* exclude a rectal carcinoma or proctitis
• Anaemia should never be attributed to haemorrhoidal bleeding without investigation

Haemorrhoidal prolapse
• Prolapse is recognized by the patient, but has to be distinguished on rectal examination from a polyp, rectal prolapse, anal cancer, or skin tag of Crohn's disease
• Permanent prolapse often causes discomfort from venous engorgement, or mucous discharge and pruritus. Pain does not occur without a fissure, thrombosis or infection

Thrombosis
• Rapid onset; severe perianal pain may take several days to resolve
• Severe pain from a thrombosed haemorrhoid may justify direct admission to hospital
• Anal carcinoma must be considered in the differential diagnosis of a painful, thrombosed haemorrhoid of long duration (several weeks)
• A perianal haematoma is due to thrombosis of a venous saccule

Management
• A serious cause of rectal bleeding must be excluded by sigmoidoscopy, and colonoscopy or a flexible sigmoidoscopy with a barium enema if aged >40 years
• A high-fibre diet is suitable for most patients, to soften the stool (p. 416)
• Persistent hard stools suggest that dietary fibre intake remains insufficient

Table 9.7 Management of haemorrhoids.

Situation	Management
All patients	High-fibre diet (p. 416)
Severe bleeding	Proctoscopic band ligation, or haerronhoidectomy
Prolapse	Proctoscopic band ligation
Thrombosis	Local ice pack to relieve oedema
	Lignocaine 1% gel (no more than 3 days)
	Lactulose 30–100 mL/day
	Injection or ligation after recovery
Recurrence	Haemorrhoidectomy, if injection or ligation is unsuccessful (< 10%)

(possibly due to poor tolerance) and can be temporarily relieved by lactulose 30–100 mL/day
• Surgical intervention is only indicated for persistent symptoms (Table 9.7)

Fissures and fistulae

Anal fissure
• A linear breach in the anal mucosa, often associated with a skin tag (sentinel pile) or anal polyp
• Pain during defaecation or acute constipation is characteristic, often with bleeding
• Diagnosis is made by inspection of the anal margin when gently parting the buttocks. Rectal examination is painful, but may be possible after applying lignocaine 2% gel perianally and into the anal canal
• Management is directed at relieving constipation (dietary fibre, with lactulose). Direct admission may be needed in the acute stage, if symptoms are very distressing. Surgical division of the internal anal sphincter (lateral sphincterotomy), or anal stretch, is then indicated

Perianal fistulae
• Perianal fistulae result from chronic infection. Acute infection causes an abscess
• Most are non-specific, but an underlying cause should be suspected for extensive, bilateral (horseshoe) or recurrent fistulae. Crohn's disease and rarely diabetes or tuberculosis should be considered
• Types of fistulae are shown in Fig. 9.7
• The track of the fistula should be identified by MRI (p. 292) when fistulae are recurrent or potentially complex as in Crohn's disease

- Surgery aims to lay open the fistulous track to allow healing by gradual granulation. Biopsies *must* be taken at every opportunity to exclude Crohn's disease. Complex or deep fistulae may need insertion of a Seton of monofilament nylon along the track that prevents premature closure

Pruritus ani

Perianal itching has many causes (Table 9.8). Questions about cleansing, rectal or vaginal discharge, local ointments (for 'piles'), skin disorders, or family members with the condition are relevant.

- Examination must include inspection for skin disease, digital assessment of sphincter tone and proctosigmoidoscopy
- Urine testing for glycosuria, Sellotape slide for threadworm (*Enterobius . vermicularis*) and skin scrape for fungi are often helpful. Skin biopsy, high vaginal swab or anorectal manometry (for sphincter dysfunction) are rarely indicated
- Treatment is directed at the cause. Careful washing after defaecation is most important. Topical hydrocortisone 1% twice daily for 2 weeks provides symptomatic relief, but reassessment rather than re-prescription is indicated for persistent symptoms

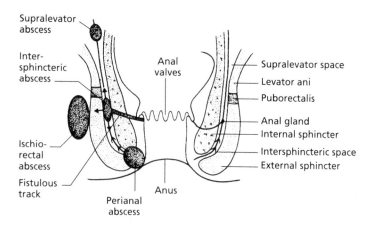

Infection   **Normal anatomy**

Fig. 9.7 Perianal fistulae and abscesses. Infection starts in the anal glands and may spread vertically, horizontally or circumferentially. An abscess is an acute, localized collection of pus, whilst a fistula, which connects two epithelial surfaces, is the chronic phase of the same disease process.

Table 9.8 Causes of pruritus ani.

Common	Uncommon	Rare
Poor hygiene	Rectal discharge	Eczema
Haemorrhoids	(sphincter dysfunction)	Lichen sclerosus
Fissure	Fistula	Paget's disease
Threadworm	Fungal infection (diabetes)	Bowen's disease
Skin sensitivity to	Vaginal discharge	
'haemorrhoid' ointment	Spurious diarrhoea	

Proctalgia fugax

Paroxysmal perineal pain lasting a few minutes, often felt deep in the rectum or after defaecation and perhaps waking the patient at night, has no organic cause. Rectal or puborectalis spasm have been suggested as causes. Avoidance of constipation and temazepam 10–20 mg at night may be helpful.

9.7 Investigation of iron-deficiency anaemia

Patients with iron-deficiency anaemia, often detected during a full blood count for non-specific symptoms, are a common gastroenterological problem and generally inadequately investigated. Investigation of the oesophagus, stomach, duodenum and whole colon is fundamental. In one health district of 290 000 population, 130 new cases of iron deficiency were identified in a 6-month period. In 21 patients the source was clearly not gastrointestinal, but of the remaining 109, only 19% had investigation of the upper and lower gastrointestinal tract. 50% had no investigation performed. 18 months after presentation, nine colorectal cancers, five gastric cancers and 11 peptic ulcers had been diagnosed.

- Endoscopy, distal duodenal biopsy (to exclude villous atrophy) and barium enema are the minimum investigations and can be relied upon to exclude serious pathology, although the cause may not be identified in a third of patients
- Iron deficiency should not be attributed to an uncomplicated peptic ulcer, hiatus hernia, NSAIDs, oesophagitis or haemorrhoids without investigation of the colon
- Iron deficiency in postmenopausal women, or men beyond middle age, suggests a caecal neoplasm until proven otherwise
- In teenagers suspected of having anorexia nervosa, iron deficiency should provoke a search for Crohn's disease

- Recurrent iron deficiency over some years should always raise the suspicion of coeliac disease

Essential investigations

History

A careful history is mandatory. Ask about:
- Evidence of bleeding—menstrual loss in women
- Diet—frequency of meat intake, vegetarian (no meat), vegan (no dairy products either)
- Weight loss—suggests carcinoma, malabsorption
- Diarrhoea—coeliac, Crohn's disease, but by no means universal
- Easy bruising—bleeding diathesis
- Mouth ulcers—coeliac, Crohn's disease

Examination

- Signs of iron deficiency—cheilosis, koilonychia (Table 12.4, p. 403)
- Mouth and lips—for telangiectases (hereditary haemorrhagic telangiectasia usually presents as iron deficiency in adults)
- Abdominal mass—neoplasm, Crohn's disease
- Rectal—faecal occult blood
- Sigmoidoscopy and rectal biopsy (p. 443)

Blood tests

- A hypochromic (MCH < 27 pg), microcytic (MCV < 80 fL) anaemia (Hb < 14 g/dL in men, < 12 g/dL in women) can be due to chronic disease, thalassaemia trait or sideroblastic anaemia, as well as iron deficiency
- Full blood count and film—hypochromic microcytosis and target cells when severe; thrombocytosis indicates inflammation, or acute on chronic bleeding; occasional macrocytes (dimorphic film) or Howell–Jolly bodies (hyposplenism) strongly suggests coeliac disease
- Serum ferritin (< 30 µg/L), or iron and total iron binding capacity—low serum iron (< 10 µmol/L) and high total iron binding capacity (> 70 µmol/L) confirms iron deficiency; low iron and low total iron binding capacity (< 45 µmol/L) suggests chronic disease; normal values suggest a haemoglobinopathy and is an indication for measuring HbA_2 (normal < 2%). Serum ferritin is an acute phase reactant and may not be reduced in inflammatory disease with iron deficiency (Crohn's disease, rheumatoid arthritis)

- Folate, B$_{12}$, albumin—if malabsorption suspected
- Prothrombin time (13–15 s) or ratio (INR 1.0–1.1)—should be within 30% of normal range before jejunal biopsy

Upper gastrointestinal endoscopy

Distal duodenal biopsies should *always* be taken to exclude coeliac disease when any patient with iron deficiency is endoscoped. Otherwise coeliac disease is frequently overlooked and the diagnosis delayed.

Barium enema

- More readily available in most (UK) hospitals than colonoscopy and more reliably images the caecum, as well as the terminal ileum if Crohn's is suspected
- Patients are, however, potentially subjected to a further procedure (colonoscopy and polypectomy), should polyps be detected

Colonoscopy

- More appropriate than barium enema if there is visible rectal bleeding or diarrhoea, and can be performed immediately after upper gastrointestinal endoscopy, under the same sedation
- Allows biopsies to be taken of any colonic lesions and the cause to be treated if bleeding is due to polyps or angiodysplasia
- Usually reserved for investigating obscure causes of recurrent anaemia (Fig. 9.8)

Further investigations for gastrointestinal bleeding of obscure origin

The cause of iron-deficiency anaemia which has not been diagnosed after the investigations above, can present a very difficult problem. Before repeating any of the investigations, it is wise to retake the history and to review the results, to ensure that obvious causes (dietary insufficiency, menstrual loss, coeliac disease) or pitfalls (haemo-globinopathy, renal cell carcinoma) have not been overlooked.

All patients

Recheck history

- Dietary intake of red meat
- Menstrual history

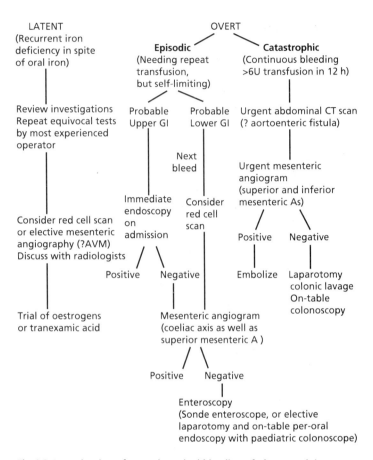

Fig. 9.8 Investigation of gastrointestinal bleeding of obscure origin.

- Associated symptoms
- Drug history (NSAIDs?)

Re-examine the patient

- Look for oral telangiectases
- Palpate for an abdominal mass
- Check urine for haematuria—if positive, perform an intravenous urogram to exclude renal carcinoma

Review results

- Ferritin—iron deficiency confirmed and haemoglobinopathy considered?
- Coagulation—bleeding diathesis excluded, including von Willebrand's disease?
- Endoscopy—by an experienced endoscopist?
- Distal duodenal biopsy—result of histology seen and reviewed?
- Barium enema—complete examination?
- Colonoscopy—good preparation, with views of proximal colon, by an experienced colonoscopist?
- Abdominal ultrasound—any evidence of portal hypertension?

Asymptomatic patients

- Stop iron therapy and repeat the full blood count after 3–6 months
- If anaemia recurs, the next investigation is small bowel radiology, preferably by a small bowel enema to obtain optimal mucosal definition
- In young people (age < 30 years) a Meckel's scan should be performed, although false-negative results are disappointingly frequent
- Regular iron therapy is then appropriate, with regular checks on full blood count

Symptomatic patients

This includes those needing repeat transfusions, or in whom there is clear evidence of gastrointestinal blood loss (recurrent melaena, rectal bleeding or positive faecal occult blood).

The sequence in Fig. 9.8 is recommended, but judgement is needed according to the age and condition of the patient. Whilst catastrophic bleeding is not the province of iron-deficiency anaemia, it helps to discriminate between the types of obscure gastrointestinal bleeding in the same algorithm.

- Isotope tests are frequently advocated, but almost as frequently disappointing
- Mesenteric angiography is usually only performed when there is brisk bleeding (1 unit/4 h, p. 24), but experienced radiologists can also detect mesenteric arteriovenous malformations, or intestinal varices from portal hypertension as an elective procedure. There may also be an inclination to ignore the coeliac axis if upper gastrointestinal endoscopy is normal, but this neglects the possibility of rare hepatic, biliary or pancreatic sources of bleeding. Careful discussion with the appropriate radiologist is essential
- Oestrogens are highly effective in recurrent bleeding from angiodysplasia (p. 14)

• 'Blind' right hemicolectomy is no longer appropriate for bleeding of obscure origin, now that on-table colonoscopy can be performed

• Enteroscopy is fashionable, but not widely available. It is time-consuming (4–8 h per procedure) and purely diagnostic. On the rare occasions that the source of recurrent bleeding is not detected by other means, elective laparotomy and on-table endoscopy by an experienced endoscopist is rewarding and potentially therapeutic. The surgeon initially excludes a Meckel's diverticulum, then feeds the small bowel over the endoscope to identify a lesion

10 Irritable Bowel Syndrome

10.1 Clinical features

The term 'irritable bowel syndrome' is used to describe a heterogeneous group of abdominal symptoms for which no organic cause can be found. This does not mean that the symptoms are all psychological; most are probably due to disorders of bowel motility, or of different sensory pathways from the alimentary tract, which are poorly defined because diagnostic tests are lacking, or insufficiently sensitive. Symptoms may involve organs outside the digestive tract, including the bladder. Although the group is distinguished by the lack of pathology or mortality, the morbidity from persistent symptoms is often substantial.

Typical features

The diagnosis can be made with confidence if five or more features are present in the presence of normal full blood count and inflammatory markers (ESR, C-reactive protein, plasma viscosity):

- Age 20–40 years
- Abdominal pain
- Duration >6 months
- Bloating
- Erratic bowel habit (constipation alternating with looseness)
- Pellety or ribbon-like stools
- Sensation of incomplete evacuation (tenesmus)
- Obsessional personality
- Unremarkable examination, although abdominal tenderness, especially over the sigmoid, is common
- Insufflation of air on sigmoidoscopy reproduces pain

Less common, but consistent features

- Nausea
- Dyspareunia
- Pain in the back, thigh or chest
- Malaise after defaecation
- Urinary frequency (irritable bladder)
- Depression

Symptom patterns

Symptoms occasionally follow an episode of acute gastroenteritis ('postinfective irritable bowel syndrome'). More commonly there is no obvious precipitating factor, although stress frequently exacerbates the condition.

Pain predominant
- Central, right or left iliac fossa pain, less commonly in several sites. It is often poorly localized
- Daily pain for > 6 months is rarely organic
- Persistent ache, often with sharp exacerbations
- Relieved by defaecation, but sometimes follows defaecation
- Worse at times of stress, or during menstruation in women

Diarrhoea predominant
- Morning frequency, often with urgency
- Usually with pain, but often relieved by defaecation

Constipation predominant
- Especially women
- Sensation of incomplete evacuation
- Associated with the passage of mucus, but never blood

Non-ulcer dyspepsia
See p. 90.

Markers of organic disease

See Table 10.1.

Investigations

The aim is to exclude organic disease by minimal appropriate tests.

Table 10.1 Markers distinguishing organic disease from irritable bowel syndrome.

Onset age > 40 years
History < 6 months
Episodic pain, with periods of complete relief
Anorexia
Weight loss
Mouth ulcers
Rectal bleeding
Abnormal clinical signs or investigations

All patients

- Urine test for protein or blood caused by renal tract disease
- Full blood count, ESR (or C-reactive protein, plasma viscosity) and liver enzymes will identify most organic causes of similar symptoms
- Haematinics (ferritin, folate, B_{12}) if diarrhoea predominates
- Stool culture if diarrhoea is present
- Sigmoidoscopy and rectal biopsy are always indicated if diarrhoea predominates
- Proctoscopy, to identify anterior mucosal prolapse, is always indicated if there is a sensation of incomplete evacuation after defaecation (p. 331)

Indications for a barium enema

- Typical features with any marker of organic disease (Table 10.1, p. 368) (especially if age > 40 years)
- Typical features with rectal bleeding at any age
- Barium enema may be deferred until diet or drugs are found to be ineffective if the history is < 6 months *and* age < 40 years

Further investigations

- Additional tests should be avoided unless there are unusual features or markers of organic disease: there is no need to arrange an ultrasound just because the pain is in the right upper quadrant, nor an endoscopy just because the pain is epigastric. Gall stones, hiatus hernia or colonic diverticulosis may be incidental to the patient's symptoms
- Endoscopy may be justified when the pain is clearly related to meals (dyspepsia), retrosternal (heartburn) or periodic (p. 85). It is essential if there is iron or folate deficiency to obtain distal duodenal biopsies
- Ultrasound of the pancreas and biliary tree is appropriate when upper abdominal pain is episodic and the endoscopy is normal. Pelvic ultrasound is indicated for lower abdominal pain related to periods
- Small bowel radiology is necessary when there is weight loss or abdominal pain and diarrhoea, to exclude Crohn's disease
- Diarrhoea without pain is investigated as in Fig. 7.1 (p. 237). Mild symptoms from hypolactasia, coeliac disease or small intestinal bacterial overgrowth may be misattributed to an irritable bowel, especially after an episode of gastroenteritis. Colonoscopic biopsies may show collagenous or lymphocytic colitis
- Motility tests (such as transit studies or intestinal manometry) are not diagnostic of irritable bowel syndrome, probably because the condition represents more than one motility disorder. Many show increased sensitivity to rectal balloon distension, but this also occurs in proctitis and other diseases

10.2) **Management**

Approach

Taking the history and examining the patient in a careful, sympathetic and thorough manner makes subsequent explanation and reassurance very much easier. The 'there's nothing wrong, it's all in the mind' approach helps nobody.

Explanation

Initial

A provisional diagnosis and initial explanation can usually be given on the first visit. Helpful descriptions (unfortunately without much objective pathophysiological evidence) include:

- Explaining that small volume, hard faeces cause the bowel muscle to contract harder
- Describing the pain as bowel spasm, similar to muscle cramp
- Suggesting that the bowel is more sensitive than normal, and that some foods may trigger spasm in many patients (Section 13.2, p. 421)
- Describing the typical features of an irritable bowel (often recognized by the patient, with relief) and relation to stress in some people (like pre-examination diarrhoea)
- A diagram illustrating colonic segmentation (haustra) may assist explanation

Subsequent

On a subsequent visit, with the results of normal investigations, it is important to make a definitive diagnosis of irritable bowel syndrome, to acknowledge the symptoms and explain the likely pattern of symptoms.

- Symptoms often continue for months or years, but ultimately usually resolve
- Symptoms can be relieved, but not always cured
- There is no risk of cancer or serious disease
- Explain that there is something wrong, but that it is not a disease and the bowel is 'out of tune' or 'more sensitive' than normal
- Emphasize that a combination strategy (dietary manipulation, fibre, antispasmodics, anticholinergic agents) is often needed, rather than to expect a single treatment to work. For intractable symptoms, aim to help the patient cope with the symptoms rather than expect a cure

Diet

Food intolerance

- Many patients have a specific food intolerance (terminology explained on p. 260) that can be reproducibly identified by an exclusion diet (p. 421). An exclusion diet is said to improve symptoms in about two-thirds of patients, but is not easy to implement in practice
- Once the food has been identified (often wheat, milk, caffeine, onions, chocolate or salad vegetables), avoidance brings relief. The food can often be reintroduced without relapse after 12 months, for unexplained reasons
- Coffee, tea, milk or alcohol may exacerbate diarrhoea
- 'Food allergy' tests waste time and money

High-fibre diet

- Only indicated when constipation is a prominent feature
- Fibre intake should be increased gradually. Mixed unrefined sources of fibre (fruit, vegetables, wholemeal bread) is more palatable than adding bran to food (p. 327), but may not be sufficient
- A high-fibre diet (p. 416) may make flatulence, diarrhoea or bloating worse
- Patients who already have a high dietary fibre intake may benefit from a reduction, especially if symptoms of bloating or diarrhoea predominate

Drugs

Drugs are only used to treat symptoms and none are universally successful. About a third of patients will get better on any particular drug. Many patients prefer to manage without drugs. The efficacy of one drug in an individual often varies with time.

Pain

- Antispasmodics have an anticholinergic action and are less likely to work when constipation predominates
- Mebeverine 135–270 mg three times daily is dramatically effective in a few, gives some relief to many, but may have no effect. Other drugs (alverine citrate 60–120 mg, or dicyclomine 20 mg, three times daily) may help different patients
- Peppermint oil (1–2 capsules three times daily) is useful for patients who have constipation and bloating, since it has no anticholinergic action, or for those patients who dislike 'drugs'

• It is worth trying different drugs, because benefit is often temporary, or unpredictable

• Amitriptyline 10–30 mg daily, or Motival 1–3 tablets daily are helpful for persistent pain, especially when associated with diarrhoea

Constipation

• A high-fibre diet (p. 416) is preferable to commercial fibre preparations (Fybogel, Regulan), or 1–2 tbs of coarse bran daily, but these can be tried if the diet does not produce a soft stool

• An osmotic laxative (lactulose 30–100 mL/day) can be added if bran alone is ineffective. Stimulant laxatives (p. 328) may make pain worse

Diarrhoea

• Loperamide, up to 12 mg/day, relieves frequency and urgency. The dose can be calibrated using liquid loperamide

• Codeine phosphate is best avoided, because long-term use may cause dependency

• Amitriptyline 10–30 mg, or Motival 1–3 tablets daily may help persistent diarrhoea, partly through its anticholinergic effect. It is important to start with small, 'paediatric' doses and to increase these gradually, as well as emphasizing their peripheral effect on enteric nerves, even though they were originally developed as 'antidepressants'

• Diarrhoea that is not readily controlled is an indication for investigation (Fig. 7.1, p. 237)

Other drugs

• Dyspeptic symptoms may respond to metoclopramide or antacids (p. 92)

• Anxiolytics or antidepressants (see above) may benefit some patients (such as amitriptyline 10 mg at night)

Alternative therapy

• There are some patients who remain symptomatic, or who cannot tolerate or will not take conventional medication

• It is often helpful to discuss the limits of conventional ('Western' medicine) in these poorly understood disorders and to acknowledge the role of complementary medicine

• Some treatments (hypnotherapy, acupuncture) have been subjected to comparative trials and shown to benefit some patients with intractable symptoms. It is unclear how reproducible the response is with different practitioners using different techniques, but the trials with medically qualified hypnotists indicate that prolonged remission can be induced. Not

everyone can be hypnotized. Treatment is time-consuming and not widely available at present
- Advise patients to beware claims of a single cause or cure for symptoms
- Aloe vera, slippery elm and other herbal remedies have their adherents and are unlikely to do any harm

Prognosis

- Symptoms disappear or improve in about half after 12 months; <5% become worse and the remainder remain unchanged
- Intermittent symptoms are likely, but these are usually due to identifiable stress or a change in diet and can be controlled
- There is no mortality

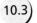

Clinical dilemmas

Persistent symptoms

- Usually due to a failure to treat constipation adequately, or to alter the diet
- Personality is important. Psychologically distressed patients select themselves by presenting for treatment. Explanations to provide insight and assistance in coping with symptoms are more likely to reduce visits than a dismissive approach. Clinical depression may be present and should be treated
- Further investigation is not justified unless the symptom pattern has changed or clinical signs (such as weight loss) have developed

Clinical psychology

- Irritable bowel syndrome should not be considered a psychological disorder, but there are some patients who are particularly anxious, or whose symptoms are a feature of bereavement, or stress-related illness
- A high prevalence of sexual abuse in childhood has been reported in patients with irritable bowel syndrome. Time to develop a rapport is essential before these issues are explored. It may be best done by the patient's general practitioner, although some patients who know their general practitioner particularly well may prefer to discuss such problems outside the primary care setting
- Referral to a clinical psychologist depends on individual interest, local availability and resources, which are often overwhelmed in the UK. Sensitive

discussion about psychological factors that are exacerbating symptoms should identify those patients most likely to be helped by referral
- Some general practice surgeries have a stress counsellor to help teach coping strategies

Symptoms with identifiable disease

- Features of irritable bowel syndrome remain common in patients with identifiable gastrointestinal disorders, such as gall stones, gastro-oesophageal reflux, ulcerative colitis or Crohn's disease
- Whilst judgement is necessary to decide which symptoms are related to the known disease, continuous abdominal discomfort, bloating or symptoms that do not fit with the common pattern of the disease are more likely to be due to an irritable bowel and are best treated with sympathetic explanation and reassurance

(10.4) **Somatization disorder**

Somatization disorder is a term used to denote a chronic condition characterized by a history of numerous, recurrent physical complaints that begin in early life (before the age of 30 years) and persist for many years. If no single person takes responsibility for overall management of the patient, then the complaints are likely to continue, with multiple unnecessary referrals, investigations and treatment.

Diagnosis

Establishing the diagnosis is time-consuming, requiring careful scrutiny of hospital and primary care notes. All four criteria (A, B, C and D) in Table 10.2 must be present for diagnosis.

An alert clinician will recognize the 'frequent attender' and a liaison psychiatrist, working alongside the clinical colleagues in the main hospital, is best placed to confirm the diagnosis as well as helping with management. General psychiatrists can frequently find no treatable psychiatric disorder.

Management

After establishing the diagnosis, the general practitioner and psychiatrist should implement a care plan to reduce hospital and primary care visits.
- Proactive care, with arrangements to see the patient at fixed intervals

Table 10.2 Diagnostic criteria for somatization disorder.

Criterion	Explanation or examples
A A history of many physical complaints beginning before age 30 years	
B Four pain symptoms	Pain in four sites (e.g. head, abdomen, back, joints, chest, or rectum)
and two gastrointestinal symptoms	Symptoms other than abdominal pain (e.g. nausea, bloating, diarrhoea, food intolerance)
and one sexual symptom	Not dyspareunia (e.g. sexual indifference, impotence, irregular menses)
and one neurological symptom	(e.g. impaired coordination/balance, dysphonia, numbness without neuropathy)
C *Either* none of the symptoms can be explained by disease or drug misuse	
Or when disease exists, the symptoms or disability are greater than explicable by the organic findings	
D The symptoms are not intentionally produced or consciously feigned	

- The doctor and not the patient should determine the frequency of these visits
- Make the patient feel understood, with the help of supportive listening, acceptance and interest
- Broaden the agenda by discussing previously elicited psychological and social factors (e.g. 'I am reminded of the troubles at home that have been worrying you')
- Make a possible link between symptoms and psychological problems (e.g. 'overbreathing can cause chest pain', 'depression lowers the threshold for pain')
- Negotiate graded withdrawal of psychotropic and/or analgesic drugs
- Treat any coexisting psychiatric disorder in the normal way
- Interview nearest relative and try to involve him/her as a therapeutic ally
- Minimize contact with other specialists to avoid over-investigation and iatrogenic harm
- Talk to the patient in terms of 'coping' not 'curing'

11 Gastrointestinal Infections

11.1 Acute gastroenteritis

Gastroenteritis is caused by infection in the gastrointestinal tract which usually results in diarrhoea and abdominal pain of acute onset and short duration, commonly with vomiting. It is often not possible or necessary to identify the organism, but it is important to recognize when investigation is indicated (p. 382).

Causes

Viruses are the commonest cause of gastroenteritis worldwide, whilst many bacteria exert their effect through toxins (Table 11.1). In adults in the UK, the causes are:

- Non-specific (culture-negative)—50%
- *Campylobacter* spp.—20%
- *Salmonella* spp.—15% (zoonotic organisms, spread from infected animals to humans, not those causing enteric fever)
- *Shigella* spp.—5%
- *Clostridium difficile*—5%
- Miscellaneous—5%

Clinical features

- History of travel, or eating unusual or suspect food (reheated chicken, seafood, take-away food, mass catering, conference dinners)
- The incubation period depends on the cause (Table 11.2)
- Other people are often affected

Table 11.1 Common causes of acute gastroenteritis.

Bacterial	Viral	Toxins	Other
Salmonella spp.	Rotavirus	*E. coli*	*G. lamblia*
Shigella spp.*	Echovirus	*Staphylococcus aureus*	*Cryptosporidium* spp.
Campylobacter spp.	Norwalk	*Cl. difficile*	*Isospora belli*
*Y. enterocolitica**	agent	*Vibrio cholerae*	Alcohol†
Clostridium		*B. cereus*	Heavy metals†
*perfringens**		*Vibrio parahaemolyticus*	
E. coli		*Clostridium botulinum*	
Aeromonas spp.		*G. breve*	

*Action partly through toxin production.
†Symptoms may be similar to infective causes.

Table 11.2 Bacteria involved in food poisoning.

Organism	Incubation (h)*	Food at risk	Duration
B. cereus†	1–5	Fried or reheated rice	12–24 h
Staphylococcus aureus	2–6	Unrefrigerated meat, milk	6–24 h
Vibrio parahaemolyticus	12–18 (< 48)	Crabs, shellfish	2–5 days
Clostridium perfringens	8–22	Cooled stewed meat	12–48 h
Salmonella spp.	12–24 (< 48)	Undercooked poultry, eggs	1–7 days
Clostridium botulinum‡	18–36 (< 96)	Fermented canned food	Months

*All times are very approximate.
†A non-vomiting type, causing diarrhoea, has a longer (8–20 h) incubation and may be acquired from ice cream, meat or vegetables.
‡Paralysis progresses rapidly after initial gastrointestinal upset. Antitoxin 20 mL intramuscular injection and 20 mL intravenously, after an intradermal test dose of 0.1 mL, is given when the diagnosis is suspected, with intravenous penicillin 2 MU four times daily to kill remaining bacteria. Ventilation is indicated if vital capacity < 1000 mL.

- Diarrhoea—may be bloody (*Shigella* spp., *Campylobacter* spp., enteroinvasive *Escherichia coli*, Table 7.3, p. 244)
- Crampy abdominal pain—often severe in the young or elderly, especially with *Campylobacter* spp.
- Vomiting—particularly with *Bacillus cereus*
- Systemic features (fever, headache, myalgia) are common in *Shigella* spp., *Campylobacter* spp., or *Yersinia enterocolitica* infections
- Resolution usually within 24–96 h

Susceptible patients
- Elderly or very young
- Hypogammaglobulinaemia
- Gastric hypoacidity—but does not appear to be a major problem with H_2-receptor antagonists, or proton-pump inhibitors
- Total gastrectomy
- Immunocompromised—chemotherapy, AIDS (p. 393)
- Hyposplenic—invasive salmonellosis is more common

Sequelae
Sequelae are uncommon.
- Persistent diarrhoea may be due to:

- secondary hypolactasia (especially postviral, in children)
- persistent infection (*Giardia lamblia*, immunocompromised)
- unmasked latent disease (ulcerative colitis, coeliac disease)
- postinfective irritable bowel syndrome (particularly common)
- Asymptomatic carrier—following *Salmonella* spp. enteritis
- Reactive arthritis:
  - or a full Reiter's syndrome (asymmetrical polyarthritis, orogenital ulceration, conjunctivitis) can occur after *Yersinia enterocolitica* or *Campylobacter* spp. infection and may be confused with ulcerative colitis or Crohn's disease
  - may also occur after *Salmonella* spp. and rarely after *Shigella* spp. infection in the susceptible
  - *Salmonella* spp. osteomyelitis may occur in hyposplenic patients
- Erythema nodosum:
  - after *Yersinia enterocolitica*
  - after *Campylobacter* spp. infection
- Haemolytic uraemic syndrome—renal failure and haemolysis after *Escherichia coli* 0157 occurs particularly in children
- Septicaemia:
  - in the immunocompromised, elderly or functionally hyposplenic (sickle cell disease, coeliac disease, splenectomy)
  - usually the cause of *Salmonella*-associated deaths
  - focal infections (cholecystitis, meningitis) are very rare
- Infective colitis:
  - diffuse mucosal changes may mimic ulcerative colitis, but glandular architecture is preserved
  - *Campylobacter* spp., *Yersinia enterocolitica*, *Shigella* spp. or *Escherichia coli* 0157 are often the cause
- Toxic dilatation—more commonly due to undiagnosed ulcerative colitis than *Campylobacter* spp., *Yersinia enterocolitica* or *Esherichia coli* 0157 enteritis
- Neuropathy—may complicate *Clostridium botulinum* (12–72 h), tetrahydropurine toxin (*Gymnodinium breve*) from shellfish or heavy-metal poisoning. Guillain–Barré syndrome rarely complicates *Campylobacter* spp.

Investigations

Uncomplicated acute gastroenteritis does not need investigation, because it usually resolves rapidly and spontaneously. When investigation is indicated (see below), stool culture and microscopy for cysts and trophozoites of *Giardia lamblia* and *Entamoeba histolytica* must be performed, with subsequent tests depending on the circumstances. Formed stool is unlikely to harbour pathogens. Investigation may be necessary for public health reasons (such as contact with a *Salmonella* carrier in the food industry).

Indications for investigation
- Elderly
- More than one person affected
- Symptoms persisting for more than 4 days
- Associated bleeding or other sequelae (see above)
- Acute gastroenteritis in a residential establishment or institution

Subsequent investigation
- Repeat stool culture if the first specimen is negative and symptoms persist, including faecal assay for *Clostridium difficile* toxin
- Stool examination for virus by electron microscopy is not necessary, except in outbreaks of culture-negative diarrhoea in institutions, or in children
- Persistent diarrhoea (> 3 weeks) is an indication for sigmoidoscopy, biopsy and referral to a gastroenterologist (Fig. 7.1, p. 237)
- Arthritis is an indication for joint aspiration if there is a fever or leucocytosis, rheumatoid factor to confirm a seronegative arthropathy, antibodies to *Yersinia enterocolitica* and X-ray if a large joint is involved
- Severely ill patients need admission to hospital, full blood count, electrolytes to assess dehydration, blood cultures and plain abdominal X-ray to exclude colonic dilatation

Management of specific infections

- Encourage fluid intake
- Oral rehydration solutions (Dioralyte, 500–3000 mL/day) for the elderly, very young, dehydrated, or if diarrhoea is severe
- Meticulous hand hygiene and a personal towel
- Personal eating and drinking utensils probably do little to prevent the spread of infection, except in *Shigella* spp. infections, but remains customary advice
- Antidiarrhoeal agents should be avoided if possible, although clearance of pathogens is probably not delayed. Loperamide 4 mg, then 2 mg after each loose motion, usually relieves diarrhoea if symptom control is needed, but should never be given to children because fatal paralytic ileus has been reported

- Metoclopramide 10 mg intramuscular injection up to three times a day controls vomiting. Dystonic reactions (more common in the elderly and adolescents) do not occur with rectal domperidone, 30–60 mg three times daily
- Intravenous 0.9% saline, alternating with 5% dextrose, each with 20 mmol/L KCl, is indicated for rehydrating severely ill patients. Judge adequate hydration by good urine output, but watch for possible fluid overload in the elderly
- *Suspected* food poisoning is a notifiable disease (p. 398)

Salmonella spp.

- Standard advice is *not* to give antibiotics, unless there is extraintestinal infection. Ciprofloxacin is *not* appropriate for ordinary infection causing self-limiting gastroenteritis, except in the elderly, immunocompromised or young
- Faecal excretion continues for 4–8 weeks and very rarely up to 6 months, usually from a gall bladder reservoir of infection. This is part of the natural history of infection and antibiotics for acute infection, including ciprofloxacin, may prolong excretion
- Repeat stool samples are no longer advised, even in jobs such as food handlers or nurses. The risk of crossinfection from a patient with formed stools is negligible. Good education in personal hygiene is equally important
- Septicaemia or invasive salmonellosis is treated with ciprofloxacin 750 mg twice daily for 1 week (or intravenous 200 mg twice daily over 30 min if too sick for oral medication). Trimethoprim 200 mg twice daily (orally, or by slow intravenous infusion) is the alternative drug of choice
- Treatment of asymptomatic carriers is unnecessary because such patients represent a very small risk to public health and no risk to themselves. Gall stones may be a nidus of infection and cholecystectomy is then advisable, with antibiotic cover (ciprofloxacin 500 mg twice daily, for 48 h) to kill spilled organisms

Shigella spp.

- It is often possible to manage patients without antibiotics
- Ciprofloxacin 500 mg orally twice daily is appropriate for patients with virulent species (*Sh. shigae* or *Sh. dysenteriae*), the severely ill, or those at the extremes of life, in whom the dose of antibiotics should be adjusted
- Repeat stool samples are needed for the same reasons as *Salmonella* spp. enteritis
- Bacteria can survive for several hours on hands or towels. Outbreaks in residential establishments are an indication for disposable towels, and disinfection of hands, lavatory seats and taps

Campylobacter spp.
- Antibiotics are usually unnecessary. Ciprofloxacin 750 mg twice daily for 1 week is probably only effective if started very early in the infection, or in the severely ill, but there is increasing resistance: currently 10% in the UK, but over 60% in parts of Europe and even higher in Asia. Erythromycin 500 mg four times daily for 1 week is an alternative
- Excretion often continues for weeks after recovery, but no treatment is needed

Yersinia enterocolitica
- Stool culture is positive in the acute stage, but antibody titres are necessary to confirm the diagnosis if presentation is delayed for more than 2 weeks. It may closely mimic Crohn's disease
- Tetracycline 250 mg four times daily for 2 weeks is indicated (but not in pregnancy, lactation or childhood), but this does not affect established postinfective arthritis

Escherichia coli 0157
- Haemorrhagic colitis caused by this organism is treated with ciprofloxacin 750 mg twice daily (or 200 mg intravenously over 30 min twice daily in the severely ill)
- It is the cause of haemolytic–uraemic syndrome in children and can be virulent in the elderly

Cryptosporidium spp.
No treatment is needed, since infection is usually self-limiting except in the immunocompromised.

Cyclospora spp.
- Increasingly recognized cause of persistent diarrhoea after foreign travel
- Co-trimoxazole 960 mg twice daily for 1–2 weeks is usually effective

Giardia lamblia
Tinidazole 2 g as a single dose (p. 258) or metronidazole 800 mg three times daily for 3 days.

Viruses
- Cause 60% of children's infectious diarrhoea and probably account for many episodes of culture-negative infectious diarrhoea in adults
- General measures alone are sufficient

Clostridium difficile

• Causes acute or persistent diarrhoea after antibiotic treatment, sometimes with no bleeding or systemic upset. Pseudomembranous colitis represents the severe end of the spectrum (p. 321)

• Metronidazole 400 mg three times daily for 1 week is indicated. Vancomycin 125–250 mg four times daily for 1 week can be used for resistant or recurrent infections

• Other antibiotics must be stopped immediately, if possible

Other toxins

Food poisoning (Table 11.2, p. 380) and travellers' diarrhoea (p. 244) need general supportive measures alone, except at the extremes of life.

Food poisoning

• Bacteria either produce a toxin in food and rapidly cause symptoms, or cause enteric infection after ingestion (Table 11.2, p. 380)

• Other organisms may also be transmitted through food (hepatitis A, *Listeria monocytogenes*, parasites)

11.2) Other gastrointestinal infections

Postinfective and tropical enteropathy

A variety of infections, including *Giardia lamblia*, *Escherichia coli*, *Klebsiella pneumoniae* and some viruses, may be followed by enterocyte damage that can be asymptomatic. It may progress to partial villous atrophy and cause malabsorption (postinfective tropical malabsorption or tropical sprue), but this is due to no specific organism. Clinical features, investigations and treatment are covered on pp. 256–258.

Tuberculosis

Intestinal tuberculosis is caused by *Mycobacterium tuberculosis* or *M. bovis* after direct ingestion (swallowed sputum or infected milk), or after blood-borne spread from another focus. Atypical mycobacteria (such as *M. avium-intracellulare*) is an AIDS-defining infection.

Clinical features

The diagnosis should always be considered in Indian, African, South-East Asian or South/Central American patients with chronic gastrointestinal symptoms, even in second-generation immigrants. Presentation several years after the patient arrives from abroad is common.

Ileocaecal tuberculosis

• Clinically similar to Crohn's disease (p. 284), with recurrent abdominal pain, pyrexia, weight loss or diarrhoea
• A mass is palpable in 40% and lymphocytosis is common, but by no means always present

Tuberculous peritonitis

• Ascites, weight loss and ill health. A 'doughy' feeling on abdominal palpation is rare
• Clinical suspicion and a diagnostic tap are essential, although laparotomy is often needed to establish the diagnosis (p. 285)

Tuberculous adenitis

Mesenteric adenitis may cause acute abdominal pain, similar to appendicitis.

Perianal tuberculosis

• Similar to Crohn's disease
• Colonic tuberculosis is very rare

Diagnosis

• About 30% have an abnormal chest X-ray; sputum samples may then be diagnostic. Most have no pulmonary disease. Gastric washings for *Mycobacterium* spp. are overrated and unpleasant
• A positive Mantoux test simply indicates previous exposure or vaccination. A strongly positive test (> 10 mm induration following 0.1 mL 1:10000 tuberculin) favours active infection, but is often negative in peritonitis
• Small bowel radiology will demonstrate ileocaecal tuberculosis, but cannot distinguish this from Crohn's disease, lymphoma, or severe *Strongyloides stercoralis* infection
• Laparotomy is indicated to establish the diagnosis when doubt exists. In an African or Indian patient with radiological ileocaecal distortion, tuberculosis can be assumed to be the cause unless there is no response to treatment after 2 months
• Culture of biopsy specimens is necessary to determine drug sensitivities. *Mycobacterium bovis* is insensitive to pyrazinamide
• Ascitic fluid adenosine deaminase levels (p. 168), or peritoneal biopsy

with an Abrams needle may be diagnostic for tuberculous peritonitis, but laparotomy is often necessary to establish the diagnosis

Management

- The same regimen as for pulmonary tuberculosis is used, although evidence for efficacy is not as certain
- Triple therapy for 2 months (isoniazid 300 mg/day, rifampicin 600 mg/day, pyrazinamide 2 g/day, for an average patient), followed by isoniazid and rifampicin alone for 4 months
- *M. bovis* should be treated with rifampicin and isoniazid for 9 months, and ethambutol for the initial 2 months
- Pyridoxine 10 mg/day is unnecessary, unless higher doses of isoniazid are used or paraesthesiae occur
- Response is judged by clinical improvement, weight gain, reversal of anaemia and fall in ESR. Intestinal parasites often coexist and may contribute to anaemia
- Routine liver function tests are unnecessary during antituberculous chemotherapy, unless there is pre-existing liver disease, or results are borderline at the start of treatment
- Abnormal liver function tests may be due to drugs (isoniazid, rifampicin), tuberculosis or other disease (cirrhosis). Drugs should be continued unless deterioration occurs (threefold elevation in AST). Biopsy is then indicated to establish the cause
- Follow-up for 2 years after recovery and stopping treatment is recommended, in case of relapse
- Notification and contact tracing are essential (p. 398)

Typhoid and paratyphoid (enteric fever)

About 200 cases a year of *Salmonella typhi*, *S. paratyphi A* or *S. paratyphi B* infection occur in Britain. Paratyphoid produces similar, but less severe features than typhoid.

Clinical features

- Fever—stepwise progression is characteristic, but rare
- Headache is typical
- Constipation—initially, but diarrhoea develops later
- Relative bradycardia—rarely in brucellosis too
- Rash ('rose-spots')—after a few days, often overlooked

- Complications, in the third week or before, include intestinal haemorrhage, perforation and death. Asymptomatic carriers are rare

Diagnosis

- Leucopenia is common, but may also occur with dengue fever and rarely in brucellosis
- Blood cultures in the first week, but bone marrow culture is the most reliable test and may be positive even after prior antibiotic treatment
- Urine or faecal culture in the second week
- Serology (Widal test) is of no value in acute illness

Management

- Ciprofloxacin 750 mg twice daily (or 400 mg by slow intravenous injection twice daily)
- Chloramphenicol 1 g (oral or intravenous) four times daily for 2 weeks. Multiple antibiotic resistance is increasing, especially from the Indian subcontinent. Care is necessary in children, for whom alternatives are trimethoprim or amoxycillin
- Isolation of excreta (urine, faeces), to prevent cross-infection
- Notification is necessary (Table 11.7, p. 397) and contacts must be traced
- Three negative stool cultures are necessary before the patient returns to work. The district consultant for communicable diseases will advise (p. 398)

Amoebiasis (Entamoeba histolytica infection)

Amoebiasis is prevalent throughout the tropics and sub-tropics, and asymptomatic cyst excretion is common (> 10% worldwide, 1% in Europe).

Clinical features

- > 90% of infections are asymptomatic
- Amoebic dysentery—clinically similar to ulcerative colitis (p. 301), with proctocolitis or, rarely, a fulminant course which has a bad prognosis
- Non-dysenteric colonic disease—strictures, an inflammatory mass (amoeboma), appendicitis, abscess, perianal or skip lesions are less common, but can simulate Crohn's disease (p. 284)
- Invasive amoebiasis—hepatic abscess (acutely or focally tender hepatomegaly in an ill patient, p. 206) may rupture into the pleural, peritoneal or pericardial cavities, with serious consequences. Other organs are rarely affected

Diagnosis

- Microscopy of fresh, warm stools to identify red-cell consuming (haematophagous) amoebae is diagnostic. Cyst excretion alone may be incidental. Three negative stool specimens virtually exclude the diagnosis
- Biopsies or mucosal scrapings should also be examined for trophozoites (amoebae with pseudopodia adjacent to the mucosa)
- Negative serology (several methods) is common in early disease and should not negate a clinical diagnosis of amoebiasis. Serology is never positive in asymptomatic cyst carriage. A positive test confirms previous exposure rather than active disease, although antibodies may be markedly elevated in invasive amoebiasis
- Ultrasound and markedly elevated antibodies to *E. histolytica*, or trophozoites in a fresh faecal sample, establish the diagnosis of amoebic liver abscess. Percutaneous aspiration of viscous, reddish ('anchovy sauce') fluid is characteristic of an amoebic liver abscess, but is rarely needed and may be complicated by a pyogenic abscess

Management

- Metronidazole 800 mg three times daily for 5 days is effective for all types of amoebiasis, but should always be followed by diloxanide furoate 500 mg three times daily for 10 days, because recurrent invasive disease sometimes occurs
- Three repeat stool specimens, to confirm clearance, are advisable
- Asymptomatic cyst excretors should receive a full course of metronidazole, with diloxanide for persistent excretors

Schistosomiasis

Schistosomiasis is endemic in Asia, much of the Middle East, Africa, the Caribbean and South America. Chronic schistosomiasis usually affects the indigenous population, who may then travel and present to doctors in non-endemic areas.

Visitors to endemic areas do not develop severe chronic schistosomiasis as a heavy worm burden takes many years to accumulate, but may suffer schistosome dermatitis, or rarely acute schistosomiasis (Katayama fever). Swimming in sea water or chlorinated swimming pools is safe, even in endemic areas, because the parasite needs the freshwater snail to develop. It is not infectious, for the same reason.

Diagnosis is made by detecting excretion of ova in faeces. As a rule schistosomiasis does not cause symptoms unless there is heavy excretion of ova, even if serological tests are positive, which only indicates previous exposure.

Schistosome dermatitis

An itchy papular rash affects exposed skin (swimmers' itch) within 24 h and resolves within 72 h, but is most unusual after primary exposure.

Acute schistosomiasis (Katayama fever)

• Fever, rigors, anorexia, diarrhoea, hepatosplenomegaly and cough develop 20–60 days after heavy initial exposure

• Diagnosis is suspected because of eosinophilia and confirmed by finding schistosome ova in faeces; serology becomes positive later. Steroids have been used in conjunction with praziquantel

Chronic schistosomiasis

• *Schistosoma japonicum* in Asia, and *S. mansoni* in other areas, may cause bloody diarrhoea or hepatosplenomegaly and portal hypertension

• *S. haematobium* in the Middle East predominantly affects the urinary tract

• Schistosomal colitis causes granulomatous inflammatory nodules, visible on sigmoidoscopy and confirmed by rectal biopsy, which also shows ova

• Portal hypertension may cause recurrent haematemesis, but not encephalopathy except in the terminal stages, because hepatic fibrosis is presinusoidal and hepatocellular function is preserved until very late in the disease (p. 173). Chronic liver disease in an Asian patient with light excretion of ova may still be due to hepatitis B, but granulomas on liver biopsy suggest schistosomiasis

• Treatment is indicated for chronic schistosomiasis with praziquantel, but is best undertaken by specialists, preferably following quantitative egg counts. Praziquantel 40 mg/kg as a single dose is effective in *S. mansoni*, and 25 mg/kg for 3 days in *S. japonicum*. Portal hypertension is likely to improve and surgical portosystemic shunting should be a last resort, although surgery gives a better prognosis than in patients with cirrhosis

11.3 Other parasitic infections

Infection by parasites, often several, is the norm in many parts of the world. Classification can be confusing (Table 11.3).

Clinical features

General

• Infections are usually asymptomatic, but can cause low-grade debility or specific features (see below)

Table 11.3 Classification of common gastrointestinal parasites.

Protozoa	Nematodes	Cestodes	Trematodes
G. lamblia	Roundworm	Tapeworm	Liver flukes
Cryptosporidium	*A. lumbricoides*	*T. solium*	*Clonorchis sinensis*
spp.	Hookworm	(cysticercosis)	*Opisthorchis viverrini*
E. histolytica	*Necator americanus*	*T. saginata*	*Fasciola hepatica*
Leishmania spp.	*A. duodenale*	*Hymenolopsis*	*Schistosoma* spp.
	Threadworm	*nana*	*S. mansoni*
	E. vermicularis	*D. latum*	*S. japonicum*
	Whipworm	Hydatid	
	T. trichiura	*E. granulosus*	
	S. stercoralis		
	Trichinella spiralis		

• Gastrointestinal upset—nausea, bloating or diarrhoea are common but non-specific when symptoms occur; this affects a minority only
• Weight loss—sindicates heavy infection or a complication, but this is unusual

Specific

• Anaemia: iron deficiency (*Necator americanus*, *Ancylostoma duodenale*, *Trichuris trichiura*), B$_{12}$ deficiency (*Diphyllobothrium latum*, from raw fish)
• Asthma—during larval migration (*Ascaris lumbricoides*, *Strongyloides stercoralis*)
• Colitis—often with granulomas (*Entamoeba histolytica*, *Trichuris trichiura*, *Schistosoma mansoni* or *S. japonicum*)
• Cutaneous: urticaria (*Strongyloides stercoralis* 'cutaneous larva migrans'), dermatitis (*Schistosoma* spp. 'swimmer's itch')
• Encystment—muscle, brain (*Taenia solium*, *Trichinella spiralis*)
• Fever: transient (*Trichinella spiralis*, *Schistosoma* spp.) fulminant septicaemia (*Strongyloides stercoralis* hyperinfection in immuno-compromised patients)
• Obstruction: intestinal, biliary (*Ascaris lumbricoides*, hydatid)
• Portal hypertension: *Schistosoma* spp., *Clonorchis sinensis*
• Pruritus ani: *Enterobius vermicularis*
• Steatorrhoea: *Strongyloides stercoralis*

Visible faecal worms

This may be the only manifestation of infection and usually prompts a rapid visit to the doctor in the UK. The worm may have been retained for inspection.

- 0.5 cm long and 0.1 cm diameter, thicker at one end than the other: *Trichuris trichiura* (whipworm) or *Enterobius vermicularis* (threadworm)
- 10–30 cm long, like a white earthworm: *Ascaris lumbricoides*
- Between 2 and over 20 cm long, segmented: *Taenia saginata* or *T. solium*. *Diphyllobothrium latum* is a single, long (up to 25 m) worm that is very rare in Britain
- All other worms excreted in faeces are microscopic

Diagnosis

Eosinophilia
- $> 0.44 \times 10^9$/L. The number of eosinophils should be expressed in absolute terms, not as a percentage
- Common marker of infection, usually $> 0.8 \times 10^9$/L in active infection
- Other causes include:
  - drug hypersensitivity
  - atopy
  - bronchopulmonary aspergillosis
  - pulmonary infiltrates and eosinophilia
  - vasculitis (polyarteritis)
  - lymphoma (rarely)
  - chronic active hepatitis (rarely)
  - Crohn's disease (rarely)
  - eosinophilic gastroenteritis
  - eosinophilic leukaemia (very rarely)

Examination of faecal sample
- Faecal examination of ova or cysts is the only way of differentiating infections, but ova or cyst excretion may be difficult to detect. Repeated stool samples and concentration techniques should be discussed with the laboratory
- Perianal skin is heavily infected during *Enterobius vermicularis* infection, which can be detected by a Sellotape slide (Sellotape applied to the anal margin and examined under a microscope for 0.5–1 cm long worms)

Serological tests
- Not available for most parasitic infections
- ELISA tests for *Entamoeba histolytica*, *Schistosoma* spp., *Echinococcus granulosus* (hydatid disease), *Leishmania* spp. and *Trichinella spiralis* virtually exclude the disease if negative, except in the early stages

Serological tests are not a reliable index of active infection. Treatment is, however, indicated in the UK for patients with positive serology and a compatible clinical history

Management of specific parasites

• The recommendations in Table 11.4 are for sporadic infection in non-endemic areas. General measures, including hand hygiene for nematode infections (especially *Enterobius vermicularis*), or treatment of anaemia, are also important. Other members of the patient's family should have stools examined for parasites
• Treatment of complications (such as *Strongyloides stercoralis* hyperinfection) should be in consultation with specialists

11.4 Immunocompromised patients

HIV-1 or -2 are now the predominant cause of acquired immune deficiency in all parts of the world, but other immunocompromised patients (following chemotherapy) are also susceptible to opportunistic gastrointestinal infections.

Detailed consideration of the gastrointestinal and hepatobiliary manifestations of HIV infection are beyond the scope of this text. Readers are referred to further reading (Appendix 2, p. 485).

AIDS

Acute HIV infection has unusual, specific gastrointestinal features, but most opportunistic infections that become pathogenic (*Cryptosporidium* spp., CMV; Tables 11.5, 11.6) suggest AIDS.

The term 'gay bowel syndrome' is no longer used, but referred to infections causing proctocolitis or diarrhoea in homosexual men who were not necessarily immunocompromised. Any infection with an organism in Tables 11.5 or 11.6 is an indication for measuring immunoglobulins and HIV status, *after* counselling.

Specialist combination treatment for HIV infection with antiretroviral agents and protease inhibitors is appropriate.

HIV enteropathy

Diarrhoea for which no causative organism can be found is common in AIDS

Table 11.4 Drugs for gastrointestinal parasites.

Parasite	First choice	Second choice
Protozoa		
G. lamblia	Tinidazole 2 g *stat.*	Mepacrine 100 mg t.d.s. 7 days
E. histolytica	Metronidazole 800 mg t.d.s. 5 days	Diloxanide furoate 500 mg t.d.s. 10 days
Cryptosporidium spp.	None	
I. belli	Co-trimoxazole 960 mg b.d. 21 days	Metronidazole
Cyclospora spp.	Co-trimoxazole 960 mg b.d. 7 days	
Leishmania spp.	Sodium stibogluconate 20 mg/kg 20 days	Pentamidine†
Nematodes		
A. lumbricoides	Mebendazole 100 mg b.d. 3 days	Levamisole†
Necator americanus	Mebendazole 100 mg b.d. 2 days	†
A. duodenale	Same	†
E. vermicularis	Mebendazole 100 mg *stat.* (repeated after 2 weeks)	†
T. trichiura	Mebendazole 100 mg b.d. 3 days	Albendazole 4 mg/kg *stat.**
S. stercoralis	Thiabendazole 1.5 g b.d. 3 days	†
Trichinella spiralis	Thiabendazole 25 mg/kg for 3 days	
Cestodes		
Taenia spp.	Niclosamide 2 g *stat.*	Praziquantel 10–20 mg/kg *stat.**
D. latum	Same	†
Hymenolepsis nana	Same	†
Echinococcus spp.	Albendazole 800 mg daily for 28 days†	Praziquantel†
Trematodes		
Clonorchis sinensis	Praziquantel 25 mg/kg t.d.s. 2 days*	
Opisthorchis viverrani	Same	
Fasciola hepatica	Same	
S. japonicum	Same	
S. mansoni	Praziquantel 40 mg/kg*†	

*Named patients only, from SmithKline Beecham (albendazole), or Bayer (praziquantel).
†Specialist advice required; general measures (hygiene) are as important.
Stat., single dose; b.d.; twice daily; t.d.s.; three times daily.

Table 11.5 Differential diagnosis of diarrhoea in AIDS.

Moderate	Severe/malabsorption	Bloody
G. lamblia	Cryptosporidium spp.	Herpes simplex virus
Salmonella spp.	I. Belli	Chlamydia trachomatis
Campylobacter spp.	Cytomegalovirus	Cytomegalovirus
Mycobacterium spp.	Enterocytozoon bieneusi	Campylobacter spp.
Gonorrhoea	Cyclospora spp.	E. histolytica
HIV enteropathy		Shigella spp.

Table 11.6 Gastrointestinal complications of AIDS.

Clinical problem	Site	Cause
Sore mouth	Oropharyngeal	Candida spp.
		Gonorrhoea
		Herpes simplex
Mouth ulcer(s)	Oropharyngeal	Herpes simplex
		Syphilis
		Kaposi's sarcoma*
		Acute HIV infection
Painful dysphagia	Oesophageal	Candida spp.
		Cytomegalovirus*
		Acute HIV infection
Diarrhoea (Table 11.5)		
Constipation	Rectal stricture	Chlamydia spp.
		Lymphogranuloma venereum
Abdominal pain	Subacute obstruction	Mycobacterium spp.*
		Intestinal lymphoma*
		Kaposi's sarcoma*
	Gall bladder	Cytomegalovirus*
Rectal bleeding	Ulcer/tumour	Syphilis
		Lymphogranuloma venereum
		Kaposi's sarcoma*
		Anorectal carcinoma
	Other	Thrombocytopenia
		(drug-induced)
Jaundice	Livers	Hepatitis B, B + D or C
		Sclerosing cholangitis
		(microsporidia)
		Drugs

*Diagnostic of AIDS in the presence of immunodeficiency for which no other cause can be found.
†Systemic infection is common in immunodeficiency.

and AIDS-related complex (ARC). This is attributed to HIV enteropathy causing partial villous atrophy, with histological crypt malabsorption, weight loss or susceptibility to infection.

A lactose-free diet will diminish symptoms associated with hypolactasia, but there is no other specific treatment apart from antidiarrhoeal agents. Severe diarrhoea is usually caused by a superimposed infection.

Candida *spp.*

• Oropharyngeal candidiasis causes a sore mouth or painful dysphagia if there is oesophageal involvement (p. 80)
• Diagnosis is by sight (white oral plaques, not to be confused with oral hairy leucoplakia) and confirmed by swab (hyphae, demonstrated by Gram stain)
• Oral candidiasis is treated with nystatin suspension 1 mL four times daily, or oral fluconazole 50 mg daily for 7 days, which should be given prophylactically in AIDS after an episode of oral candidiasis
• Oesophageal or systemic candidiasis is treated with oral fluconazole 50 mg daily for 7–14 days, or ketoconazole 200 mg daily for 14 days. Specialist advice is recommended

Herpes simplex virus type 1

• Proctitis occasionally occurs. Extensive oropharyngeal ulceration or disseminated herpetic infection is more common in the immunocompromised. There is often a past history of genital herpes (herpes simplex virus type 2)
• Cellular inclusion bodies in a rectal biopsy specimen distinguish herpetic proctitis from Crohn's disease
• Antibodies to herpes simplex virus (and other viruses, including hepatitis B) may be absent in immunodeficiency. This is a poor prognostic sign
• Oral acyclovir (200–400 mg five times daily for 5 days) is effective, but intravenous treatment (5–10 mg/kg over 1 h, three times daily) is needed for sick patients. Maintenance therapy (same oral dose, long term) is indicated for frequent relapse

CMV

• Proctocolitis is recognized by bloody, watery diarrhoea and superficial mucosal ulceration at sigmoidoscopy, in association with choroidoretinitis or pneumonitis. Oesophagitis causes odynophagia (p. 81)

- Diagnosis is confirmed by intranuclear eosinophilic inclusion bodies in a rectal biopsy specimen
- Treatment with ganciclovir is more effective but more toxic than acyclovir. Foscarnet intravenously is indicated in life- or sight-threatening circumstances, but causes renal impairment in 50%. Disseminated infection is usually fatal

Chlamydia *spp.*

- Chlamydial proctitis closely resembles Crohn's disease
- Biopsy occasionally demonstrates chlamydial inclusion bodies, which can be distinguished from CMV or herpes simplex virus inclusion bodies by electron microscopy. Microimmunofluorescent antibody tests establish the diagnosis
- Tetracycline 500 mg four times daily is effective, but may have to be continued for several weeks

Cryptosporidium *spp. and* Isospora belli

- Intractable watery diarrhoea causes malabsorption, weight loss and dehydration in the immunocompromised patient. *Cryptosporidium* spp. in normal individuals is a cause of travellers' diarrhoea, which is severe but transient (Table 7.3, p. 244)

Table 11.7 Notifiable and prescribed gastrointestinal disorders.

Common	Rare
Hepatitis—any type*	Tuberculosis*
Food poisoning—any type or suspected	Leptospirosis*
Dysentery—bacillary (*Shigella* spp.)	Amoebiasis
	Typhoid
	Paratyphoid
	Cholera
	Lead poisoning*
	Toxic jaundice (hydrocarbons)*
	Ancylostomiasis†
	Brucellosis†
	Vinyl chloride portal fibrosis†
	Hepatic angiosarcoma†
	Beryllium (hepatic granuloma)†
	Arsenic and other heavy metals†

*Statutorily notifiable, but a prescribed disease in certain occupations.
†Prescribed disease in certain occupations.

- Oocysts are readily identified in stool
- Spiramycin 1 g three times daily for 3 weeks (not available on UK market) is sometimes effective for cryptosporidiosis; there is no alternative. Co-trimoxazole 960 mg twice daily for 2–3 weeks is indicated for *Isospora belli*

11.5 Notification

Diseases affecting the gastrointestinal tract that are notifiable by law are shown in Table 11.7. The Director of Public Health (telephone number and address on the notification form, or from the area health authority offices) should first be telephoned and then sent the notification form, for which a small fee is payable. Some districts in Britain now have a consultant in communicable diseases; the local microbiology department will know. The environmental health department of local councils in Britain deal with commercial establishments, rather than patients.

Prescribed diseases have an industrial origin for which compensation may be payable, if the claimant has worked in a specified occupation. The Employment Medical Adviser at the Health and Safety Executive (Appendix 1, p. 475) will advise.

12 Nutrition

Nutritional assessment

Nutritional assessment of any patient, particularly one with gastrointestinal disease, is essential. Dietary inadequacy, appetite disorders and general or specific malabsorption all contribute to nutritional deficiency. Neglecting the nutritional status of ill patients compromises survival. Starvation in hospital may follow surgery, prolonged investigation or gastrointestinal symptoms, combined with apprehension and unappetizing food (see below).

The aim of assessment is to recognize general (protein–calorie) malnutrition (Table 12.1), as well as specific deficiencies (Tables 12.2–12.4).

Table 12.1 Assessment of protein–calorie malnutrition.

Readily assessed	Objective measurements
History	Weight loss > 10% in < 3 months
anorexia	Blood tests
dietary history (dietitian)	albumin < 35 g/L
calorie intake (dietitian)	lymphocytes < 1.5 × 10^9/L
food and fluid chart (inpatient)	transferrin < 2 g/L
Examination	Skin tests
muscle wasting	mid-triceps skin fold
oedema	< 8 mm (M)
angular stomatitis	< 17 mm (F)
Weight and height (Appendix 3, p. 486)	mid-arm circumference
below minimum weight for height	< 30 cm (M)
body mass index < 19 kg/m^2	< 26 cm (F)
	negative tuberculin test

F, female; M, male.

Table 12.2 Recognition of fat-soluble vitamin deficiencies in adults.

Substance	Clinical	Diagnostic tests
Vitamin A	Night blindness Xerophthalmia, keratomalacia	Dark adaptation time
Vitamin D	Bone pain, proximal myopathy	Alkaline phosphatase Low Ca, low P Pelvic X-ray (Looser's zones), bone biopsy
Vitamin K	Bruising	Prothrombin time, or INR > 1.3
Vitamin E	Spinocerebellar degeneration	White cell vitamin E

Table 12.3 Recognition of water-soluble vitamin deficiencies in adults.

Substance	Clinical	Diagnostic tests
Thiamine (B_1)	Neuropathy, ophthalmoplegia, psychosis, cardiac failure All alcoholics admitted to hospital	Red cell transketolase
Riboflavin (B_2)	Angular stomatitis, mucosal fissures (lips, genitalia) Normochromic anaemia, apathy, ataxia	Red cell glutathione reductase activity
Pyridoxine (B_6)	Sideroblastic anaemia, neuropathy, hyperoxaluria	Aminotransferase activity
Nicotinamide (Niacin)	Dermatitis, diarrhoea, dementia, weight loss	Urinary metabolites
Folate	Macrocytic anaemia Alcoholic patients	Red cell folate < 120 ng/L
B_{12}	Macrocytic anaemia, painful neuropathy, ataxia, poor proprioception, paresis	Serum B_{12} < 150 ng/L
Vitamin C	Poor wound healing, gum hyperplasia, bleeding, perifollicular or subperiosteal haemorrhages	White cell ascorbic acid, or urinary excretion < 10% after 1 g ascorbate

General malnutrition

- No single measurement is sufficient
- Height, weight and serum albumin (or total protein) may be the simplest measures available, but do not accurately reflect nutritional status. Hepatic, renal or intestinal disease will contribute to a low albumin or total serum protein
- Malabsorption, which may occur in the absence of diarrhoea, must not be overlooked (p. 248)
- The body mass index (Quetelet index) is most often used to assess obesity—the malnutrition of affluence. It is calculated according to the formula: body mass index = weight (kg)/height^2 (m)
- The relation to mortality is shown in Fig. 12.1

Malnutrition in hospital patients

- Frequently not recognized, although treatment of malnutrition has a major effect on length of hospital stay, postoperative complications and

Table 12.4 Recognition of mineral deficiencies in adults.

Substance	Clinical	Diagnostic tests
Iron	Microcytic anaemia, glossitis, cheilosis, koilonychia	Serum iron < 11 µmol/L (F) < 14 µmol/L (M), iron binding capacity > 75 µmol/L, serum ferritin < 15 µg/L
Calcium	Weakness, proximal myopathy, perioral paraesthesiae, tetany, Chvostek (jaw), Trousseau (arm) signs	Serum calcium < 2.20 mmol/L add 0.02 × (40-serum albumin) to correct for albumin level)
Phosphate	Proximal myopathy	Serum phosphate < 0.80 mmol/L
Magnesium	Myopathy not responding to calcium replacement	Serum magnesium < 0.70 mmol/L
Zinc	Anorexia, crusting red rash, diarrhoea, depression, anaemia, candidiasis	Serum zinc < 6 µmol/L (may be low in any acute illness)
Copper	Hypochromic anaemia not responsive to iron, low white cell count, osteoporosis	Red cell superoxide dismutase activity
Selenium	Cardiac failure	Glutathione peroxidase activity, serum Se

F, female; M, male.

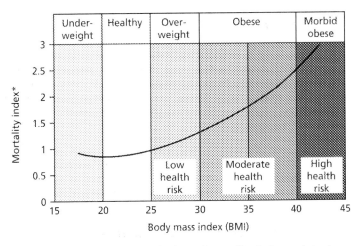

Fig. 12.1 Relationship between obesity and mortality. Body mass index is explained in the text. Adapted from Bray GA. *International Journal of Obesity* 1978; **2**: 99–114, with permission. *Excess mortality from life insurance statistics.

survival. Malnutrition demonstrably affects the immune response, respiratory function and comorbidity in surgical patients
- Six studies on hospital admissions have shown a 20–53% prevalence of malnutrition
- In one study of 112 patients (Appendix 2, p. 485) assessed on discharge from hospital, 66% had lost weight in hospital and those undernourished on admission had lost a greater proportion of weight whilst in hospital
- In another study of 501 patients with a fractured neck of femur, those receiving oral nutritional supplements stayed in hospital 24 days, compared to 40 days in a control group receiving no supplements. Mortality was also reduced by 19% in those receiving supplements
- A nutritional support team is a cost-effective way of reducing complications related to total parenteral nutrition in hospital, coordinating purchasing policy of enteral feeds and educating hospital staff

Specific deficiencies

- Deficiencies of vitamins and minerals are usually mixed, so clinical presentation is rarely classic (Tables 12.2–12.4 and p. 422)
- Diagnosis depends on the clinical context. Clues to the type of nutritional deficiency may be provided by chronic hepatic disease, malabsorption or malnutrition due to inadequate diet in housebound elderly, alcoholics, vegans (B_{12}) or Asians (vitamin D)
- Normal values of many of the less common tests vary between laboratories and the technique used. It is often unnecessary to do specific vitamin or

Table 12.5 Indications for nutritional support.

General	Specific
Weight loss > 10%	Multiple injuries
Albumin < 35 g/L	Burns
No food intake > 3 days	Inadequate dietary intake > 5 days
	Chronic sepsis (abscess)
	Acute pancreatitis
	Intestinal fistulae
	Short bowel syndrome
	Crohn's disease (adolescents)
	Complications of major surgery
	Dysphagia
	Persistent vomiting
	Malignancy
	Children or adolescents with chronic disease

Table 12.6 Daily nutritional requirements.

Catabolic states	Low	Intermediate	High
Energy			
kJ/kg/24 h*	125	125–150	150–250
kcal/kg/24 h	30	30–35	35–60
Nitrogen			
g/kg/24 h†	0.16	0.2–0.3	0.25–0.35
K (mmol/L/g N)	5	5	7
Phosphate (mmol/24 h)	20	20–30	30–50

Requirements for all catabolic states	Enteral	Parenteral
Electrolytes		
Na	1 mmol/kg/24 h	1 mmol/kg/24 h
K	5 mmol/kg/24 h	5 mmol/kg/24 h
Ca	20 mmol/24 h	7–14 mmol/24 h
Mg	14 mmol/24 h	3–28 mmol/24 h
Trace elements (µmol/24 h)		
Fe	180–320	20–70
Zn	230	100
Mn	45–90	5–10
Cu	30–45	20
Cr	1–4	0.2–0.4
F	80–200	50
I	1–2	1
Se	0.6–2.6	0.4
Mo	0.2	0.2

*Energy is also measured in kilocalories (1 cal = 4.2 J), but kcal is frequently shortened to cal, which is confusing.
†The non-protein energy: nitrogen ratio is not widely used any more, but is approximately 1000 kJ/g N (250 kcal/g N) in low catabolic and 550 kJ/g N (135 kcal/g N) in high catabolic states.

trace element tests, but simply to treat suspected deficiency generously (Tables 12.5, 12.6)

Indications for nutritional support

The decision to provide nutritional support depends on the nutritional status (Table 12.1, p. 401) and nature of the illness (Table 12.5, p. 404). A decision concerning nutritional support is mandatory if eating has not been possible for 3 days or dietary intake has been inadequate for 5 days.

Nutritional requirements

- Four factors must be considered:
  - energy
  - nitrogen
  - electrolytes
  - trace elements/vitamins
- The nutritional status of the patient, severity of disease and catabolic rate determine the energy/nitrogen balance required (Table 12.6, p. 405). High energy and nitrogen intakes are not needed in most situations, unless the patient is profoundly catabolic or has major nutrient losses, as in burns
- In low catabolic states such as starvation, paralysis or disease preventing an adequate oral intake, replacement with a normal energy/nitrogen balance is needed, with electrolyte, trace element or vitamin supplements if specific deficiencies are present
- In high catabolic states, including fever, sepsis, major surgery, trauma and burns, energy expenditure and hence requirements are increased by 10–100%
- Protein is 16% nitrogen, so 1 g N = 6.25 g protein

Feeding route

- Enteral feeding is the preferred method and should always be used if the gut is functioning, by whatever access is possible (sip feed supplements, fine-bore nasogastric tube, percutaneous endoscopic or surgical gastrostomy, or jejunostomy)
- Parenteral feeding should only be used when enteral feeding is impossible due to gut failure (Table 12.9, p. 411)

12.2 Enteral feeding

Enteral feeding includes feeding with specially formulated feeds by sips, fine-bore nasogastric tube or by enterostomy (gastro- or jejunostomy).

Indications

See Table 12.7.

Table 12.7 Indications for enteral nutrition.

Gastrointestinal disease
  malabsorption
  short bowel
Catabolic states
  burns
  sepsis
Anorexia
  any prolonged (> 5 days) illness
  especially after a stroke
  other neurological illness (bulbar palsy, motor neurone disease)
  before/after surgery
  cancer and its therapy

Choice of feed

- There are either general purpose (polymeric) or elemental (monomeric or oligomeric) feeds, with many proprietary preparations. Elemental feeds are only indicated for severe malabsorption (short bowel, pancreatic insufficiency)
- Energy and nitrogen balance (Table 12.6, p. 405), volume, osmolality, palatability and cost must be considered
- Most preparations contain appropriate amounts of vitamins (except folate) and trace elements, unless there are specific deficiencies, when supplements will be needed. Most are also gluten and lactose free
- Other modifications include variations in fat content (for steatorrhoea), fibre (purported to reduce the incidence of feed-associated diarrhoea) and glutamine content (ostensibly to enhance small intestinal integrity)
- Disease-specific formulas have been marketed for patients with hepatic, renal or pulmonary disease for various theoretical reasons, but are expensive and of little demonstrable benefit
- Careful studies have not shown any difference in nutrient absorption or clinical benefit between polymeric, oligomeric or monomeric feeds and it is difficult to show any consistent benefit from the various modifications
- The choice of feed can be limited to a polymeric feed for almost every patient and is reasonably guided by a local prescribing policy taking cost into account

General purpose (polymeric) feeds
- Fresubin (3.8 g protein, 420 kJ energy/100 mL) is a suitable preparation. It is palatable as a sip feed and appropriate for fine-bore tube feeding
- 1500–2000 mL/day is needed for moderately catabolic patients

• Many hospitals have a local prescribing policy to limit the choice of enteral feeds and other preparations on account of cost. Ensure, Osmolite or Clinifeed Favour have a similar balance of protein, energy, vitamins and trace elements to Fresubin and are competitively priced

Elemental feeds

• Elemental feeds are predigested, containing nutrients in a directly absorbable form
• Monomeric elemental feeds (such as Elemental 028 powder) are unpalatable and hyperosmolar, although considerable advances have been made in palatability with Elemental 028 cartons. They are expensive and the indications for their use are extremely limited (such as active Crohn's disease refractory to steroids, p. 286), especially now that active Crohn's disease has been shown to respond as well to polymeric feeds
• Oligomeric elemental feeds (such as Peptisorb, Perative) are more palatable and seem designed to appeal to those who cannot decide between elemental and polymeric feeds. In these circumstances, a polymeric feed should be selected
• A fine-bore tube is usually needed and the feed must be introduced slowly to avoid side-effects (diarrhoea, abdominal cramps, nausea)
• Elemental 028 cartons (1550 kJ/100 mL) are a suitable choice of elemental feed (about 500 mL/day). Vitamins and trace elements are included, but folate may be insufficient

Oral supplements

Sip feeds, in addition to meals

• Suitable for most patients needing nutritional supplements. Any nutritious drinks, cooled or warmed for palatability, are suitable. Proprietary preparations (such as Fortisip, Fortimel) have a wide variety of flavours and whilst expensive, it is worth experimenting to find the most palatable preparation because poor compliance is likely to lead to higher costs
• Patients who cannot eat are unlikely to drink sufficient liquid supplements (1500–2000 mL/day) for all their nutritional requirements. Fine-bore nasogastric feeding is then needed, with a balanced proprietary preparation (such as Fresubin, Ensure or Osmolite)

Nasogastric and nasojejunal tube feeding

• Polyurethane tubes with a stylet are easily inserted (p. 445) and neither

impair the swallowing reflex in patients with a stroke, nor cause oesophagitis
- Nasogastric feeding can be used for up to 6 weeks, but if feeding is needed for longer than 2 weeks then a percutaneous gastrostomy is usually appropriate
- Bolus feeding should not be used: this promotes gastro-oesophageal reflux and risks aspiration
- Weighted tubes offer little advantage, except for nasojejunal feeding for patients with impaired gastric motility
- Combined nasojejunal feeding tubes with a gastric aspiration channel are available and useful in an intensive care setting

Regimen
- Continuous drip feeding enhances absorption and reduces complications. A pump should be used to regulate the feed
- Start at a slow rate (30 mL/h) and increase to 125 mL/h over 3 days (by 10 mL/h every 6 h)
- Starter regimens are not necessary. Additional water to maintain fluid balance, is better than diluting the feed. Bolus feeding causes aspiration, diarrhoea or unpleasant abdominal distension

Gastrostomy and jejunostomy feeding

Percutaneous endoscopic gastrostomy (PEG)
- PEG is now widely available and the technique of choice for longer-term (> 2 weeks) feeding of patients with neurological dysphagia, most commonly following a stroke
- Complications are unusual, but may follow sedation during the procedure, aspiration pneumonia after feeding has commenced, or a blocked tube

Home enteral feeding
- Increasing exponentially, but needs careful liaison between hospital and community nurses, dietitians and doctors
- PEG feeding should be well established before discharge (usually 125 mL/h for 16 h/day
- Arrangements for supplies of feed, plastic connectors, infusion pump and a contact number for the carer to call if there are problems with the pump are essential, as well as agreement about who is to pay. Plastics and feed can usually be supplied by the local chemist, who should be given the regimen and product order numbers by the hospital before discharge

Table 12.8 Potential complications of enteral nutrition.

Problem	Prevention
Aspiration	Feed in semi-recumbent position
Diarrhoea	Do not give feed directly from the refrigerator
	Introduce feed slowly (increase rate over 3 days)
	Stop antibiotics if possible
Abdominal distension	Reduce rate of infusion
Tube obstruction	Inject water (1 mL syringe), or replace tube
Tube misplacement	X-ray position in unconscious patients
Oesophagitis	Use a soft, fine-bore, polyurethane tube
Hyperglycaemia	Insulin s.c. (common in septicaemia)
Electrolyte imbalance	Check serum K weekly, phosphate and zinc after 3-weeks
Low folate	Folate supplements after 3 weeks

Complications (Table 12.8)

Diarrhoea with enteral feeding is usually due to excessive bolus feeding or antibiotics. It can be alleviated by continuous feeding (if necessary at a slow rate to start with) and loperamide 8–16 mg/day, or codeine phosphate 60–180 mg/day.

12.3 Parenteral feeding

Parenteral feeding is much more demanding and hazardous than enteral feeding, unless it is done well. Meticulous asepsis and care of the catheter are essential, if life-threatening complications are to be avoided.

Indications

The gastrointestinal tract is inaccessible in unusual circumstances (Table 12.9). The indications for nutritional support are the same as for enteral feeding (Table 12.5, p. 404; Table 12.7, p. 407), when associated with gut failure.

Choice of feed

All-in-one bags

• All-in-one bags are much safer and easier to use than separate bottles of lipid emulsion and glucose/amino acid solutions, because the risk of infection is lower. This is especially true for occasional users
• Many hospitals make up their own 2.25–3 L bags and 70% of patients should be suitable for a standard bag

Table 12.9 Circumstances requiring parenteral nutrition.

Problem	Comment
Complete dysphagia	Fine-bore tubes pass most strictures
	Tube placement with a paediatric endoscope is sometimes necessary, pending definitive treatment
Intestinal obstruction	
mechanical	Perioperative
ileus	Postoperative
Short bowel	When enteral feeding is insufficient
intestinal fistulae	
extensive disease	Elemental feeds may be an alternative for Crohn's disease (p. 286)
resection	Home parenteral feeding is for specialist centres
Acute pancreatitis	Fig. 1.4 (p. 37)

- Ready made bags are available commercially and can be adapted to a patient's daily nutritional requirements (Appendix 1, p. 478)

Individual constituents

Nitrogen is provided by an amino acid solution, with equal proportions of energy from glucose and a fat emulsion. There are four steps in calculating the constituents for an individual patient:

- Daily nitrogen requirements must be decided first (Table 12.6, p. 405), in broad terms. 12–14 g nitrogen per day is sufficient for the majority. Hypercatabolic patients may need 16 g nitrogen per day, but greater amounts of nitrogen are not utilized. Patients with renal failure may need only 8 g nitrogen per day
- The amount of energy required must then be calculated, depending on the weight of the patient and the underlying disease (p. 406, and Table 12.6, p. 405)
- Additional electrolytes are added according to the daily results of electrolyte monitoring (Table 12.10). In unstable patients it is often easier to use a separate peripheral line to infuse additional fluids and electrolytes
- Soluble insulin (1–2 U/h by separate subcutaneous infusion) may be needed if hyperglycaemic. Adding insulin to the bag prevents adjustment of the rate and may lead to wastage of the feed
- Vitamins and trace elements are added (such as Solvito N 1 vial daily for water-soluble vitamins, Vitlipid N 10 mL/24 h for fat-soluble vitamins and Addamel 10 mL/24 h for trace elements). Many amino acid solutions are low in phosphate and this needs to be corrected (Addiphos contains 40 mmol phosphate, but also contains 30 mmol K and 30 mmol Na/20 mL)

Table 12.10 Monitoring during parenteral nutrition.

Measurement	Daily	Twice weekly	Weekly	Monthly
Electrolytes	+			
Urea	+			
Full blood count	+			
Glucose	+			
Check entry site	+			
Fluid balance	+			
Weight		+		
Albumin		+		
Liver function tests		+		
Calcium		+		
Magnesium			+	
Phosphate			+	
Zinc			+	
Iron				+
Folate				+
Trace elements				+

Techniques

Tunnelled central venous lines

• The cannula is inserted under local anaesthetic, in the operating theatre or anaesthetic room. The catheter runs subcutaneously for about 5 cm before entering the subclavian or internal jugular vein

• The cannula is connected to a 10 cm extension tube, which is both sutured and taped onto the skin, to avoid tugging directly on the cannula

• The position is checked by X-ray (catheters are faintly radio-opaque). The tip should lie about 1 cm proximal to the atrium

Catheter care

• The skin entry site and any connections must be checked and cleaned aseptically daily

• 1 cm wide Elastoplast strips should be used to secure the extension tube, but should not cover the connections or entry site

• A dressing is unnecessary. Dressings hide the entry site, create a warm, moist environment for bacterial growth and, when changed, increase the risk of infection. Some transparent dressings (such as Opsite) adhere tenaciously to plastic tubing. No dressing at all is preferable if the site is checked and cleaned daily

• The catheter must only be used for parenteral feeding and not for giving drugs or taking blood. A triple-lumen catheter is advisable for sick patients

• The giving set must be changed daily. A three-way tap is sometimes

inserted between the extension tube and giving set, to lock off the catheter, but this increases the temptation to inject drugs through this route
- Should a pyrexia develop and other causes have been excluded, the catheter must be removed and the tip sent for culture

Peripheral parenteral nutrition
- Peripheral intravenous nutrition is useful when it is desirable to maintain nutrition, but when enteral feeding is temporarily inappropriate and can be expected to start within the next 10 days. 75% of patients receive parenteral nutrition for < 14 days
- Lower osmolality feed, sometimes with heparin or hydrocortisone, reduce thrombophlebitis, which is the main problem. Complications associated with central venous cannulation are avoided
- Special long, soft catheters (such as Hydrocath) inserted into the basilic vein have a good patency rate. A nitrate patch applied over the vein distal to the cannula may also decrease thrombophlebitis
- Additives cannot currently be given, although peripheral parenteral nutrition is much better than no nutrition at all

Monitoring

- Guidelines are shown in Table 12.10. More frequent estimations (especially of electrolytes and glucose) are often necessary in the first week, but when feeding is stable the frequency can be reduced
- Baseline measurements must be taken before treatment; measurement of magnesium, folate and zinc are often forgotten
- Microbiology specimens (sputum, urine, drains, blood, faeces, catheter tips) are done as clinically indicated
- Accurate fluid balance is vital
- It is no longer considered necessary to perform 24-h urine collections for nitrogen balance. Nitrogen loss calculated from 24-h urinary urea (1 mol urea contains 28 g nitrogen) is inaccurate

Complications

- The complication rate depends on the experience of the person inserting the line, and especially on subsequent catheter care (Table 12.11). Designated people should be responsible for inserting feeding lines and checking catheter care
- Refeeding syndrome is a particular complication of electrolyte imbalance (hypokalaemia, hypophosphataemia) induced by too rapid reintroduction of

Table 12.11 Complications of parenteral nutrition.

Mechanical
  pneumothorax
  air embolus
  catheter displacement
  major venous thrombosis
  pulmonary embolus
Septic
  septicaemia
  endocarditis
Metabolic
  refeeding syndrome
  fluid overload
  hyperglycaemia
  electrolyte imbalance
Hepatic
  abnormal liver function tests*
  jaundice
Deficiencies
  phosphate
  trace elements
  essential fatty acids (linoleic, arachidonic)
  vitamins, especially folate

*Usually mild, transient and predominantly cholestatic.

feed after a prolonged period of starvation. Patients weighing < 40 kg should be fed slowly to start with, at a rate of a standard all-in-one bag over 36–48 h for the first 3–5 days

• Too few British hospitals have a nutritional support team consisting of a doctor, nurse, dietitian and pharmacist (Appendix 2, p. 485). The advantages are that a nutritional team can agree on standard procedures and policy, as well as offering expertise, advice and training throughout the hospital

12.4 Therapeutic diets

Badly planned, badly presented or poorly understood diets result in poor compliance and are not worth prescribing. An imaginative dietitian is invaluable for helping patients maintain special diets.

Weight reducing diet

Obesity contributes to the cause of osteoarthritis, diabetes, cardiovascular disease and many other diseases, directly increasing the risk of death

(Fig. 12.1, p. 403). Mortality in patients more than 25% overweight is increased by 500% in diabetics, and 160% in patients with ischaemic heart disease.

Principles

- Indicated for overweight (> 110% recommended weight for height; Appendix 3, p. 486) and obese (> 120%) patients (body mass index > 25 kg/m^2)
- A realistic target weight should be set (Appendix 3, p. 486) and steady, moderate weight loss planned (about 0.5 kg/week)
- Low fat and sugar, but high complex carbohydrate (fibre) intake is recommended. Fat has more than twice the energy density of protein or carbohydrate
- Early weight loss is largely due to loss of body water due to breakdown of glycogen. Inappropriately low carbohydrate intake can lead to a breakdown of lean body mass (protein)
- Sustained, steady dieting is necessary for any substantial loss of body fat
- Energy expenditure must exceed intake until the target weight is reached
- Eating patterns must be permanently changed, or weight will be regained
- Regular supervision, a weight chart posted in a prominent place, support from a skilled dietitian or slimming organizations (especially those that charge) improve success
- The minimum daily energy intake that includes essential nutrients without supplements is about 3000 kJ (700 kcal)
- Patients > 120 kg usually have a *high* metabolic rate (> 8000 kJ) and even higher food intake, despite frequent denials about excessive eating

Constituents of 4700 kJ (1100 kcal) diet

- Daily allowance:
  - skimmed milk 1 pint
  - butter or margarine 15 g, or low-fat butter substitute 25 g
  - as much vegetables/salad as wanted
  - three pieces of fruit (but no bananas)
  - unlimited water, tea, coffee, low-calorie fizzy drinks/squashes
- Protein—any two of the following, each day:
  - lean meat 100 g (liver, pork, veal, steak, beef, lamb, no fat)
  - fish or shellfish 100 g (not in batter)
  - beans or pulses 175 g
  - cottage cheese 100 g
  - hard cheese 50 g

- two eggs (no more than six eggs/week)
- Carbohydrate (unrefined, high fibre—a total of 6–10 portions of any of the following:
  - one slice wholemeal bread
  - one medium-sized potato
  - 25 g breakfast cereal (not sugar coated)
  - one Weetabix or Shredded Wheat
  - 25 g pasta or rice (before cooking)

Other approaches to obesity

- Dietary compliance is invariably required with any antiobesity drug treatment
- Appetite suppressants—only when excessive appetite limits the effect of diet, for a maximum of 6 months. All have serious side-effects (diarrhoea, blood disorders, pulmonary hypertension). D-fenfluramine 30 mg/day was the only non-amphetamine, but has recently been withdrawn from the UK market
- Thermogenic drugs—thyroxine, ephedrine or caffeine are not recommended, because protein, rather than fat, is mobilized and side-effects are unacceptable. Lipolysis-specific β-agonists are under trial
- Mechanical devices—for patients who cannot achieve dietary compliance and only if concomitant disease requires urgent weight loss, or if obesity poses a danger to life:
  - jaw wiring—efficacious, but weight regained when jaws unwired
  - nylon waist cord—after weight loss, to prevent regain in weight
  - gastric balloon—inserted endoscopically. Initially effective, but usually poorly tolerated and deflation after several weeks is common. It is not recommended
- Surgery—same indications as for mechanical devices. The risks should be carefully discussed with the patient:
  - jejunoileal bypass has 5% mortality and >60% morbidity
  - gastroplasty is effective, but mortality is 4% and morbidity 33%

High-fibre diet

Indicated for diverticulosis, most patients with constipation and some with irritable bowel syndrome. The potential for reducing the risk of colorectal cancer, cardiovascular disease or gall stones has yet to be confirmed. A higher fibre intake (aiming for 30 g/day) is suitable for most Western people as a pattern of healthy eating.

Principles

- Fibre provides bulk, absorbs water and satisfies hunger. Intake should be increased gradually to minimize adverse symptoms, e.g. flatulence or bloating
- Insoluble fibre is characteristically particulate and is found in cereal husks, bran, etc. It is particularly effective in regulating colonic function by increasing stool bulk. Soluble fibre is viscous in the form of gums and mucilages, derived mainly from legumes and oats. It modifies digestion and absorption, thus helping lower cholesterol and stabilize diabetes
- Excessive flatulence from bacterial fermentation is the main disadvantage, but only intestinal strictures or neurogenic constipation (p. 327) are contraindications
- Additional bran is rarely needed if fibre-rich foods are eaten regularly and in sufficient quantity
- Fluid intake must be increased (to 1500 mL/day or more) to compensate for water retained by increased fibre

Guidelines

- Good sources of fibre are:
  - wholemeal (not ordinary brown) bread
  - wholegrain cereals (muesli, All Bran, Bran Flakes, Weetabix, Shredded Wheat)
  - porridge oats
  - wholemeal flour
  - wholemeal pasta
  - fresh vegetables (beans, peas, green leafy vegetables)
  - pulses (dried beans, lentils)
  - fresh fruit (oranges, apples, peaches)
- Vegetables should be lightly cooked
- Unprocessed coarse bran can be added if dietary changes are insufficient: 1 tbs/day, added to soups, cereals, stewed fruit, home baking
- Bran tablets are available, but not prescribable. Isphagula husk granules (Regulan, Fybogel) are more convenient and expensive than dietary changes or unprocessed bran, but much less preferable

Gluten-free diet

Indicated for coeliac disease (p. 251).

Principles

- An *absolute* gluten-free diet is the only way to treat coeliacs. Non-compliance is the commonest cause of persistent symptoms (p. 255)

- Gluten ingestion increases the risk of lymphoma and ulcerative jejunitis in coeliac disease, so the diet must be continued for life
- The Coeliac Society (Appendix 1, p. 473) provides an excellent recipe book, with the gluten content of most foods

Guidelines

- Avoid:
  - wheat, barley, oats, rye
  - any products of these cereals (bread, cakes, biscuits, pastry, crispbread)
  - wheat cereals (Weetabix, Puffed Wheat)
  - pasta
  - packet soups
  - gravy, Oxo cubes, curry powder, mustard, sauces
  - chocolate, ice cream, sweets
- Allowed:
  - any fish, meat, poultry, game (no breadcrumbs/batter)
  - any cheese, eggs, milk, dairy products
  - any vegetables, potatoes, rice or fruit
  - Cornflakes, Rice Krispies
  - bread, cakes or biscuits made from gluten-free flour
- Essential gluten-free products are prescribable, including bread (Juvela, Rite Diet), pasta (Aglutella, Aproten), biscuits (Nutricia) and flour (see British National Formulary for comprehensive list)

Lactose-free diet

Indicated for hypolactasia, especially when diarrhoea persists after acute gastroenteritis (p. 243), Crohn's disease (p. 296), ulcerative colitis (p. 315) or coeliac disease (p. 256).

Principles

- Milk and liquid milk products are the only appreciable source of lactose. Many dairy products contain insufficient lactose to cause symptoms
- Hypolactasia may be temporary, so milk can be reintroduced later
- Variable tolerance to milk is often due to changes in colonic absorptive capacity (p. 237)

Guidelines

- Avoid:
  - milk of any sort (cows, goats, sheeps, cream), except soya milk

- yoghurt
- cottage cheese
- ice cream
- Allowed—anything else, including butter and cheese

Elemental diet

See p. 286.

Low-residue diet

Indicated when intestinal strictures cause symptoms, or in preparation for investigations (colonoscopy, barium enema, small bowel radiology), or colorectal surgery. Occasionally beneficial in patients with poor anal sphincter control.

Principles
- Indigestible fibrous foods are kept to a minimum
- Nutritional supplements (p. 408) are often necessary for strictures in association with Crohn's disease

Guidelines
- Avoid high-fibre foods (p. 417)
- Allowed any meat, fish, poultry or game (no stuffing) milk, dairy products

Low-fat diet

Indicated for steatorrhoea due to chronic pancreatitis, cholestasis or severe malabsorption, as well as hyperlipidaemia. No benefit has been shown for other types of hepatobiliary disease, although avoiding fatty foods (rather than a specific low-fat diet) decreases postprandial discomfort in some patients with gall stones or hepatitis.

Principles
- Reduce total fat intake to 30–50 g/day, or until steatorrhoea is controlled
- Substitute unsaturated for saturated fats in hyperlipidaemia
- Fat is important for palatability and the diet must be prescribed carefully. Medium-chain triglyceride supplements are indicated if calorie intake is insufficient following fat restriction (shown by continued weight loss)

Guidelines

- Avoid:
  - all fried food
  - butter, margarine (in moderation)
  - any cheese (except cottage cheese)
  - whole, evaporated or condensed milk, cream
  - fatty meat (goose, duck, sausages, pâté)
  - fatty fish (salmon, halibut, herrings)
  - salad cream, mayonnaise, salad dressing
  - any pastry or cakes
  - chocolate, marzipan, Ovaltine, nuts, olives
- Allowed:
  - skimmed milk
  - low-fat spreads
  - cottage cheese
  - chicken, turkey, liver, game (not roasted)
  - white fish, haddock, smoked fish
  - any vegetables or fruit
  - any bread or pasta and most cereals
  - Marmite, Oxo, herbs, spices

Low-protein diet

Indicated in acute hepatic encephalopathy (p. 166) or renal failure, but only continued if encephalopathy relapses after treatment of the provoking cause. Not indicated for cirrhosis without encephalopathy.

Principles

- The aim is an intake that avoids encephalopathy but maintains adequate nutrition (usually 40–50 g/day)
- The purpose is to decrease toxic products of bacterial action on nitrogenous compounds (protein) which are ammonia, mercaptans, aromatic amino acids

Guidelines

- Limit meat, fish, cheese, peas, lentils, nuts eggs
- Allowed:
  - other vegetables (potatoes, greens, tomatoes, marrow)
  - 200 mL/day milk (0.5 pt)
  - butter
  - bread

Low-salt diet

Indicated for refractory ascites or fluid retention in hepatic, cardiac or renal failure, although it is usually sufficient to avoid adding salt to food.

Principles
- Normal intake often exceeds the recommended daily allowance (1 mmol/kg/day), because most salt is added to food to improve palatability
- The aim is to restrict intake to 40–60 mmol/day
- KCl (such as 'Lo salt') is best avoided, especially if potassium-sparing diuretics are prescribed, and re-education about salt intake given

Guidelines
- Avoid:
  - any salt added before, during or after cooking
  - convenience foods (ready-made meals)
  - bacon, gammon, ham, sausages, pâté, cheese
  - Oxo, Marmite, bottled sauces
  - crisps, savoury biscuits, peanuts, savoury snacks
- Allowed:
  - bread (in moderation)
  - butter or margarine (in moderation)
  - any meat, fish, eggs, vegetables, fruit
  - pasta, cereals
- Palatability is improved by lightly cooking vegetables, using herbs (dill, garlic, rosemary, chives) or sauces (onion, apple)

Exclusion diet (Table 12.12)

Indicated for irritable bowel syndrome, especially if symptoms appear related to food. About half respond well and more are improved (p. 370). An experienced dietitian is needed to motivate the patient and to provide a systematic approach.

Principles
- The diet is continued for 2 weeks, with a diary kept of food eaten and symptoms experienced
- Foods are reintroduced one at a time after 2 weeks, if improvement has occurred. Further items are tried at intervals of 2 days
- Foods should be fresh or frozen, since many tinned or packet foods contain preservatives
- Intelligent cooperation by the patient is clearly essential

421

Table 12.12 Constituents of an exclusion diet.

	Not allowed	Allowed
Meat	Preserved tinned meats Corned beef, pâté, salami Bacon, sausages	All other meats Chicken, lamb
Fish	Smoked fish (haddock, kippers) Shellfish (mussels, prawns)	White fish (cod, sole)
Vegetables	Potatoes (any kind) Onions (fresh or dried) Sweetcorn	All other vegetables Cabbage, sprouts, beans, carrots, peas
Fruit	Citrus (lemons, grapefruit, oranges, limes), including fruit juice	All other fruits
Cereals	Wheat (bread, cakes, biscuits) Rye (crispbreads) Oats (porridge) Pulses Corn (Cornflakes, cornflour)	Rice Tapioca Millet, buckwheat
Oils	Corn oil, vegetable oil	Sunflower, olive, soya oil
Dairy	Cows' milk Butter Cheese Eggs Yoghurt	Goats', soya milk Goats', sheeps' milk cheese
Drinks	Tea Coffee (fresh, decaffeinated) Alcohol Squashes	Apple, pineapple, tomato juices
Others	Chocolate Yeast Marmite Nuts Preservatives	Spices Herbs Sea salt

Mineral and vitamin supplements

Indicated when there are specific deficiencies (Table 12.4, p. 403), or unexplained symptoms in association with severe malabsorption. Prophylaxis is indicated in profound cholestasis (primary biliary cirrhosis), short bowel syndrome or parenteral nutrition. Optimum amounts are often uncertain, but Tables 12.13–12.15 provide guidance.

Table 12.13 Treatment of fat-soluble vitamin deficiencies in gastrointestinal disorders.

Substance	Acute deficiency	Prophylaxis
Vitamin A	Retinol 100 000 U i.m. weekly	100 000 U i.m. monthly
Vitamin D	Calciferol 100 000 U i.m. weekly Oral alfacalcidol 1 µg daily is indicated in severe primary biliary cholangitis	Calciferol 100 000 U i.m. monthly
Vitamin K	Phytomenadione 10 mg i.v. for 3 days	10 mg i.m. monthly
Vitamin E	Vitamin E suspension 5 mg daily	No parenteral preparation

i.m., intramuscular injection; i.v., intravenous injection; o.d., once daily; b.d., twice daily; t.d.s., three times daily

Table 12.14 Treatment of water-soluble vitamin deficiencies in gastrointestinal disorders.

Substance	Acute deficiency	Prophylaxis
Thiamine (B_1)	Parentrovite HP 10 mL slowly i.v. for 3 days	Parentrovite weak 4 mL i.m. monthly
Riboflavin (B_2)	Same	Same (although deficiency still possible despite Parentrovite)
Pyridoxine (B_6)	Same	Parentrovite weak 4 mL i.m. monthly, or oral pyridoxine 10 mg
Nicotinamide (niacin)	Same	Parentrovite weak 4 mL i.m. monthly
Folate	Folic acid 15 mg daily for 1 month, then 5 mg for 3 months to replenish stores	5 mg daily; 15 mg daily in malabsorption; no parenteral preparation
B_{12}	Hydroxycobalamin 1000 µg i.m. daily for 5 days	1000 µg i.m. every 3 months
Vitamin C	Ascorbic acid 300 mg i.m. daily	Parentrovite weak 4 mL i.m. monthly

Parenteral administration is usually necessary, since deficiencies in gastrointestinal disease are due to failure of absorption (p. 248).

Principles

- Diagnostic tests are complicated or unreliable for many substances (Table 12.3, p. 402). Iron, B_{12} and folate are exceptions

Table 12.15 Treatment of mineral deficiencies in gastrointestinal disorders.

Substance	Acute deficiency	Prophylaxis
Iron	Ferrous sulphate 200 mg t.d.s. for 3 months Total dose iron infusion if oral iron not absorbed or tolerated	200 mg daily
Calcium	Calcium gluconate 10 mL i.v. (tetany) then 40 mL i.v./day	Calcium gluconate 2 tabs* three times daily
Phosphate	50 mmol/L i.v. over 12 h	Phosphate-Sandoz 2 tabs o.d.†
Magnesium	50 mmol $MgCl_2$ i.v. over 12 h	Magnesium glycerophosphate 1 g twice daily
Zinc	200 mg tab three times daily for 2 weeks	200 mg daily
Trace elements (see above)		

*Effervescent calcium tablets contain 4.5 mmol Na. Calcium should be monitored every 2 weeks, especially if vitamin D is given as well.
†Rarely required.

- Mixed deficiencies are common
- Fat-soluble vitamins are deficient in cholestasis, but all vitamins and some trace elements become deficient in severe malabsorption
- Vitamins A or D, iron, calcium, zinc and copper are toxic in overdose, so response should be checked every 1–2 weeks

Guidelines for trace elements

- Copper, manganese, iodine, fluoride, chromium, selenium, molybdenum, nickel, cobalt, vanadium are ubiquitous
- Additrace 10 mL contains the daily requirements (including Ca, Mg but not P, and relatively deficient in Fe) for parenteral nutrition
- Supplementation is rarely necessary even in severe chronic malabsorption, but copper, iodine or selenium deficiency may occur
- If zinc or magnesium supplements are required, monthly infusions (40 mL Addamel/L over 12 h) are justifiable
- 500 mL Intralipid 20% should then also be given to provide essential fatty acids

13 The Gut in Systemic Disorders

Most systemic disorders have gastrointestinal manifestations, which may sometimes be the presenting feature of the condition. More commonly, gastrointestinal symptoms present in a patient with a known condition which then influences the investigation or management of the symptoms. This chapter draws attention to problems that are often a cause for referral to gastroenterologists from other specialists.

13.1 Pregnancy

The most serious gastroenterological diseases in pregnancy are hepatic (HELLP syndrome and acute fatty liver), but luminal disorders are far more common. Pregnancy alters oesophagogastric and intestinal motility, as well as changing visceral anatomy, the omental response to peritoneal inflammation and influences investigations or treatment with regard to the fetus.

Nausea and vomiting

- Nausea and vomiting affect up to 50% of pregnant women between 5 and occasionally up to 20 weeks
- Hyperemesis gravidarum is defined as persistent severe nausea and vomiting in the first trimester, leading to 5% loss of body weight
- Consider other provoking factors, including urinary infection, gastroenteritis, gastro-oesophageal reflux, prodromal phase of hepatitis and biliary disease. Peptic ulcers are rare
- Conservative treatment is initially advisable, with reassurance, fluids and frequent small meals
- Metoclopramide (10 mg three times daily) or prochlorperazine (25 mg three times daily) have been widely used and appear to be safe. Endoscopy and treatment of reflux is appropriate for refractory cases

Gastro-oesophageal reflux

- A majority experience heartburn during pregnancy, often deteriorating in the third trimester
- General measures include elevating the head of the bed, frequent small meals, avoiding lying down after eating and symptom relief with alginates (Gastrocote or Gaviscon)
- Although not licensed, both H_2-receptor antagonists and proton-pump inhibitors appear to be safe for refractory symptoms. Endoscopy is advisable before using potent acid suppression

Acute abdominal pain (p. 39)

• In the absence of labour, biliary or renal colic, appendicitis and pancreatitis should be considered

• Amylase, full blood count and liver function tests should be checked and ultrasound arranged

• Management depends on the stage of pregnancy and severity of illness. The most experienced advice should be sought. Early surgery is appropriate if appendicitis is suspected

• ERCP and sphincterotomy have been performed successfully during pregnancy for gall stone related pancreatitis or obstructive jaundice, but definitive management of gall stones in uncomplicated biliary colic is best delayed until after delivery if possible

• If pancreatitis occurs for the first time in pregnancy and if there are no gall stones, then it is likely to recur in subsequent pregnancies

Jaundice and abnormal liver function tests (p. 163)

• Consider coincidental illness (incubating hepatitis before pregnancy or gall stones), drugs (including recreational), pre-existing disease, cholestasis of pregnancy, HELLP syndrome and acute fatty liver of pregnancy. Liver function tests, viral serology, autoantibodies and abdominal ultrasound should be arranged. Specialist advice should be sought

• Cholestasis of pregnancy occurs in the third trimester, with itching, cholestatic liver function tests and resolution after delivery. It commonly recurs with subsequent pregnancy, but is of no significance

• HELLP syndrome has a spectrum of severity up to fulminant hepatic failure. It occurs in the third trimester often associated with pre-eclampsia and early delivery is essential

• Acute fatty liver of pregnancy is potentially fatal, presents with vomiting and abdominal pain in the third trimester, with elevated AST, bilirubin and INR, but no haemolysis. Early delivery is essential

• Pre-existing liver disease usually reduces fertility. Primary biliary cirrhosis may present in pregnancy. Bleeding from varices is a real risk, especially when varices have previously bled. Liver biopsy is appropriate when abnormal liver function tests persist for 3–6 months after delivery

Inflammatory bowel disease (p. 298)

• Fertility is usually normal except in women with active disease, or severe Crohn's disease, who may have tubal obstruction. Sulphasalazine causes reversible oligospermia in men

• Pregnancy is best planned during a period of sustained remission (> 6 months). Folate supplements are appropriate as for all planned pregnancies, to reduce the risk of neural tube defects. Sulphasalazine only affects folate metabolism *in vitro*, not *in vivo*

• Maintenance therapy should be continued, to reduce the risk of relapse. The risks from active disease are higher than any side-effects of medication. Azathioprine is a special case: experience suggests that it is safe and it is often not possible to stop the drug in patients with previously refractory disease. The advantages (maintaining remission) and disadvantages (theoretical concerns of immunosuppression on the fetus) should be carefully discussed with the patient

• Active disease should be promptly treated with corticosteroids as for other patients. Severe or refractory disease increases fetal mortality

13.2 Elderly

About 15% of the population of the UK and USA are aged over 65 years, compared to 5% in the Far East. Demographic predictions indicate that in the UK, the proportion is not going to change appreciably, although a greater percentage will be aged > 85 years (currently 1.5%, projected to be 2% by 2001). Although at age 65 life expectancy is 12 years, at age 85 the chance of living another year becomes even.

Investigations

Classical symptom patterns rarely occur in the elderly. Cholangitis, for example, may present as confusion and abnormal liver function tests, without pain or fever. Prompt investigation by an alert clinician allows definitive treatment such as endoscopic sphincterotomy with good results. Delay in the elderly compromises already diminished nutritional and functional reserves.

Technological advances in less invasive imaging techniques particularly benefit the elderly. Abdominal CT scanning (especially with spiral CT) has a diagnostic accuracy for colonic neoplasms of about 85–90%. Whilst this is less than contrast radiology (95%), or colonoscopy (98%), the minimal preparation and non-invasive nature of CT scans may make it the best technique for frail, elderly patients. In contrast, colonoscopy may offer a therapeutic as well as diagnostic opportunity (such as polypectomy or lasering haemorrhagic tumours). Clinical judgement is needed, guided by the need to make a diagnosis and achieve symptom relief with minimum distress to the patient.

Dysphagia

• Peptic oesophageal strictures and oesophageal cancer (p. 70) are common, but so are age-related pharyngeal and neuromuscular disorders (pharyngeal pouch, xerostomia, stroke or Parkinson's disease, Table 2.1 p. 59). Motility disorders are common, but the ageing oesophagus ('presbyoesophagus') is no longer considered a distinct entity

• A barium swallow is the initial investigation of choice, before endoscopy, to exclude a high stricture or pharyngeal pouch

• Treatment of motility disorders is difficult. Small, solid meals, avoiding drinking and eating at the same time, or prokinetic agents (cisapride 20 mg twice daily) may help

Constipation (p. 325)

• Inadequate fibre and poor mobility are common causes

• Exclude drugs (analgesics, tricyclics, calcium antagonists), hypothyroidism, hypercalcaemia and local disease (fissure, prolapse)

Diarrhoea

• Gastroenteritis (including *Clostridium difficile*) and faecal impaction should not be overlooked. Send stool culture, request *Cl. difficile* toxin assay and do a rectal examination

• Apart from malignancy, ulcerative or ischaemic colitis may cause bloody diarrhoea

• Flexible sigmoidoscopy after phosphate enema preparation takes a few minutes, is well tolerated and rapidly provides a definitive diagnosis

• Barium enema is often worse than useless: preparation may be detrimental, inadequate pictures are common due to poor mobility or faecal residue, and significant mucosal disease can be overlooked

• Jejunal diverticulosis, bacterial overgrowth, thyrotoxicosis or microscopic colitis may cause watery or malodorous diarrhoea. An empirical course of metronidazole 400 mg three times daily for 1 week may give rapid symptomatic relief

Abdominal pain (p. 39)

• Serum amylase, abdominal ultrasound, then CT scan are the most useful diagnostic tests

• Appendicitis or perforation (diverticulum or duodenal ulcer) have a high mortality, because signs of peritonitis can be minimal
• Mesenteric ischaemia should always be considered when pain is severe and signs are few
• Early laparotomy is advisable if there is doubt. Delay increases mortality when there is serious pathology and if there is not, laparotomy is usually well tolerated

Inflammatory bowel disease

• Malnutrition, especially in elderly patients with colonic Crohn's disease, is common
• Early diagnosis by flexible sigmoidoscopy and adequate treatment with corticosteroids are fundamental (p. 308)
• Joint care with a gastroenterologist is advisable, especially when patients are ill enough to be admitted. The severity of ulcerative colitis is readily underestimated (p. 301) and if colectomy is inappropriately delayed, mortality is high

13.3 Endocrine disease

Diabetes

Gastroparesis, autonomic neuropathy and concomitant disease need to be considered.

Gastroparesis
• Causes fullness, postprandial vomiting and a succussion splash
• Endoscopy or barium meal identify food residue in the stomach and also exclude pyloric stenosis. The diagnosis may be obvious in these circumstances, but lesser degrees of delayed gastric emptying can be detected by isotope studies
• Prokinetic agents (cisapride up to 60 mg daily, or erythromycin 250 mg before meals) may help. In the most severe cases, Roux-en-Y anastomosis may be necessary

Autonomic neuropathy
• Commonly presents with watery diarrhoea, but may also cause pseudo-obstruction
• Concomitant disease (villous atrophy, thyrotoxicosis, hypolactasia, microscopic colitis) should be excluded

- Postural hypotension or peripheral neuropathy are clues to autonomic dysfunction
- Bacterial overgrowth or decreased adrenergic tone may cause the diarrhoea
- Metronidazole 400 mg three times daily (repeated if necessary), anticholinergic agents (amitriptyline), clonidine 500 µg three times daily, subcutaneous octreotide and careful diabetic control can be tried
- Pseudo-obstruction with constipation and severe abdominal pain can be intractable. Prokinetic agents, stool softening laxatives and meticulous diabetic control may help

Concomitant disease

Diseases associated with diabetes include coeliac disease (iron deficiency is a clue), acute pancreatitis (may present with ketoacidosis), chronic pancreatitis (consider alcohol or haemochromatosis), fatty liver (10% of diabetics have abnormal liver enzymes) and mesenteric ischaemia.

Thyrotoxicosis

- Diarrhoea is a well-recognized feature and can be the presenting feature
- Mildly abnormal liver function tests are also common and return to normal when euthyroid
- Occasionally frank malabsorption, abdominal pain or jaundice can occur
- Ulcerative colitis is said to be associated

Hypothyroidism

- Constipation of recent onset should always raise the possibility of myxoedema. Pseudo-obstruction or spurious diarrhoea due to faecal impaction may occur in hypothyroidism
- Ascites occurs in extreme cases, but hypothyroidism is also associated with primary biliary cirrhosis

Addison's disease

Anorexia, weight loss and abdominal pain are common non-specific symptoms in gastroenterology outpatients. If common causes are excluded, Addison's should be considered before symptoms are attributed to a functional disorder.

Multiple endocrine neoplasia

See p. 148.

13.4 **Neoplastic and paraneoplastic disorders**

• Intestinal metastases occur in up to 20% of all non-gut cancers. Breast, lung, ovarian cancer and melanoma are the commonest source. Serosal metastases may cause pain, ascites, obstruction or recurrent gastrointestinal bleeding

• Paraneoplastic pseudo-obstruction is a rare feature of small cell lung cancer

• Chemotherapy can cause diarrhoea due to *Cl. difficile* (especially with neutropenia, also termed 'typhlitis'), mucositis (malnutrition may be critical and require parenteral nutrition) or autonomic neuropathy

13.5 **Connective tissue disease**

Rheumatoid arthritis

• Dysphagia may be due to impaired mastication (temporomandibular arthritis) or oesophageal dysmotility

• Anaemia is common. Consider NSAID-induced peptic ulceration (p. 126), enteropathy or colitis, coincidental colonic pathology (such as caecal carcinoma) or small intestinal villous atrophy (very rarely due to NSAIDs), anaemia of chronic disease, and drug-induced haemolysis or marrow suppression (sulphasalazine, penicillamine, gold). Essential investigations include haematinics, reticulocyte count and Coombs' test, endoscopy with distal duodenal biopsy, and barium enema or colonoscopy

• Abdominal pain may be due to a peptic ulcer, but acalculous cholecystitis, appendicitis and mesenteric vasculitis must be considered. Small intestinal obstruction can very rarely be caused by NSAID-induced strictures, which are best detected by small bowel enema

• Malabsorption may rarely be caused by amyloidosis, or drugs (NSAIDs, gold)

• Bloody diarrhoea may be due to ischaemic colitis, gold or NSAID-induced colitis, or infection (*Cl. difficile*). Stool culture, toxin assay, plain abdominal X-ray, colonoscopy and serial biopsies should identify the cause

Systemic sclerosis

- Dysphagia is characteristic, often with severe oesophagitis, a peptic stricture and aperistalsis on oesophageal manometry. High dose omeprazole (40–80 mg daily and cisapride) usually help. Specialist advice should be sought. Surgery (Roux-en-Y anastomosis) is a last resort
- Diarrhoea may be due to bacterial overgrowth and often responds to antibiotics on an intermittent or cyclical basis (p. 259). Small bowel radiology shows characteristic pseudosacculation
- Constipation is also due to intestinal dysmotility and is often progressive, ultimately causing pseudo-obstruction. Treatment is difficult. Stool softening and stimulant laxatives are often needed in combination
- Malnutrition is common, often due to dysphagia and intestinal dysmotility. Nutrition supplements are appropriate at an early stage. A smaller mouth may need a smaller spoon. Any decision to start parenteral nutrition should be carefully considered, since by this stage the patient usually has poor manual dexterity and is entering the terminal phase of a progressive disease

Systemic lupus erythematosus

- Dysphagia, abdominal pain and bloating are common, due to oesophageal and intestinal motility. Active disease should be controlled and prokinetics, antispasmodics or tricyclic agents may help
- Mesenteric vasculitis affects about 2%. Severe pain (exclude pancreatitis), intestinal haemorrhage or peritonitis suggest the diagnosis. Mortality is high. Cyclophosphamide may be more effective than steroids as an adjunct to surgery for perforation or ischaemic bowel

Polymyositis

- Dysphagia is common and may be the presenting feature. The association of dysphagia with a systemic illness suggests the diagnosis, confirmed by elevated muscle enzymes (creatine kinase, aldolase)
- Up to 10% of patients with polymyositis–dermatomyositis have an underlying malignancy, which may be gastric or colonic

Vasculitis

- Behçet's syndrome is a rare cause of ileocaecal disease. An abdominal

bruit suggests a vasculitis rather than Crohn's disease, but the two conditions can be similar and occasionally overlap
- Henoch–Schönlein purpura is characterized by abdominal pain, purpuric rash on the extensor surfaces and renal impairment. Melaena or rectal bleeding may occur; adults of any age, as well as children, may be affected

NSAIDs and dyspepsia

See p. 126.

13.6 Renal disease

Chronic renal failure

- Anorexia, dyspepsia and reflux are common, often with a normal endoscopy, although peptic ulcers are more common in patients on haemodialysis. Acid suppression, domperidone or cisapride can be tried for symptomatic relief if a peptic ulcer is excluded
- Gastrointestinal bleeding is common. Once a peptic ulcer has been excluded, angiodysplasia and uraemic platelet dysfunction are common causes. Anecdotal reports suggest that oestrogen therapy (p. 14) may help. Colonic haemorrhage may be due to isolated caecal or rectal ulcers, diverticula or stercoral ulcers and may be life-threatening. Active resuscitation, diagnosis and definitive treatment should be the approach. The temptation to delay colonoscopy or surgery (because the patient is 'too ill') should usually be resisted, because delay increases mortality
- Diarrhoea is commonly due to *Cl. difficile* ('uraemic colitis' is an obsolete term, before the prevalence of pseudomembranous colitis was recognized). Occasionally, chronic diarrhoea can be due to bile salt malabsorption. Cholestyramine is worth trying, but consider other systemic causes of renal failure that may affect the gut (vasculitis, amyloid)

Transplantation

- Up to half of early post-transplant deaths are gastrointestinal-related. Haemorrhage from peptic ulcer is frequent, but perforation and enteritis occur
- CMV oesophagitis, enteritis or colitis should be considered. Diagnosis is by endoscopy (aphthoid or diffuse ulceration), biopsy (inclusion bodies) and serology

- Colonic or small bowel perforation is common, possibly due to ischaemia, immunosuppression or faecal impaction

Anaemia

Anaemia should not be attributed to renal failure without considering gastrointestinal blood loss. Active investigation (endoscopy, distal duodenal biopsy, barium enema or colonoscopy) is cost-effective, since treatment of blood loss reduces the dose of expensive erythropoietin.

13.7 Cardiorespiratory disease

Myocardial infarction and acute gastrointestinal bleeding

- Haematemesis or melaena in the immediate postinfarct period is not that uncommon (between five and 10 cases/year in a hospital serving 500 000). Active resuscitation is essential, but endoscopy is potentially dangerous, since it may provoke dysrrhythmias. If the bleeding is minor and self-limiting, endoscopy is best delayed for 6 weeks after infarction and empirical acid suppression (proton-pump inhibitor) given meanwhile
- If bleeding continues, endoscopy should be performed by an experienced endoscopist on the coronary care unit, with supplemental oxygen, adequate sedation, ECG, blood pressure and oximetry monitoring. The cardiology registrar should be present to monitor the ECG during the procedure. The aim is to find and inject a bleeding point. A combination of 1:10 000 adrenaline and thrombin appears to be most successful. Surgery is avoided if possible, because mortality in the postinfarct period is very high

Chronic gastrointestinal bleeding

- An association between aortic stenosis and intestinal angiodysplasia has long been speculated. Portal hypertension in tricuspid regurgitation is another unusual cause
- Gastroduodenal and colonic lesions must be excluded by endoscopy and colonoscopy, in the first instance, followed by a small bowel enema (Fig. 9.8, p. 362)
- Valve replacement with a xenograft which will not require anticoagulation is usually advisable, but has an unpredictable effect on blood loss. If regular iron does not maintain the haemoglobin, oestrogens can be tried (p. 14)

Thrombolysis or anticoagulation in dyspeptic patients

- Dyspepsia or a history of peptic ulceration is *not* a contraindication to thrombolysis or starting heparin, *unless* there has been a documented ulcer within the past month
- Endoscopy is sensible prior to starting warfarin if there is a history of dyspepsia

Reflux and asthma

Nocturnal asthma may be a symptom of reflux (p. 62), but the association is often difficult to define. An empirical trial of a proton-pump inhibitor for 4 weeks with monitoring of peak flow rates is appropriate when treating nocturnal symptoms.

Miscellaneous disorders

Osteoporosis

- Coeliac disease, ulcerative colitis and Crohn's disease all increase the risk of osteoporosis independently of corticosteroids, although steroids hasten bone loss within 3–6 months of use
- HRT delays or abolishes bone loss in controlled trials of women with inflammatory bowel disease or malabsorption. This alone is sufficient indication for advising HRT in postmenopausal women with these conditions
- Calcium supplements have a debatable role in preventing osteoporosis. Premenopausal women should be encouraged to maintain an 'adequate' calcium intake, but recommended daily allowances are confusing. 50–100 mmol calcium/day (1–2 g calcium) is often advised when there is intestinal disease. Milk is the only appreciable source of calcium and contains 1.02 g/L, or 0.58 g/pint. Very few patients will drink or tolerate 1–2 L of milk/day. A sensible balance is to supplement clearly inadequate intake (< 15 mmol/day, or < 250 mL milk/day)
- Bone densitometry (dual emission X-ray absorptiometry, DEXA) is the best way of evaluating osteoporosis and is indicated in men or premenopausal women who have taken or are likely to take steroids for long periods (6 months or more). If bone density is < 66% age- and sex-matched controls, biphosphonates should be considered. There are no adequate controlled trials of biphosphonates in intestinal disease, because the

pharmaceutical companies are wary about side-effects (nausea, diarrhoea). However, biphosphonates are often well tolerated

Bone marrow transplantation

• Three principal causes of intestinal and hepatic disease after transplantation are: chemotherapy, infections and graft-versus-host disease
• Pretransplant chemo/radiotherapy causes symptoms (diarrhoea, abdominal pain) by day 10 due to 'mucositis' damaging crypt cell proliferation, but resolves by day 30. It may also cause veno-occlusive disease, with painful hepatomegaly and jaundice, especially in patients with pre-existing hepatitis B or C. Post-transplant chemotherapy (cyclosporin, methotrexate) may promote intestinal lymphoma
• Infections occur during the recovery phase from transplant—bacterial or fungal before day 30, viral thereafter. Diarrhoea due to *Cl. difficile*, *Candida* oesophagitis, CMV colitis or hepatitis are among the common infections
• Graft-versus-host disease is an immunological phenomenon causing rashes, diarrhoea with sloughing of the intestinal mucosa, protein-losing enteropathy, or cholestasis in the acute phase (1–3 months). Chronic graft-versus-host disease at 3–15 months causes cholestasis with bile duct obliteration and malabsorption due to sub-mucosal fibrosis and a scleroderma-like syndrome. Diagnosis is made by hepatic or endoscopic intestinal biopsy. Treatment with nutritional support and immuno-suppression is difficult

Blood coagulation disorders

• Haemophiliacs may bleed from a peptic ulcer or develop acute abdominal pain from intramural haemorrhage, but chronic liver disease due to hepatitis C (p. 189) and AIDS (p. 393) are more serious problems
• von Willebrand's disease quite frequently causes chronic iron deficiency without an identifiable source of blood loss. Iron supplements are appropriate, with oestrogen therapy for women, or tranexamic acid for men if anaemia persists. Desamino-D-arginine vasopressin (dDAVP) is rarely effective for chronic loss
• Thrombotic thrombocytopenic purpura causes thrombocytopenia, microangiopathic haemolytic anaemia, fever, renal insufficiency and confusion, often with abdominal pain. Pancreatitis, mesenteric infarction and acalculous cholecystitis are complications. Plasmapheresis and FFP or

cryosupernatant (with high molecular weight von Willebrand factor removed) infusion are appropriate

Neuromuscular disease

• Dysphagia commonly complicates cerebrovascular or progressive neurological disease. Endoscopy is often normal, but necessary to exclude other pathology. Prokinetic agents rarely help. When nutrition is compromised, percutaneous gastrostomy is appropriate (p. 408)

• Constipation is a major problem after spinal injury, or progressive neuromuscular disease such as motor neurone disease, Parkinson's disease, mitochondrial myopathy, other myopathies, or multiple sclerosis. Fibre often makes symptoms worse. Early use of stool softening agents and occasional stimulant laxatives should be given. When constipation is intractable, vigorous bowel clearout with Picolax and high doses of lactulose (40–80 mL daily) to prevent silting up again may help. Spurious diarrhoea from constipation is best treated by keeping the rectum empty with a Micralax on alternate days. Faecal impaction can also be treated with polyethylene glycol (Movicol 8 sachets in 6 h) (p. 328). Effective treatment of constipation, however, may lead to faecal incontinence

• Chronic abdominal pain and pseudo-obstruction can become intractable. Treatment is unsatisfactory. Analgesics, laxatives, tricyclic agents or serotonin-reuptake inhibitors can be tried, often without success. Faecal impaction can be a cause of confusion or apparent neurological deterioration

Autonomic dysreflexia

Severe hypertension and tachycardia with subsequent subarachnoid haemorrhage or seizures in tetraplegic patients can be provoked by faecal impaction or urinary retention. Prevention by avoiding constipation and routine catheterization is the key.

14 Procedures and Investigations

14.1 Practical techniques

Rectal examination

Rectal examination is an essential part of every complete physical examination and fundamental when there is a history of rectal bleeding, melaena, abdominal pain, altered bowel habit or anaemia. It is all too often cursorily performed.

- Explain the procedure. It often helps to sympathize with the embarrassment and discomfort
- Position the patient in the left lateral position
- Part the buttocks to inspect the perineum for skin tags (violaceous and oedematous in Crohn's) or excoriation. If there is a history of incontinence or neurological disorder, test perineal sensation with an orange stick
- Gently insert the lubricated, gloved right index finger and assess anal sphincter tone, then introduce it to its fullest extent
- Sweep the finger round in a full circle, consciously feeling anterior, lateral and posterior walls of the rectum. Cancer of the rectum (15% of all colorectal cancers can be felt on digital examination) is felt as an indurated ulcerating lesion, a stenosis or proliferating tumour. Faecal residue may sometimes be confused with polyps. A villous tumour has a characteristic feel, somewhat like plastic bubble-packing
- Clean the anus after examination. Inspect the material on the glove, which can also be used for microscopy or testing for occult blood

Rigid sigmoidoscopy

Proctosigmoidoscopy should always be performed before referring a patient for barium enema.

- A rigid 25 cm instrument with a fibreoptic light source is commonly used. Before starting, check that the light source fits the instrument and works, that the air insufflator is connected, that the obturator fits, that there are biopsy forceps, formalin, gloves, tissues and lubricant jelly
- Explain sympathetically to the patient that the procedure may cause some discomfort and a desire to defaecate, but should not be painful. Deep breathing often relieves the discomfort. No bowel preparation is necessary
- Position the patient in the left lateral position, lying almost transversely across the bed or couch. Unsuccessful examination is often the consequence of faulty positioning

- Perform a careful rectal examination before introducing 5 cm of the lubricated sigmoidoscope through the anal sphincter in the direction of the umbilicus
- Remove the obturator and close the eyepiece. Gently insufflate air and introduce the sigmoidoscope under direct vision. The tip has to point posteriorly along the sacral curve, so the examiner's head must move forward
- If mucosa occludes the lumen, withdraw the sigmoidoscope 1 cm, insufflate a little more air (too much is uncomfortable and can be dangerous) then move the tip further posteriorly, or laterally. Faecal residue can be moved out of the way with the tip of the sigmoidoscope, but if stool occludes the lumen, it can usually be displaced by swab-holding forceps
- Examine the mucosa up to the rectosigmoid junction (15 cm) and beyond if not too uncomfortable for the patient
- Biopsies should routinely be taken if the patient has had diarrhoea, because they may detect unexpected pathology and also provide an objective record of the procedure. The St Mark's pinch biopsy forceps with 2 mm cups are safest and easiest to use. Most other biopsy forceps with larger cups were originally designed to remove rectal polyps or tumour tissue and take too deep a biopsy from flat mucosa. It is following a biopsy with these larger forceps that a barium enema should be delayed for 3 days to reduce the risk of perforation
- Continue to inspect the mucosa when withdrawing the instrument. Clean the anus and document in the notes the distance examined, appearance of the mucosa and stool, and whether a biopsy was taken

Abdominal paracentesis

Diagnostic paracentesis ('ascitic tap') is essential in any patient with ascites (p. 168). Therapeutic paracentesis is increasingly used in the management of tense ascites (p. 170).

Diagnostic paracentesis

- An aseptic technique performed at the bedside
- Clean the right flank around the site midway between the umbilicus and the anterior superior iliac spine. Cover the area with a dressing towel with a hole torn in the middle, over the paracentesis site
- Infiltrate 2 mL 2% lignocaine through a 21 gauge needle intradermally and more deeply to anaesthetize the peritoneum. Some consider anaesthetic unnecessary, but reflect on how you would like the procedure performed on yourself

- Aspirate ascites through a 19 gauge needle attached to a 20 mL syringe. If unsuccessful, ask the patient to lie a little further on the right side, or use a longer needle (lumbar puncture needle). Inspect the fluid (Table 5.8, p. 169) send it for protein estimation, culture and cytology (p. 169)

Therapeutic paracentesis

- Performed in the same site as diagnostic paracentesis, but it is important to make sure the patient has an empty bladder
- No 'paracentesis kit' is readily available, but the best technique is to use the soft catheter designed for suprapubic bladder aspiration. Alternatives are a wide-bore intravenous cannula, but this almost always blocks unless tediously held in position, or a peritoneal dialysis catheter. This has the disadvantages of being large and rigid with connections designed not to fit catheter bags or ordinary intravenous giving sets
- After cleaning and anaesthetizing the skin, make a small stab incision with a no. 15 surgical blade to allow easy introduction of the cannula into the right flank midway between the umbilicus and anterior superior iliac spine
- Insert the suprapubic catheter, remove the trocar, connect the catheter bag and secure the catheter with a suture and tape
- Give 100 mL 20% salt-poor albumin for every 5 L of ascites drained to avoid intravascular volume depletion

Nasogastric tube insertion

Fine-bore (8 French gauge) nasogastric feeding has transformed enteral nutritional support (p. 405) and does not interfere with the swallowing reflex in stroke patients. Fine-bore tubes have a wire stylet to help introduction and the procedure is explained below; ordinary nasogastric tubes (12 or 14 French gauge) do not have a stylet, but are otherwise inserted in a similar way.

- Explain the procedure to the patient
- Sit the patient up, with neck slightly flexed
- Ensure the stylet can be inserted and removed easily from the tube (lubricate with water)
- Lubricate the end of the tube with gel and gently insert through the nose into the back of the throat (nasopharynx)
- Allow the patient to rest and give a sip of water to hold in their mouth
- Ask the patient to swallow and gently advance the tube
- If coughing occurs, stop and withdraw the tube into the nasopharynx before starting again

- Once the tube is half-way down, withdraw the stylet a few centimetres to make sure it runs freely
- Continue insertion until about 10 cm remains. Withdraw the stylet. If it sticks, carefully pull the tube back until the stylet can be withdrawn before reintroducing the tube
- Confirm the tube is in the stomach by aspirating gastric contents or the bubble test (sharply inject 20 mL air whilst listening for bubbling over the epigastrium with a stethoscope)
- Obtain an X-ray to check position if the conscious level is impaired or if there is any doubt about position after aspirating or using the bubble test
- Tape the tube securely to the nose and along the skin under the cheek bone

(14.2) Houseman's checklist

The explanation given in each section is designed to help those unfamiliar with the procedures to describe them to patients. The history and examination must be documented in the notes before any invasive procedure. A preprinted history sheet saves time when there is direct access to endoscopy from general practitioners. Resuscitation equipment must be immediately available for any procedure that involves sedation.

Upper gastrointestinal endoscopy

Indications

Diagnostic
- Dyspepsia or abdominal pain, especially when age >45 years or after gastric surgery (p. 86)
- Haematemesis or melaena (p. 10)
- Weight loss
- Iron-deficiency anaemia (always take distal duodenal biopsies to look for villous atrophy, p. 359)
- Persistent vomiting (p. 95)
- Biopsy of gastric lesions detected by barium meal (p. 86)
- Biopsy of distal duodenal mucosa for coeliac disease (p. 251)
- Surveillance of Barrett's oesophagus (p. 66)
- Follow-up of gastric ulcer

Therapeutic
- Sclerotherapy of bleeding oesophageal varices (p. 15)

- Injection, thermocoagulation or laser photocoagulation of other bleeding lesions (p. 14)
- Dilatation of oesophageal or pyloric strictures
- Palliation of oesophageal cancer with plastic or self-expanding metal stents, alcohol injection or laser therapy (p. 73)
- Positioning of percutaneous gastrostomy or nasojejunal feeding tubes

Preparation

- Nil by mouth for at least 4 h (longer after a large meal)
- Water only for 12 h and nil by mouth for 8 h, if pyloric obstruction is suspected
- Delay for 24 h after any upper gastrointestinal barium study (such as a barium swallow for dysphagia): barium can block the suction channel of the endoscope
- Written consent, after explanation

Explanation

- Intravenous sedation (often midazolam 2.5–10 mg) is usually given. The procedure can readily be performed without sedation, only using local anaesthetic spray to the pharynx, but requires good cooperation between endoscopist and patient. Many patients prefer light sedation; some choose heavier sedation so that they have no recall
- The pharynx is sprayed with lignocaine 1% to reduce the gag reflex
- The flexible endoscope, the diameter of a small finger, is gently passed into the oesophagus and steered through the stomach into the duodenum (a diagram helps patients to understand)
- Breathing is not impaired, but a probe (from a pulse oximeter) is strapped to a finger to measure blood oxygen saturation. Supplemental oxygen through a nasal cannula should be routine
- The procedure takes 5–10 min
- Eating or drinking is allowed 30–60 min after the procedure if local anaesthetic spray has been used, when pharyngeal sensation has recovered
- Findings and instructions should be given after the procedure in the presence of a friend, or written down, because amnesia often follows sedation

Complications

- Sore throat occurs, but is transient. Occasionally nasal oxygen dries out the nasal mucosa, which later results in hypersecretion for 24 h
- Amnesia following sedation sometimes persists for hours, even though the patient appears to have recovered. Patients must not be allowed to

drive or perform a responsible job without assistance for 24 h (looking after children, driving, operating machinery, signing legal documents)
- Perforation (< 0.1%)
- Cardiorespiratory arrest or death (< 0.01%) are very rare and mainly affect the very sick or elderly, but remain a risk which must be considered when requesting the procedure

Antibiotic prophylaxis for endoscopy, sigmoidoscopy, colonoscopy and barium enema

Indications
- Prosthetic heart valves
- Previous endocarditis
- Synthetic vascular graft < 1 year old
- Severe neutropenia (< 100×10^9/L)
- Surgically constructed systemic–pulmonary shunt

Recommendations

Patients not allergic to penicillin
Patients not allergic to penicillin, and who have not had penicillin more than once in the previous month:
- Adults: 1 g amoxycillin and 120 mg gentamicin intravenously over 3–4 min before the procedure
- Children under 10 years: 500 mg amoxycillin and gentamicin 2 mg/kg body weight intravenously as above

Patients allergic to penicillin
Patients allergic to penicillin, or who have had penicillin more than once in the previous month
- Adults: vancomycin 1 g infusion over 2 h followed by gentamicin 120 mg intravenously before the start of the procedure; or teicoplanin 400 mg and gentamicin 120 mg before the start of the procedure
- Children under 10 years: vancomycin 20 mg/kg infusion and gentamicin 2 mg/kg as above; or teicoplanin 6 mg/kg and gentamicin 2 mg/kg as above

Patients with severe neutropenia
Add metronidazole 7.5 mg/kg intravenously to any of the above regimes.

Jejunal biopsy

- Two distal duodenal biopsies (from the third part of the duodenum) at upper gastrointestinal endoscopy are satisfactory for most purposes (p. 249). Whilst a normal biopsy excludes coeliac disease, duodenal villi can appear stunted when overlying Brunner's glands: repeat biopsy, sometimes using a paediatric colonoscope instead of a gastroscope to reach the jejunum, or a jejunal biopsy with a Crosby–Watson biopsy capsule is then indicated if there is any doubt about the diagnosis
- Unusual causes of malabsorption, including giardiasis, lymphoma, Whipple's disease or amyloidosis can also be diagnosed by jejunal biopsy (p. 265). Multiple jejunal biopsies can be obtained with a Quinton hydraulic biopsy instrument at specialist centres; this is helpful if there is doubt about the diagnosis after using simpler techniques

Indications

Diagnostic
- Diagnosis of coeliac disease and repeated, after 3–6 months on a gluten-free diet, to confirm response (p. 252)
- Iron-deficiency anaemia, at the time of the first upper gastrointestinal endoscopy
- Persistent diarrhoea (Fig. 7.1, p. 237)
- Folate deficiency
- Weight loss
- Diagnosis of *Giardia lamblia* infection, if stool examination normal (p. 258)
- Occasionally for diagnosis of small bowel bacterial overgrowth or hypolactasia (p. 260)

Preparation
- Platelet count $> 100 \times 10^9$/L
- Coagulation studies (INR < 1.3, or prothrombin time < 22 s)
- Nil by mouth for 4 h
- Consent, after explanation

Explanation
- Performed in X-ray department, or where fluoroscopy is available
- The pharynx is sprayed with lignocaine 1%. Sedation is sometimes necessary
- A fine-bore tube (3 mm diameter) attached to the biopsy capsule is swallowed, whilst the patient is standing. When 60 cm has been swallowed,

the patient lies down and the position is checked fluoroscopically. The tube is steered into the jejunum (Meditech catheter), or passes spontaneously (Crosby–Watson capsule) and the biopsy is triggered by suction, after which it is removed

- The procedure takes between 15 min (Meditech) and 60 min (Crosby–Watson)
- The biopsy is painless, although swallowing the capsule is often unpleasant
- Eating or drinking after completion is allowed at least 30 min after the anaesthetic spray

Complications

- Sore throat occurs, but is transient
- Bleeding occurs in <0.1%. Perforation has been reported in malnourished patients, but is extremely rare
- Retained capsule is extremely uncommon. The tube is cut as short as possible and the remainder should pass spontaneously

Colonoscopy

Indications

Diagnostic

- Investigation of bloody diarrhoea, in preference to a barium enema
- Rectal bleeding, especially when recurrent, or after a normal or inadequate barium enema (p. 240)
- Persistent diarrhoea (Fig. 7.1, p. 237), to obtain serial mucosal biopsies
- Assessing the distribution of disease in patients with Crohn's disease (p. 279) or ulcerative colitis (p. 302)
- Biopsy of a lesion detected by barium enema
- Iron-deficiency anaemia (p. 361)
- Surveillance for colorectal cancer in selected patients (p. 335)

Therapeutic

- Polypectomy
- Diathermy or laser photocoagulation of angiodysplasia or rectal tumours
- Dilatation of colonic strictures in selected patients (p. 290)

Preparation

Regimens vary enormously between endoscopy units. The following is a simple and widely available approach.

- Low-residue diet (no fruit, vegetables or bread) for 48 h and nothing solid for 24 h before the procedure. Stop iron supplements
- Sodium picosulphate and magnesium citrate (Picolax), 1 sachet at 8 a.m. and another at 4 p.m. on the day before the procedure, with a cup of water every hour to ensure a good fluid intake (inadequate fluid is usually the cause of poor preparation)
- Consent, after explanation

Explanation

- Sedation is given (such as intravenous midazolam 2.5–10 mg), often with intravenous pethidine 25–50 mg or hyoscine butylbromide as well
- The flexible colonoscope (diameter of a large finger) is passed per rectum, around the colon. Fluoroscopy is sometimes helpful
- The procedure takes 10–20 min
- The patient goes home accompanied, an hour or two after the procedure

Complications

- Abdominal discomfort after the procedure is common, but rarely persists for more than a few hours. It can be reduced if air, which is insufflated during the procedure, is aspirated during withdrawal of the colonoscope, or if carbon dioxide is used instead of air for insufflation. Faecal soiling can occur, which can be distressing
- Incomplete examination occurs in 5–20%, depending on operator experience. A barium enema or repeat examination is then indicated
- Perforation is rare (0.2%), but more common in acute colitis, severe diverticulosis or ischaemic colitis, which are relative contraindications to colonoscopy. Haemorrhage after biopsy or polypectomy is even less common

Flexible sigmoidoscopy

Indications

- Investigation of bright red rectal bleeding, especially in young patients (< 30 years), when a distal source of bleeding is suspected and full examination of the colon is unnecessary
- Investigation of choice in acute colitis in hospitalized patients, when full colonoscopy is unsafe
- An alternative to rigid sigmoidoscopy for initial examination of the distal colon in outpatients, if the equipment and facilities for preparation are available. Up to 75% of colorectal tumours are accessible at flexible sigmoidoscopy

Preparation

- Phosphate enema 30–60 min before the procedure
- Can be performed without any preparation at all, but views are usually sub-optimal and a phosphate enema is safe and reasonably well tolerated even in acute colitis

Explanation

- Usually performed without sedation, although sedation can be given if necessary as long as appropriate facilities are available (on an endoscopy unit, rather than outpatients)
- An ordinary colonoscope (see above) is usually used to examine the rectum and sigmoid colon. Short (60 cm) flexible sigmoidoscopes are available, but are less versatile than a colonoscope and cost only slightly less
- The procedure takes 5 min

ERCP

Indications

See p. 224; Fig. 4.2, p. 137; Fig. 6.5, p. 225.

Preparation

- Platelet count $> 100 \times 10^9$/L
- Coagulation studies (INR < 1.3, prothrombin time < 22 s)
- Nil by mouth for 4 h
- Premedication policy differs between units. Some always use parenteral sedative and antibiotic premedication; others only use oral antibiotics and perform diagnostic ERCP as an outpatient
- Parenteral premedication with intramuscular fentanyl 50–100 µg and droperidol 5 mg, with intravenous piperacillin 4 g or gentamicin 120 mg 1 h before the procedure is one regime for inpatients
- Oral ciprofloxacin 750 mg 60–90 min before the procedure is as effective as intravenous antibiotic prophylaxis
- Consent, after explanation

Explanation

- The procedure is performed in the X-ray department
- Effective sedation (intravenous midazolam 5–10 mg with pethidine 50 mg) is given, depending on premedication and individual needs of the patient
- A side-viewing endoscope is passed into the duodenum. A fine catheter is inserted through the ampulla, into the pancreatic duct and then into the bile duct. Contrast is injected and X-rays taken

- Therapeutic procedures include sphincterotomy (5–15 mm incision through the ampulla), precut sphincterotomy (when the bile duct cannot be cannulated), stent insertion (through a stricture) or stone retrieval (by basket, balloon, lithotripsy or occasionally dissolution)
- The procedure takes 20–60 min
- The patient can go home the same day, unless a therapeutic procedure has been performed

Complications

- Complete examination is possible in >90%, but more than one attempt may be needed, especially for therapeutic procedures
- Acute pancreatitis (2%; the serum amylase always rises after ERCP, but in the absence of abdominal pain and vomiting can be ignored)
- Haemorrhage after sphincterotomy (1%), requiring prompt surgery since it rarely stops spontaneously. If haemorrhage is haemodynamically significant, it is rarely possible to obtain adequate views to perform effective endoscopic haemostasis
- Cholangitis (2%)
- Death (<0.5%)

Liver biopsy

Indications

Diagnostic

- Persistently elevated (>twofold) liver enzymes 6 months after viral hepatitis (p. 183)
- Asymptomatic elevation of liver enzymes (Fig. 5.7, p. 208), especially in alcohol abuse (p. 200)
- Clinical suspicion of cirrhosis (p. 197), chronic active hepatitis (p. 185) or carcinoma (p. 204)
- Biopsy of hepatic lesions detected by ultrasound or CT scan
- Investigation of unexplained pyrexia (to detect granulomas, p. 196, miliary tuberculosis, lymphoma or systemic vasculitis)
- Abnormal liver function in relatives of patients with familial hepatic disease (haemochromatosis, Wilson's disease)
- Contraindications include a bleeding diathesis, ascites, extrahepatic biliary obstruction, suspected hydatid disease, hepatic peliosis or haemangioma, or emphysema

Preparation

- Platelet count > 100×10^9/L
- Coagulation studies (INR < 1.3, prothrombin time < 22 s). Give a single dose of vitamin K 10 mg and recheck clotting 48 h later if coagulation is disordered; otherwise infuse 2–4 units of FFP immediately prior to biopsy
- Consent, after explanation
- Liver biopsy should not be performed after 2 p.m., so that observations can be done when staff are readily available and complications recognized
- Ultrasound or CT scan guided liver biopsy is helpful for focal lesions, but need to be discussed and coordinated with a radiologist
- Biopsy can safely be performed as an outpatient if performed before 10 a.m. (to allow 8 h observation), in patients who have normal coagulation and platelet count, and who live within 10 miles of the hospital, as long as the biopsy is successful in a single pass

Explanation

- The procedure is usually performed on the ward, but in some hospitals is always performed by a radiologist under ultrasound control. Sedation is not usually necessary
- Lignocaine 2% is carefully infiltrated down to the capsule between the eighth and 10th ribs, where there is dullness to percussion in the mid-axillary line. Effective local anaesthesia is essential. Always use at least 10 mL 2% lignocaine and use a long needle (sometimes a spinal needle) in obese patients. The patient should not experience pain and this dose of lignocaine will not cause cardiac depression
- A 2 mm nick in the skin is made with a scalpel
- Breathing is rehearsed (breath must be held in full expiration during biopsy)
- Biopsy with a fine needle (Trucut or Menghini) takes a few seconds
- After the biopsy the patient lies on the right side for 2 h and then in bed for 6 h. Pulse and blood pressure are measured every 15 min for 1 h, every 30 min for 2 h and then hourly up to 8 h
- If being performed on an outpatient, the patient must be seen by a doctor before discharge and given the ward telephone number to call if there are problems overnight
- Transjugular or laparoscopic biopsy are specialist techniques when percutaneous biopsy is contraindicated due to disordered coagulation or ascites, or impossible

Complications

- Local pain (often pleuritic or in the shoulder) is common, but usually

relieved by oral paracetamol 2 tablets every 4 h. Severe pain may indicate a sub-capsular haematoma: ultrasound will detect a significant haematoma, but resolution of pain with analgesics within 24–48 h is usual
- Pneumothorax is rarely clinically apparent and does not need drainage unless breathing is compromised
- Bleeding, requiring transfusion (< 0.5%) or operation (very rarely)
- Death (< 0.1%) may follow inappropriate biopsy (colon, pancreas, gall bladder, inferior vena cava), or a tear in the liver capsule

Percutaneous biliary procedures

Percutaneous transhepatic cholangiograms are rarely performed now that ERCP is the procedure of first choice. The technique is, however, occasionally useful.

Indications

Diagnostic
Cholestatic jaundice with a dilated biliary tree (Fig. 6.4, p. 223) when ERCP is unavailable or impossible (p. 224)

Therapeutic
- When ERCP is initially unsuccessful in cannulating an obstructed biliary tree: performed in conjunction with ERCP by insertion of a wire which is then retrieved endoscopically, so that a stent can be inserted (p. 224)
- Insertion of a percutaneous self-expanding metal stent across biliary strictures (especially at the bifurcation) which cannot be cannulated at ERCP
- External decompression of an obstructed biliary tree is rarely performed now, because of the high incidence of infection

Preparation
As for ERCP.

Explanation
- The procedure is performed by a radiologist. Sedation is often helpful
- A fine needle is inserted into the liver, in the eighth or ninth intercostal space. Contrast is gently injected as the needle is withdrawn under fluoroscopy, until an intrahepatic duct is delineated. Contrast is then injected to outline the biliary tree and X-rays taken
- The procedure takes 15–30 min
- Observation after the procedure is the same as for liver biopsy

Complications

- Local pain is relieved by paracetamol
- Biliary leak is rare, even in obstructive jaundice, and resolves spontane-ously. Analgesia (intramuscular pethidine 50–100 mg) may be necessary
- Cholangitis is very rare, except when an external drainage catheter is left *in situ*

14.3 Radiology

Requests

Salient clinical features, rather than a statement of the suspected diagnosis, help the radiologist interpret X-rays. Stating the specific question to be answered by the radiological investigation is also helpful. Potential complicating factors (diabetes, epilepsy, allergies, pacemakers) should be mentioned, especially for contrast or invasive procedures.

Discussion with the radiologist about the most appropriate imaging technique saves the patient unnecessary investigation and allows the radiologist to proceed at his or her discretion, depending on the findings (e.g. from ultrasound to CT scan). A visit to the X-ray department and 'please' or 'thank you' on the request form are simple courtesies that pay dividends!

Plain film checklist

Plain, supine abdominal and erect chest X-rays are indicated for any patient with acute abdominal pain (p. 28). Erect abdominal X-ray is only needed to detect fluid levels when there is doubt about the diagnosis of intestinal obstruction.

On a plain abdominal X-ray
Look for:
- Sub-diaphragmatic gas, or clear delineation of liver, kidneys or spleen (perforated viscus, p. 31)
- Faecal distribution:
  - throughout the colon (constipation)
  - distal extent (identifies the proximal distribution of active ulcerative colitis, or stricture)
- Intestinal diameter:
  - small intestine > 2.5 cm (obstruction)
  - colon > 6.0 cm (obstruction, toxic dilatation, Fig. 1.6 p. 48)

- Mucosal pattern:
  - thickened wall (acute ulcerative colitis or Crohn's disease)
  - mucosal islands (small radio-opaque projections into the lumen in acute colitis, p. 47)
  - thumbprinting (large radio-opaque projections, ischaemic colitis, Fig. 9.6, p. 354)
  - gas in the wall (impending perforation, pneumatosis coli)
- Gas pattern:
  - displaced or separated loops of small bowel (mass effect, inflammation)
  - segment of jejunum ('sentinel loop' in acute pancreatitis)
  - fluid levels (obstruction, on an erect abdominal film)
  - central distribution of normal small bowel (ascites)
  - gas in the biliary tree (cholangitis, recent passage of stone)
- Calculi:
  - along the line of the transverse processes (renal/ureteric)
  - right upper quadrant (gall stones)
  - phleboliths, calcified lymph nodes, foreign bodies or artefacts may be included in the differential diagnosis

Contrast studies

Double contrast studies of upper and lower gastrointestinal tract are routinely performed. Single contrast studies have few indications (p. 458). In a double contrast study, barium coats the mucosa and gas provides the contrast. Effervescent tablets are swallowed, or air is insufflated, to put the mucosa under slight tension. Barium is used unless perforation is suspected, when Gastrografin or non-ionic agents are indicated.

Endoscopy (p. 86) is usually preferable to a barium meal except when pyloric stenosis is suspected and colonoscopy is the procedure of choice instead of a barium enema for investigating bloody diarrhoea or visible rectal bleeding (p. 240). In elderly patients, abdominal CT scan may be more appropriate than a barium enema (p. 429).

Oesophagus

Figures 1.1 (p. 7), 2.3 (p. 69), 2.4 (p. 75), 2.5 (p. 77).

Stomach and duodenum

Figures 3.1 (p. 88), 3.3 (p. 111).

Small bowel

- Barium follow-through is better tolerated and more widely used than small bowel enema, but gives inferior mucosal definition
- Large films of the abdomen are taken at 10–30-min intervals until the barium reaches the caecum. Enhanced films of areas of interest (terminal ileum) are then taken (Fig. 7.3, p. 246; Fig. 8.1, p. 280). Much depends on how closely the procedure is supervised by a radiologist using fluoroscopy if lesions are not to be missed
- Small bowel enema is more troublesome and needs bowel preparation and duodenal intubation, but produces better mucosal definition. It is indicated when mucosal changes may be subtle (Crohn's disease, polyps, diverticula), or if a follow-through examination is unsatisfactory
- Reflux of barium through the ileocaecal valve on a barium enema sometimes defines the terminal ileum very well and should not be overlooked
- A peroral pneumocologram (drinking barium, after bowel preparation, with rectal air insufflation) gives the best views of the caecum and terminal ileum

Large bowel

- Barium enema should only be done after digital rectal examination, sigmoidoscopy and biopsy. It is sensible to wait 72 h after rectal biopsy before a barium enema, but the risk of perforation with modern biopsy forceps is minimal
- Preparation is the same as for colonoscopy. Elderly patients (> 80 years) may need admission for the preparation and procedure
- A smooth muscle relaxant (intravenous hyoscine butylbromide 20 mg or glucagon 1 mg) are usually administered to decrease colonic spasm
- Large films are taken every 10–15 min until the barium reaches the caecum, followed by films of areas of interest (lateral views to show the rectum and posterior rectal space, enhanced views of the flexures or caecum). The procedure takes 20–30 min
- A single contrast enema, without preparation ('instant enema'), is only indicated when there is doubt about the diagnosis of acute colitis, or level of obstruction. The extent of colitis shown by a single contrast barium enema can be misleading. Although it should help distinguish ulcerative, Crohn's and ischaemic colitis (Fig. 9.6, p. 354), a flexible sigmoidoscopy usually gives more information
- If the caecum is not clearly shown, a peroral pneumocologram is indicated

Abdominal and endoscopic ultrasound

Abdominal ultrasound

- Indicated for the investigation of abdominal pain (gall stones, pancreatitis), jaundice, abnormal liver function tests (Fig. 5.7, p. 208), hepatomegaly, ascites or abdominal masses. Doppler examination of blood flow in portal or hepatic veins is appropriate in portal hypertension (p. 175) and of mesenteric blood flow when intestinal ischaemia is suspected (p. 352). These are specialist techniques. Diagnostic biopsy or therapeutic aspiration can be performed under ultrasound control
- An ideal, non-invasive investigation for thin patients
- Whilst reliable in experienced hands, the interpretation is subjective and intestinal gas can prevent adequate views, especially of retroperitoneal structures including the pancreas
- Preparation involves nothing to eat for 4 h if the gall bladder is to be imaged. Failure of the gall bladder to contract after a fatty meal suggests chronic cholecystitis (p. 217) and influences non-surgical management of gall stones (p. 219)
- Ultrasound of other areas of the abdomen needs no preparation, apart from the pelvis, when the bladder should be full

Endoscopic ultrasound

- Endosonography of the rectum, oesophagus, stomach or duodenum give better resolution and more accurate information about the margins of tumour infiltration than transcutaneous ultrasound, but are confined to specialist centres
- When available and in experienced hands, they are useful for preoperative staging of oesophageal, gastric, pancreatic or rectal carcinomas, detection of common bile duct calculi and avoiding unnecessary sphincterotomy, percutaneous drainage of pancreatic pseudocysts and guiding endoscopic biopsy of submucosal lesions
- Intraoperative ultrasound is particularly useful in hepatic resection of tumours or in identifying pancreatic lesions (such as endocrine tumours)

CT scan

Standard CT scanning

- Indicated when ultrasound is not technically possible (fat patients, excessive bowel gas), when doubt about the diagnosis persists (Fig. 4.1, p. 132), for percutaneous biopsy or drainage of intra-abdominal lesions and abscesses, and sometimes as an alternative to contrast radiology in frail patients (p. 429)

- CT scan is better than ultrasound for demonstrating retroperitoneal structures, common bile duct stones or for fat patients, but still needs skilled interpretation
- Contrast (5 mL oral Gastrografin on the evening before the procedure) is given to facilitate definition. Intravenous contrast to define vascular structures is given at the discretion of the radiologist
- Preparation is otherwise the same as for ultrasound

Spiral CT scanning

- Spiral CT scanning is a relatively new technique available in some centres. It uses the same technology, but allows better spatial orientation (including three-dimensional reconstruction) of lesions
- The table moves continuously through a rotating image field, so images may be viewed from different angles and at different intervals, instead of being confined to 1 or 5 mm axial 'cuts'. This improves resolution
- Other advantages include rapid scanning (complete abdominal or thoracic imaging in a single breath hold of 15–18 s), which makes it more suitable for sick patients, and ability to image luminal structures ('virtual colonoscopy')

MRI

- In abdominal pathology, the main role is in imaging the pelvis, particularly complications of perineal Crohn's disease (Fig. 8.2, p. 293). The high signal in fistulae or abscesses allows good definition of complex fistulae, potentially avoiding the need for examination under anaesthetic
- Depending on the available software, it can detect hepatic or pancreatic lesions not identified by CT scanning (particularly endocrine tumours)
- Imaging the biliary tree (magnetic resonance cholangiography) is at an early stage of development and resolution is not yet sufficient to replace ERCP for diagnostic imaging. The patient must be able to hold their breath for long periods (30 s or more) to avoid movement artefact
- Implants of magnetic materials (clips, prosthetic valves, pacemakers) are contraindications, depending on the type of implant

Other imaging techniques

Mesenteric angiography (Fig. 1.3, p. 24)
- Intra-arterial digital subtraction angiography needs less contrast than conventional techniques, for equivalent definition

- Low ionic contrast media (such as Omnipaque) cause fewer side-effects and do not contain iodine, but are much more expensive. They are indicated for patients at increased risk of reactions (asthma, diabetes, cardiac failure, other allergies) or, with care, if there is a history of sensitivity to traditional contrast agents
- Indications include active gastrointestinal bleeding when the source cannot be identified by endoscopy or colonoscopy (p. 23), investigation of recurrent iron-deficiency anaemia when an intestinal arteriovenous malformation is suspected, and investigation of chronic mesenteric ischaemia after Doppler ultrasound studies (p. 352)
- Mesenteric anatomy is shown in Fig. 9.5 (p. 351)

Isotope studies

- The ^{13}C- or ^{14}C-urea breath test are one of the most useful tests for confirming effective eradication of *Helicobacter pylori* (p. 99)
- Potentially useful minimally invasive techniques for identifying intestinal inflammation (white cell scan), blood loss (red cell scan), acute cholecystitis (HIDA scan), protein-losing enteropathy (albumin scan) or Meckel's diverticulum and some other conditions (Table 14.1). Unfortunately, results are open to interpretation and all too frequently fail to achieve the diagnostic sensitivity and specificity of published series
- Discussion with the nuclear medicine department is advised, because not all tests may be locally available
- No preparation is necessary, but isotope studies should be avoided in children, or women of child-bearing age, especially if they may be pregnant

Table 14.1 Indications for gastrointestinal isotope studies.

Condition	Scan	Page
Acute cholecystitis	^{99}Tc HIDA	29
Active bleeding	^{99}Tc sulphur colloid	24
Obscure bleeding	^{99}Tc red cell	
	^{51}Cr red cell	361
Meckel's diverticulum	^{99}Tc pertechnate	266
Protein-losing enteropathy	^{125}I-albumin	249
Steatorrhoea	^{14}C triolein	464
Crohn's disease activity	^{111}In white cell	283
	^{99}Tc-HMPAO	282
Terminal ileal absorption	^{75}SeHCAT	465
	$^{57/58}$Co B$_{12}$	243
Budd–Chiari syndrome	^{99}Tc pertechnate	177
Gastric emptying	^{99}Tc scrambled egg	467

14.4 Function tests

The reliability of results depends on familiarity with the procedure and if such tests are necessary, the patient is best referred to a centre where they are regularly performed. Details of the tests are available in larger textbooks (Appendix 2, p. 480) and only an outline is given here.

Breath tests

Lactose hydrogen breath test

- Indication: diagnosis of hypolactasia
- Principle: lactose is normally digested (into glucose and galactose), then absorbed. In hypolactasia, lactose is incompletely digested and undigested lactose is fermented when it reaches the colon. Hydrogen is then released, absorbed and exhaled in breath
- Method: 50 g lactose is ingested after an overnight fast. Exhaled breath hydrogen measured at 0, 60 and 120 min
- Results: normal breath hydrogen is < 20 p.p.m. at 120 min. Positive breath hydrogen (consistent with hypolactasia) is > 20 p.p.m. at 120 min

Lactulose hydrogen breath test

- Indication: diagnosis of intestinal bacterial overgrowth
- Principle: lactulose is a synthetic disaccharide that is not absorbed, but can be fermented to release hydrogen by intestinal bacteria. Release of hydrogen before 120 min in a person with normal orocaecal transit is consistent with bacteria in the small intestine. However, false positives occur due to oral bacteria, intestinal hurry or elevated baseline breath hydrogen in cigarette smokers, and false negatives occur after intestinal resection or lack of hydrogen-producing bacteria
- Method: 10 g lactulose ingested after a fast and an antiseptic mouth-wash. Exhaled breath hydrogen is measured at 0, 20, 40, 60, 80 100, 120, 150 and 180 min (exact timings may vary)
- Results: normal breath hydrogen is > 20 p.p.m. at > 120 min (colonic peak, quite the opposite of the lactose breath test abovse). Positive (consistent with bacterial overgrowth) is a sustained increase in breath hydrogen > 10 p.p.m. above baseline value at a time < 120 min, but preferably < 60 min for a confident diagnosis

Other breath tests for bacterial overgrowth

- ^{14}C-xylose and ^{14}C-glycoholic acid (bile acid) breath tests
- Principle: xylose is metabolized and bile acids deconjugated by Gram-

negative aerobes (always part of overgrowth flora). Carbon dioxide released, then absorbed and exhaled. Unlike lactulose, the tests are poor in the absence of H_2-generating bacteria. Xylose is said to be the most specific and sensitive

- Results: elevated $^{14}CO_2$ levels ($> 0.3\%$) detected at 2–3 h if bacteria present in small intestine

Gastric acid secretion

- Indication: investigation of elevated serum gastrin
- Method: patients should have stopped acid suppression for 2 weeks and be fasting. A nasogastric tube inserted and gastric juice aspirated every 15 min for 1 h for basal output. Pentagastrin 6 µg/kg (0.42 mg for 70 kg) is then given by intramuscular injection to stimulate gastric acid secretion. Further aspiration continues for 2 h. Cephalic stimulation to test vagal integrity by sham-feeding, should be tested before administration of pentagastrin. Measurements of volume (mL), pH (units), titratable acidity (mmol/L), acid output (mmol/h, calculated as volume (L) × titratable acidity) are made for each collection period, by prior arrangement with the biochemistry department
- Results: normal basal acid secretion (the sum of four 15-min collections) is 0–5 mmol/h; peak acid output (sum of the two highest collections after pentagastrin) ranges from 1 to 45 (mean 22) mmol/h; maximal acid output is titratable acidity in the single highest 15-min collection
- Interpretation: high basal output and no response to pentagastrin is consistent with Zollinger–Ellison syndrome. Absent basal output and no response to pentagastrin indicates achlorrhydria or ingestion of proton-pump inhibitors

Intestinal absorption and permeability tests

Xylose absorption

- Indication: investigation of suspected carbohydrate malabsorption
- Method: ingestion of 5 g D-xylose (non-metabolized monosaccharide), followed by a 5-h urine collection or 60-min blood xylose
- Results: normal urinary excretion is $> 22\%$, or blood xylose > 0.56 mmol/L at 60 min
- Interpretation: excretion $< 22\%$ is consistent with poor mucosal absorption, but 20% untreated coeliacs have normal values and rapid gastric emptying, fast intestinal transit, renal dysfunction, or incomplete urine collection give false-positive results. The test is non-specific and

insufficiently sensitive to act as a screening test for small intestinal disease, so is rarely used

• Sensitivity is improved by adding 1.0 g 3-*O*-methyl-D-glucose and measuring the plasma 60 min xylose/3-methyl-glucose ratio, but jejunal biopsy is still necessary to define the cause of malabsorption

Intestinal permeability

• Isotonic 5 g lactulose and 0.1 g L-rhamnose in 250 mL water, followed by a 5-h urine collection and calculation of the lactulose/rhamnose ratio, detects abnormal intestinal permeability, but may not be locally available. The test is sensitive but not specific

• The normal ratio is < 0.04, and higher values indicate small intestinal disease (coeliac, Crohn's tropical sprue, malnutrition). There is increasing evidence that high permeability in Crohn's disease predicts a risk of early relapse

• Other dual sugar tests (lactulose/mannitol) depend on available assay techniques, but single marker tests (polyethyleneglycol or ^{51}Cr-EDTA) may give false results for the same reasons as the xylose absorption test

^{14}C-triolein breath test

• Indication: diagnosis of fat malabsorption
• Principle: triolein is a triglyceride that normally undergoes lipid hydrolysis and absorption of the oleic acid, before metabolism to release carbon dioxide. After ingestion of ^{14}C-labelled triolein (glycerol ^{14}C-trioleic acid), ^{14}CO$_2$ can be detected in the breath. In fat malabsorption, less oleic acid is absorbed. False positives occur when triolein metabolism is impaired for reasons other than pancreatic insufficiency (diabetes, liver disease, lung disease). The test lacks sensitivity in mild pancreatic insufficiency
• Results: normal breath ^{14}CO$_2$ rises above baseline (> 0.0005%). When positive (consistent with fat malabsorption), breath ^{14}CO$_2$ remains low (< 0.0005%). It is not specific for the cause of fat malabsorption (pancreatic insufficiency, coeliac disease, gastric surgery)

Faecal fat excretion

• Indication: originally as a test to confirm a suspicion of malabsorption, but the lack of sensitivity and specificity means that it is rarely appropriate.
• Method: 3-day faecal collection during a controlled diet (100 g fat/day)
• Results: > 6 g/day fat excretion is abnormal
• Interpretation: a high value merely confirms a clinical suspicion and does not avoid the need for further investigation. A normal result does not exclude malabsorption (e.g. coeliac disease), so the test has limited value.

Malabsorption is better evaluated via history, signs, blood tests, intestinal biopsy, small bowel radiology and pancreatic ultrasound (p. 249). Stool inspection (coproscopy) for steatorrhoea has a variable sensitivity, low specificity and poor positive predictive value

Ileal absorption SeHCAT test

• Indication: investigation of chronic watery diarrhoea (bile salt malabsorption, p. 243)
• Interpretation: requested, if available, through the nuclear medicine department who will supply the local normal range. A normal test reliably excludes disease, but specificity is poor and the test is superfluous if ileal disease is identified on small bowel radiology. A therapeutic trial of cholestyramine is easier!

Pancreatic function

The principal indication is to investigate symptoms of exocrine insufficiency (p. 135), with minimal or no changes on ultrasound or ERCP. Pancreatic supplements should be stopped 5 days before the test. Direct intubation tests have been replaced in clinical practice by the fluorescein dilaurate test.

Fluorescein dilaurate ('Pancreolauryl') test

• Principle: fluorescein dilaurate is ingested and pancreatic enzymes normally split fluorescein from dilaurate. Urinary excretion of fluorescein is measured using a spectrophotometer
• Method: the test takes 2–3 days. On the first day, 2 capsules of fluorescein dilaurate are ingested and urine collected for 10 h (accurately timed). The percentage of dye excretion is calculated. On the second day, fluorescein alone (sodium salt) is ingested and urine collected for 10 h. The fluorescein excretion ratio on days 1 and 2 is calculated
• Results: normal excretion index is > 0.3, but 90% + pancreatic function needs to be lost to be detectable. A positive result < 20 usually indicates pancreatic insufficiency, but false positives occur. An index of 20–30 is equivocal and the test should be repeated

14.5 Other tests

Oesophageal manometry

Manometry is a specialist procedure that is best performed at a referral centre. The procedure is not difficult to do, but considerable expertise is needed for useful interpretation of the results.

- Indications: all patients prior to antireflux surgery, and dysphagia or chest pain of uncertain cause (p. 81). Only patients with persistent or disabling symptoms should be referred
- Method: acid suppression and drugs affecting oesophageal motility (prokinetics, nitrates, calcium antagonists, tricyclic agents) should be stopped for 1 week before the test, which is performed on fasting patients. A tiny catheter is passed through the nose and pressure recorded by intraluminal transducers. A sleeve sensor is best for measuring lower oesophageal sphincter pressure, because focal sensors become displaced during swallowing. Provocative stimuli (edrophonium, acid perfusion) are sometimes used to trigger oesophageal contraction and elucidate unusual causes of chest pain
- Results: a normal recording shows sequential progression of the peristaltic wave (pressure is measured at 5-cm intervals) and relaxation of the lower oesophageal sphincter. Abnormalities occur in either the pressure generated (amplitude can be > 80 mmHg in oesophageal spasm) or the wave progression (failure of relaxation of the lower oesophageal sphincter in achalasia)

Oesophageal pH monitoring

As with manometry, 24-h pH monitoring is best done at a referral centre, because interpretation can be complex.

- Indications: refractory symptoms of gastro-oesophageal reflux or undiagnosed chest pain, in the absence of visible oesophagitis (p. 81)
- Method: drugs for the treatment of gastro-oesophageal reflux should be stopped 1 week before testing. A catheter with a pH-sensitive transducer is introduced through the nose and placed 5 cm above the oesophagogastric junction, attached to an electronic recorder carried at the waist. Frequency, time and duration that pH < 4 are measured. Alkaline reflux is defined as pH > 7. Symptoms and position (lying or standing) are recorded by the patient
- Results: expressed as a percentage of the total recording time that oesophageal pH is below a certain level (usually < 4). Normal individuals have about 20 episodes when pH < 4 during 24 h, totalling $< 2\%$ of the recording time, and rarely at night. Symptoms due to reflux must correlate with abnormal oesophageal pH, but biliary reflux can confound results since pH may be high during symptoms

Helicobacter pylori: ¹⁴C- or ¹³C-urea breath test

- Indication: confirmation that *H. pylori* infection has been eradicated after

treatment in patients with complicated peptic ulcer disease, or those who continue to have symptoms (p. 99)
- Principle: *H. pylori* produces urease. ^{14}C-labelled urea is metabolized by urease to release $^{14}CO_2$ (and NH_4). $^{14}CO_2$ is detected in the breath
- Method: acid-suppressing drugs, antibiotics and bismuth compounds must have been stopped for 4 weeks to avoid false-negative results. After a 6-h fast, breath is exhaled through a straw into a test tube and the top capped, to act as baseline. Labelled urea is drunk and breath collected at 20 and 40 min (exact timings vary). ^{14}C isotope is measured by a scintillation counter, or ^{13}C assayed by mass spectrometry
- Results: normal breath $^{13/14}CO_2$ does not rise above baseline. In positive results, consistent with current *H. pylori* infection, $^{13/14}CO_2$ at 20 min is more than fivefold baseline

Gastric motility

Gastroparesis due to autonomic neuropathy (diabetes, amyloidosis) occasionally causes recurrent vomiting (p. 431). A barium meal provides subjective information about gastric emptying, but isotope studies provide a quantitative measurement
- Drugs that affect motility (metoclopramide, domperidone, cisapride, anticholinergics, opiates) are avoided for 72 h. Fluids only for 12 h and nil by mouth for 4 h is usual before the test
- A radiolabelled meal (such as 100 g scrambled egg) is eaten, followed by gamma camera counting for about 90 min. Normal emptying is 20–30% solids and 40–50% liquids within 60 min, but ranges vary between laboratories

Anorectal manometry

- Indications: defaecation disorders or faecal incontinence (p. 332). Some colorectal surgeons perform anorectal manometry before ileoanal pouch surgery. It is only available at specialist centres
- Method: a multilumen tube, with a distal balloon and three side ports connected to pressure transducers, is inserted 10 cm into the rectum. The rectum is distended by inflating the distal balloon (50–200 mL air). Myoelectric recordings from the external anal sphincter or puborectalis can be measured simultaneously through needle electrodes. Perineal sensation is best assessed by measuring the current threshold at which a tingling sensation is felt between two cutaneous electrodes

- Results: normal recordings show relaxation of the internal sphincter during rectal distension and a rebound increase in pressure during deflation. Absent sphincter relaxation may be detected during rectal distension (aganglionosis, p. 326), abnormal sphincteric tone (in faecal incontinence), or abnormal rectal sensation (desire to defaecate at high or low rectal volumes)

Gut hormones

- All tests are performed after an overnight fast, most easily when the patient attends for endoscopy (p. 118), or during the assessment of secretory diarrhoea (Fig. 7.2, p. 242)
- Acid-suppressing drugs must be stopped for 2 weeks before gastrin levels are measured. High gastrin levels are otherwise impossible to interpret, although patients most likely to have Zollinger–Ellison syndrome (p. 121) are also those most likely to be taking these drugs. Symptomatic treatment with antacids for these 2 weeks is trying for the patient and doctors
- 10 mL blood is taken into an ice-cold heparinized tube with 200 μL aprotinin (Trasylol 4000 iu/mL). The sample is immediately taken to biochemistry for separation and freezing
- A supraregional assay service (Appendix 1, p. 476) measures gastrin, glucagon, VIP, somatostatin or pancreatic polypeptide. Calcitonin should be measured in patients with unexplained diarrhoea, to exclude extremely rare cases of medullary thyroid carcinoma

Appendices

1 Useful addresses

Local organizations are listed in the telephone directory (or Yellow Pages) under Social Service and Welfare Organizations, or Charitable and Benevolent Organizations. These are especially helpful for:
- Alcohol abuse
- Services for the elderly
- Services for the disabled
- Drug abuse
- Hospices
- Bereaved

Adverse drug reactions
See Committee on Safety of Medicines or Drug Information.

Al-Anon
61 Great Dover Street, London SE1 4YF (Tel.: 0171 403 0888; Fax: 0171 378 9910); 24-h telephone service.
Offers group support for close friends and relatives of problem drinkers. Local groups throughout the country.

Alcoholics Anonymous
General Service Office, PO Box 1, Stonebrow House, York YO1 2NJ (Tel.: 01904 644026) or 11 Redcliffe Gardens, London SW10 (Helpline 10 a.m. to 10 p.m.; Tel.: 0171 352 3001; Fax: 01904 629091).
Provides anonymous groups for the assistance of alcoholics and problem drinkers. Local numbers in the telephone directory: over 3200 groups in the UK.

Al-Ateen
61 Great Dover Street, London SE1 4YF (Tel.: 0171 403 0888).
In conjunction with Al-Anon, provides help for young people (12–20 years) whose lives have been affected by their own or others' problem drinking

Alcohol Concern (National Agency On Alcohol Misuse)
Waterbridge House, 32–36 Loman Street, London SE1 0EE (Tel.: 0171 928 7377).
Concerned with prevention and treatment of alcohol misuse.

Anorexia and Bulimia Nervosa Association
Harringey Women and Health Centre, Annexe C, Tottenham Town Hall, Approach Rd, London N15 4RB (Tel.: 0181 885 3936).
Provides a confidential help line, support and information. Helpline Wed. 6–9 p.m.

Association of Glycogen Storage Disease
9 Lindop Road, Hale, Altrincham, Cheshire WA15 9DZ (Tel.: 0161 980 7303 after 6 p.m.); Fax: 0161 226 3813; email: a.phillips@bbc.org.uk.
Provides information and support for all persons affected by glycogen storage disease and their families.
Acts as a focus for educational, scientific and charitable activities for this disorder.

471

Association of Cystic Fibrosis Adults (UK)
28 New Road, Ferndown, Dorset BH22 8EP
Run by people with cystic fibrosis to encourage an exchange of information and promote a full and independent life for individuals with cystic fibrosis.

British Digestive Foundation
3 St Andrews Place, Regent's Park, London NW1 4LB (Tel.: 0171 486 0341)
Produces patient-orientated leaflets and supports research.

British Association of Cancer United Patients (BACUP)
3 Bath Place, Rivington Street, London EC2A 3JR (Cancer Information Service: Tel.: 0800 181199; Cancer Counselling Service Tel.: 0171 696 9000; Fax: 0171 6969002)
Provides information and support for patients and relatives using a telephone and written answer service by experienced cancer nurses. One-to-one counselling is available from offices in London and Glasgow.

British Association for Parenteral and Enteral Nutrition (BAPEN)
The White House, Hemp Lane, Wiggington, Tring, Herts HP23 6HF
Encourages education, research and audit in hospital and community nutritional support, with courses for nutrition support groups.

British Colostomy Association (incorporating the Colostomy Welfare Group)
15 Station Road, Reading RG1 1LG (Tel.: 01734 391537)
Comprised of volunteers who are all colostomists who will visit in hospital or at home, pre- and postoperatively. Advisory leaflets are available free on request.

British Digestive Foundation
3 St Andrews Place, Regent's Park, London NW1 4LB (Tel.: 0171 486 0341; Fax: 0171 224 2012; Website: wwwbdf.org.uk) Mon.–Thurs. 10 a.m.–7 p.m.; Fri. 10 a.m.–5.30 p.m.
Produces a series of patient-orientated leaflets covering the most common digestive disorders and supports research.

British Liver Trust
Central House, Central Avenue, Ransomes Euro Park, Ipswich IP3 9QG (Tel.: 01473 276326)
Provides patient information leaflets and advice for patients with chronic liver disease.

British Nutrition Foundation
High Holborn House, 52–54 High Holborn, London WC1V 6RQ (Tel.: 0171 404 6504; Fax: 0171 4046747)
Provides information and scientifically based advice to help consumers understand the relationship between nutrition, diet and lifestyle.

British Society of Gastroenterology
3 St Andrews Place, Regent's Park, London NW1 4LB (Tel.: 0171 387 3534)

Encourages education, training and audit in gastroenterology and gastrointestinal endoscopy.

Cancer Care Society (CARE)

21 Zetland Road, Redland, Bristol, Avon BS6 7AH (Tel.: 0117 942 7419).

Does not offer professional advice, but offers counselling for those whose lives have been affected by cancer. Support groups. National telephone link line. Subsidized holiday accommodation on the south coast.

Cancer Relief MacMillan Fund

Anchor House, 15–19 Britten Street, London SW3 3TZ (Tel.: 0171 351 7811; Fax: 0171 376 3098).

Provides nursing services. Local number in the telephone directory.

Cancer-Link

17 Britannia Street, London WC1X 9JN (Tel.: 0171 833 2451; Fax: 0171 833 4963) or 9 Castle Terrace, Edinburgh EH1 2DP (Tel.: 0131 228 5557).

A resource for over 500 cancer support and self-help groups in the UK. Patient-based, offering support on all aspects of cancer.

Carers National Association

20–25 Glasshouse Yard, London EC1A 4JS (Tel.: 0171 490 8818; Fax: 0171 490 8824).

Offers information and support for all people caring for relatives and friends at home.

Children's Liver Disease Foundation

138 Digbeth, Birmingham B5 6DR (Tel.: 0121 643 7282).

Provides advice and emotional support for families with a child suffering from liver disease.

Coeliac Society of the UK

PO Box 220, High Wycombe, Bucks NG11 2HY (Tel.: 01494 437278).

Provides advice and counselling concerning the disease and diet, together with holidays and social activities.

Committee on Safety of Medicines

Market Towers, 1 Nine Elms Lane, London SW8 5NQ (Tel.: 0171 720 2188).

Notification of adverse drug reactions and regulatory matters. Dial 100 and ask for CSM Freephone.
- CSM, Freepost, London SW8 5BR
- CSM Mersey, Freepost, Liverpool L3 3AB
- CSM West Midlands, Freepost, Birmingham B15 1BR
- CSM Northern, Freepost 1085, Newcastle NE1 1BR
- CSM Wales, Freepost, Cardiff CF4 1ZZ

Crohn's and Colitis Foundation of America

386 Park Avenue South, 17th Floor, New York, NY 10016–8804 (Tel.: (212) 685 3440).

Research-orientated organization, also provides a series of information leaflets for patients.

Crohn's in Childhood Research Association (CICRA)

Parkgate House, 356 West Barnes Lane, Motspur Park, Surrey KT3 6NB (Tel.: 0181 949 6209).

Offers self-help to parents and children suffering from Crohn's disease or ulcerative colitis. Raises money for research.

Cystic Fibrosis Research Trust

Alexandra House, 5 Blyth Road, Bromley, Kent BR1 3RS (Tel.: 0181 464 7211).

Provides support for parents, their children and adults suffering from cystic fibrosis.

Department of Health

Alexander Fleming House, Elephant and Castle, London SE1 6BY (Tel.: 0171 407 5522).

Head office of the Chief Medical Officer and his staff.

Disablement Information and Advice Lines (DIAL UK)

Park Lodge, 1 St Catherine's Hospital, Tickhill Road, Balby, Doncaster, South Yorkshire DN4 8QN (Tel.: 01302 310123; Fax: 01302 310404).

Provides free, impartial and confidential advice on all aspects of disablement to help the disabled live independently in the community. Provides home helps and meals on wheels.

Drug Information (on any aspect of drug therapy)

Check details in latest BNF or Data Sheet Compendium first.

- Aberdeen Tel.: 01224 681818 ext 52316
- Belfast Tel.: 01232 248095 Direct Line
- Birmingham Tel.: 0121 378 2211 ext 2296/2297
- Bristol Tel.: 0117 282867 Direct Line
- Cardiff Tel.: 01222 759541 Direct Line
- Dundee Tel.: 01382 601 11 ext 2351
- Edinburgh Tel.: 0131 229 2477 ext 2094/2416/2443
or Tel.: 0131 229 3901 Direct Line
- Glasgow Tel.: 0141 552 4726 Direct Line
- Guildford Tel.: 01483 504312 Direct Line
- Inverness Tel.: 01463 234151 ext 288 or Tel.: 01463 220157 Direct Line
- Ipswich Tel.: 01473 712233 ext 4322/4323 or Tel.: 01473 718687 Direct Line
- Leeds Tel.: 0113 2430715 Direct Line
- Leicester Tel.: 01533 555779 Direct Line
- Liverpool Tel.: 0151 236 4620 ext 2126/2127/2128
- London:
  Guy's Hospital Tel.: 0171 955 5000 ext 3594/5892
  or Tel.: 0171 378 0023 Direct Line
  Royal London Hospital Tel.: 0171 377 7487 Direct Line
  or Tel.: 0171 377 7488 Direct Line
  Northwick Park Tel.: 0181 869 2761 Direct Line

- Londonderry Tel.: 01504 451 71 ext 3262
- Manchester Tel.: 0161 225 2063 Direct Line
or Tel.: 0161 276 6270
- Newcastle Tel.: 0191 232 1525 Direct Line
- Oxford Tel.: 01865 742424 Direct Line
- Southampton Tel.: 01703 796908 Direct Line or Tel.: 01703 796909 Direct
Line

Drug Abuse ('Release')
388 Old Street, London EC1 V 9LT (Tel.: 0171 729 5255; Fax: 0171 729 2599).
- Advice 10 a.m.–6 p.m. Tel.: 0171 729 9904
- Emergency helpline overnight Tel.: 0171 603 8654
- Drugs in schools helpline Tel.: 01345 366666
   Offers advice and information for patients charged with drug offences. It deals with the social, medical and legal problems arising from drug abuse.

Drug Abuse (Families Anonymous)
The Doddington and Rollo Community Association, Charlotte Despard Avenue, London SW11 5JE (Tel.: 0171 498 4680).
   Helps families and friends of drug abusers to relieve stress and aid recovery. Local support groups.

Eating Disorders Association
Sackville Place, 44–48 Magdalen Street, Norwich NR3 1JE (Tel.: 01603 621414; Fax: 01603 664915).
   Offers mutual support and sharing of information. Concerned to promote education and understanding about the illness.

Employment Medical Advisory Services
Director of Medical Services, Health and Safety Executive, Woodside House, 261 Low Lane, Horsforth, Leeds LS18 5TW (Tel.: 0113 2834200).
   Part of the Health and Safety Executive with local offices and a Prestel Service, which enables users to send messages as well as giving general information.

Environmental Health—Medical Officer
Local names and addresses available from District Health Authority, local Microbiology Department, or Public Health Laboratory (PHLS).

European Federation of Crohn's and Ulcerative Colitis Associations (EFCCA)
Dustere-Eichen-Weg 24, D-37073, Göttingen, Deutschland.
   Facilitates contact between patient-based groups for inflammatory bowel disease in different countries.

Familial Adenomatous Polyposis
The Polyposis Registry, St Mark's Hospital, Northwick Park, London Tel.: 0171 6017958 (direct line).
   Primarily research based, data collection and follow-up.

Appendices

1 Useful addresses

Family Cancer Clinic

Department of Clinical Genetics, Royal Free Hospital NHS Trust, Pond Street, London NW3 2QG (Tel.: 0171 794 0500 ext 3702).

Referral centre and source of advice on patients and families with multiple tumours.

Food and Chemical Allergy Association

27 Ferringham Lane, Ferring-by-Sea, West Sussex BN12 5NB (Tel.: 01903 241178 after 8 p.m.).

Supplies names of doctors specializing in this field. Gives help and advice to sufferers of allergy-induced illness.

Gastrointestinal Hormone Supraregional Assay Service

Hammersmith Hospital, DuCane Road, London W12 OHS (Tel.: 0181 740 3044).

Specialist gut hormone assays available. Discuss the problem before sending samples.

Genetic Counselling

Tel.: the department of medical/clinical genetics at many teaching hospitals.

Haemochromatosis Society

Hollybush House, Hadley Green, Barnet, Herts EN5 5PR.

Provides information and advice for patients with this condition.

Helen House Hospice

37 Leopold Street, Oxford, Oxon OX4 1QT (Tel.: 01865 728251).

A hospice for children, providing terminal and short-term relief care.

Hospice Information Service

St Christopher's Hospice, 51–59 Lawrie Park Road, Sydenham, London SE26 6DZ (Tel.: 0181 778 9252; Fax: 0181 659 3680).

A resource link producing directories of hospices in the UK and overseas.

Hollister Stoma Care Advice Service

42 Broad Street, Wokingham, Berks RG40 1AB (Tel.: 0800 521377).

Offers confidential advice on any aspect of stoma care for patients and their carers.

Ileostomy and Internal Pouch Support Group

(Formerly the Ileostomy Association of Great Britain and Ireland) Ambleside House, PO Box 23, Black Scotch Lane, Mansfield, Notts N18 4TT (Tel. and Fax: 01623 228099).

Advisory service for people with ileostomies by way of hospital and home visits. Many of the volunteers are ileostomists themselves.

Irish Society for Colitis and Crohn's Disease (ISCCD)

58 Limekiln Green, Dublin, Eire.

Sister group to NACC in Ireland.

Irritable Bowel Syndrome Network (IBS Network)
St John's House, Hither Green Hospital, London SE13 6RU.

Helps organize self-help groups to alleviate the distress and isolation felt by people suffering from IBS.

Kingston Trust
The Drove, Kempshott, Basingstoke, Hants RG22 5LU (Tel.: 01256 52320).

Provides homes for all types of stoma patients or those with other abdominal diseases in need of short stay or permanent accommodation.

Liver Transplant Units
Discuss possible transplantation as early as possible to allow full assessment.
• Birmingham: Liver Unit, Queen Elizabeth Hospital, Birmingham B15 2TH (Tel.: 0121 4721311 ext 3428)
• Cambridge: Transplant Co-ordinator, Addenbrooke's NHS Trust, Hills Road, Cambridge (Tel.: 01223 217251 direct line)
• Leeds: Transplant Co-ordinator St James' University Hospital NHS Trust, Becket Street, Leeds LS9 7TF (Tel.: 0113 2433144 ext 4553)
• London: Transplant Co-ordinator, Liver Unit, King's Healthcare NHS Trust, Denmark Hill, London SE5 9RS (Tel.: 0171 737 4000 bleep 149 or Tel.: 0171 326 3254 direct line); Transplant Co-ordinator, Liver Unit, Royal Free Hospital NHS Trust, Pond Street, London NW3 2QG (Tel.: 0171 794 0500 bleep)

Marie Curie Cancer Care
28 Belgrave Square, London SW1X 0QG (Tel.: 0171 235 3325; Fax: 0171 823 2380).

Runs 11 UK nursing homes and a nationwide domicilliary nursing service, especially night nursing. Provides urgent welfare needs in kind, advice and general information.

Medical Advisory Service
10 Barley Mow Passage, Chiswick, London W4 4PH (Tel.: 0171 994 9874).

Telephone service run by nurses offering information and advice on medical and health care by nurses, putting people in touch with the right organization.

National Advisory Service for Parents of Children with a Stoma
51 Anderson Drive, Valley View Park, Darvel KA17 ODE (Tel.: 01560 220 24).

Provides a support group for parents of children who have a stoma, ileostomy, colostomy or urostomy. Includes Hirschprung's disease.

National Association for Colitis and Crohn's Disease
98A London Road, St Albans, Hertfordshire AL1 1NX (Recorded message Tel. and Fax: 01727 844296).

Offers support and information for patients with inflammatory bowel disease and their families. Local groups throughout the country.

National Reye's Syndrome Foundation
15 Nicholas Gardens, Pyrford, Woking, Surrey GU22 8SD (Tel.: 01932 346843).

A support group for parents of children suffering from Reye's syndrome.

National Society For Phenylketonuria
7 Southend Close, Willen, Milton Keynes MK15 9LL (Tel.: 01908 691653).
Offers support for parents of children suffering from phenylketonuria concerning their medical, social and educational welfare.

Nursing Services
• Health Visitors, Community Nurses, District Nurses, Private Nursing Organizations
• Local services listed under 'Nurses' in the telephone directory

Nutrition
Medical Information (Nutrition Department), Pharmacia & Upjohn, Davy Avenue, Knowlhill, Milton Keynes MK5 8PH (Tel.: 01908 603790).
Provides a commercial parenteral nutrition service. 48-h notice is generally needed before initiating feeding, but delivery is possible throughout the UK.

Oesophageal Patients Association
16 Whitefields Crescent, Solihull, West Midlands B91 3NU (Tel.: 0121 704 9860).
Provides leaflets and support for patients with oesophageal cancer and other oesophageal disorders.

Poisons Information
Check in BNF or Data Sheet Compendium for latest details.
• Belfast Tel.: 01232 240503
• Birmingham Tel.: 0121 507 5588/9
• Cardiff Tel.: 01222 709901
• Edinburgh Tel.: 0131 536 2300
• Leeds Tel.: 0113 243 0715 or 0113 292 3547
• London Tel.: 0171 635 9191 or Tel.: 0171 955 5095
• Newcastle Tel.: 0191 2325131

Primary Biliary Cirrhosis Support Group
Mrs Collete Thain, The Dean, Long Niddry, East Lothian, EH3 20PN (Tel.: 01875 853552).
Provides patient information, advice and support.

Primary Care Society for Gastroenterology
Secretariat: Mrs Ros Aukett, The Secretariat, Primary Care Society for Gastroenterology, 16 Cheltenham Road, Gloucester GL2 0LS (Tel.: 01452 304638).
Provides a forum for doctors to address the issues of education and research in gastroenterology in primary care.

Public Health Laboratory Service
61 Colindale Avenue, London NW9 5DF (Tel.: 0181 200 4000).
Central reference laboratory with local laboratories covering all districts, giving investigation services and advice.

Share-a-Care (National Register for Rare Diseases)
8 Cornmarket, Farringdon, Oxon.

Puts people with rare diseases in contact with others with the same disorder, as well as compiling a national register.

Tropical diseases
- London: Hospital for Tropical Diseases, 4 St Pancras Way, London NW1 0PE (Tel.: 0171 387 4411)
- Liverpool: Liverpool School of Tropical Medicine, Pembroke Place, Liverpool L3 5QA (Tel.: 0151 708 9393)
  Offers clinical advice and information on immunization for foreign travel.

Tracheo-oesophageal Support Group
St George's Centre, 91 Victoria Road, Netherfield, Nottingham NG4 2NN (Tel.: 0115 9400694)
  Run by parents for parents of children born with an oesophageal disorder.

2 Further reading

A bibliography in a rapid reference book cannot be comprehensive. This section suggests general reference texts and refers to papers or reviews covering areas of controversy or particular complexity.

General texts

Bouchier IAD, Allan RN, Hodgson HJF, Keighley MRB. *Gastroenterology. Clinical Science and Practice*, 2nd edn. WB Saunders, Philadelphia, 1993.

Kumar D, Christensen J, eds. *A Diagnostic Guide to Clinical Gastroenterology.* Churchill Livingstone, Edinburgh, 1996.

Misiewicz JJ, Pounder RE, Venables CW. *Diseases of the Gut and Pancreas*, 2nd edn. Blackwell Science, Oxford, 1993.

Sleisenger MH, Fordtran JS, Scharsmidt BF, Feldman M, eds. *Gastrointestinal Disease. Pathophysiology, Diagnosis, Management*, 5th edn. WB Saunders, Philadelphia, 1993.

British Society of Gastroenterology (BSG). *Guidelines in Gastroenterology.* BSG, London, 1996. BSG Secretariat, 3 St Andrews Place, London NW1 4LB, or website: http://www.bsg.org.uk/clinical/data/gmpcd.htm. Separate guidelines (with regular updates and new titles) cover dyspepsia, antibiotic prophylaxis in gastrointestinal endoscopy, oesophageal manometry and pH monitoring, inflammatory bowel disease, initial biopsy diagnosis of suspected chronic idiopathic inflammatory bowel disease, coeliac disease, artificial nutritional support and tests for malabsorption.

Gastroenterology on the Internet

There are numerous gastroenterology websites on the Internet, many of which are excellent and also cross-refer to others. The following are useful starting points:

Journals

- *Gastroenterology*—http://www.gastrojournal.org
- *Gut*—http://www.bmjpg.com/data/gut.htm
- *European Journal of Gastroenterology and Hepatology*—http://www.ejgh.com

Organizations

- British Digestive Foundation—http://www.bdf.org.uk (provides patient information)
- British Society of Gastroenterology—http://www.bsg.org.uk (includes clinical guidelines)
- OMGE—http://www.excerptamedica.com/OMGE (sources)

Guidelines

- Avicenna—http://www.avicenna.com (includes NIH's AHCPR guidelines)
- Medscape—http://www.medscape.com (with limited free access to Medline)
- Healthgate—http://www.healthgate.com (a pro-active site)

Alimentary emergencies

Berry AR, Campbell WB, Kettlewell MGW. Management of major colonic haemorrhage. *British Journal of Surgery* 1988; **75**: 637–40.

de Beaux AC, Palmer KR, Carter DC. Factors influencing morbidity and mortality in acute pancreatitis: an analysis of 279 cases. *Gut* 1995; **37**: 121–6.

Kubba AK, Murphy W, Palmer KR. Endoscopic injection of bleeding peptic ulcer: a comparison of adrenaline alone with adrenaline plus human thrombin. *Gastroenterology* 1997; **111**: 623–8.

Mutimer DJ, Ayres RCS, Neuberger JM *et al*. Serious paracetamol poisoning and the results of liver transplantation. *Gut* 1994; **35**: 809–14.

O'Grady JC. Management of acute liver failure. In: Farthing MJG (ed). *Horizons in Medicine no. 8*. London: Royal College of Physicians of London, 1997: 83–91.

Sanyal AJ, Freedman AM, Luketic VA *et al*. Transjugular intrahepatic portosystemic shunts for patients with active variceal haemorrhage unresponsive to sclerotherapy. *Gastroenterology* 1996; **111**: 138–46.

Stanley AJ, Hayes PC. Portal hypertension and variceal haemorrhage. *Lancet* 1997; **350**: 1235–9.

Webb WA. Management of foreign bodies of the upper gastrointestinal tract. *Gastroenterology* 1988; **94**: 204–16.

Oesophagus

Gillebert G, Janssens J, Vantrappen G. Ambulatory 24 h intra-oesophageal pH and pressure recordings vs. provocation tests in the diagnosis of chest pain of oesophageal origin. *Gut* 1990; **31**: 738–44.

Kelley DJ, Shah JP. Management of Barrett's oesophagus. *Lancet* 1996; **348**: 561–2.

Lambert R. Review article: current practice and future perspectives in the management of gastro-oesophageal reflux disease. *Alimentary Pharmacology and Therapeutics* 1997; **11**: 651–62.

McDougall NI, Johnston BT, Kee F *et al*. Natural history of reflux oesophagitis: a 10-year follow up of its effect on patient symptomatology and quality of life. *Gut* 1996; **38**: 481–6.

Sturgess RP, Morris AI. Metal stents in the oesophagus. *Gut* 1995; **37**: 595–7.

Walker SJ, Baxter ST, Morris AI, Sutton R. Controversy in the therapy of gastro-oesophageal reflux disease—long term proton pump inhibition or laparoscopic anti-reflux surgery? *Alimentary Pharmacology and Therapeutics* 1997; **11**: 249–60.

Stomach and duodenum

Axon ATR. Chronic dyspepsia: who needs endoscopy? *Gastroenterology* 1997; **112**: 1376–80.

Bayerdörffer E, Miehlke S, Lehn N *et al*. Cure of gastric ulcer disease after cure of *Helicobacter pylori* infection—German gastric ulcer study. *European Journal of Gastroenterology and Hepatology* 1996; **8**: 343–50.

Craanen ME, Blok P, Dekker W, Tytgat GNJ. *Helicobacter pylori* and early gastric cancer. *Gut* 1994; **35**: 1372–4.

de Boer W, Dressen W, Jansz A, Tytgat G. Effect of acid suppression on efficacy of treatment for *Helicobacter pylori* infection. *Lancet* 1995; **345**: 817–19.

Folli S, Denti M, Dell'Amore D *et al*. Early gastric cancer: prognostic factors in 223 patients. *British Journal of Surgery* 1995; **82**: 952–6.

Harris AW, Misiewicz JJ. Eradication of *Helicobacter pylori*. In: Calam J (ed) *Helicobacter pylori* London, Baillière Tindall, 1995: 583–613.

Laheij RJF, Jansen JBMJ, Van de Lisdonk EH *et al*. Symptom improvement through eradication of *Helicobacter pylori* in non-ulcer dyspepsia. *Alimentary Pharmacology and Therapeutics* 1996; **10**: 843–50.

Lind T, Velduyzen van Zanten SJO, Unge P et al. Eradication of Helicobacter pylori using 1-week triple therapies combining omeprazole with two antimicrobials. The MACH 1 study. Helicobacter 1996; **1:** 138–44.

McGowan CC, Cover TL, Blaser MJ. Helicobacter pylori and gastric acid: biological and therapeutic implications. Gastroenterology 1996; **110:** 926–38.

Misiewicz JJ, Harris AW, Bardhan KD, Levi S, Langworthy H. One week low-dose triple therapy for eradication of Helicobacter pylori. A large multi-centre randomised trial. Gut 1998 (in press).

Pancreatic disease

Ahlgren JD. Chemotherapy for pancreatic carcinoma. Cancer 1996; **78:** 654–63.

Ammann RW, Heitz PU, Löppel K. Course of alcoholic chronic pancreatitis: a prospective clinicomorphological long term study. Gastoenterology 1996; **111:** 224–31.

Arnold R, Trautmann ME, Creutzfeldt W, Benning R, Benning M. Somatostatin analogue octreotide and inhibition of tumour growth in metastatic endocrine gastroenteropancreatic tumours. Gut 1996; **38:** 430–8.

Braganza JM. The pathogenesis of chronic pancreatitis. Quarterly Journal of Medicine 1996; **89:** 243–50.

Carter DC. Cancer of the pancreas. Gut 1990; **31:** 494–6.

Kingsnorth A. Role of cytokines and their inhibitors in acute pancreatitis. Gut 1997; **40:** 1–4.

Lankisch PG, Droge M, Gottesleben F. Drug induced acute pancreatitis: incidence and severity. Gut 1995; **37:** 565–7.

Liver disease

Batts P, Ludwig J. Chronic hepatitis: an update on terminology and reporting. American Journal of Surgical Pathology 1995; **19:** 1409–17.

Dusheiko G. Hepatitis A to Z: review in depth. European Journal of Gastroenterology and Hepatology 1996; **8:** 297–328.

Forrest EH, Jalan R, Hayes PC. Renal circulatory changes in cirrhosis—pathogenesis and therapeutic prospects. Alimentary Pharmacology and Therapeutics 1996; **8:** 147–58.

Gines A, Fernández-Esparrach G, Monescillo A et al. Randomized trial comparing albumin, dextran 70 and polygeline in cirrhotic patients with ascites treated by paracentesis. Gastroenterology 1996; **111:** 1002–10.

Hayes P. Hepatocellular carcinoma: review in depth. European Journal of Gastroenterology and Hepatology 1996; **10:** 219–32.

Lindor KD, Therneau TM, Jorgensen RA, Malinchoc M, Dickson ER. Effects of ursodeoxycholic acid on survival in patients with primary biliary cirrhosis. Gastroenterology 1996; **110:** 1515–18.

Powell LW. Hemochromatosis: the impact of early diagnosis and therapy. Gastroenterology 1996; **110:** 1304–7.

Roberts SK, Therneau TM, Czaja AJ. Prognosis of histological cirrhosis in type 1 autoimmune hepatitis. Gastroenterology 1996; **110:** 848–57.

Steindl P, Ferenci P, Dienes HP, Grimm G, Pabinger I. Wilson's disease in patients presenting with liver disease: a diagnostic challenge. Gastroenterology 1997; **113:** 212–18.

Zimmerman HJ, Ishak KG. General aspects of drug-induced liver disease. Gastroenterology Clinics of North America 1995; **24:** 739–58.

Biliary disease

Barkun JS, Barkun AN, Sampalis JS et al. Randomised controlled trial of laparoscopic vs. mini-cholecystectomy. *Lancet* 1992; **340:** 116–19.

Dalton HR, Chapman RWG. Role of biliary stenting in the management of bile duct stones in the elderly. *Gut* 1995; **36:** 485–7.

Heathcote J. Autoimmune cholangitis. *Gut* 1997; **40:** 440–2.

Heaton KW, Braddon FEM, Mountford RA et al. Symptomatic and silent gall stones in the community. *Gut* 1991; **32:** 316–20.

Hobbs KEF. Laparoscopic cholecystectomy. *Gut* 1995; **36:** 161–4.

Hussaini SH. Clinical economics review: the management of gall stone disease. *Alimentary Pharmacology and Therapeutics* 1996; **10:** 699–705.

Wehrmann T, Wiemer K, Lembcke B et al. Do patients with sphincter of Oddi dysfunction benefit from endoscopic sphincterotomy? A 5-year prospective trial. *European Journal of Gastroenterology and Hepatology* 1996; **8:** 251–6.

Small intestine

Corazza GP, Menozzi MG, Strocchi A et al. The diagnosis of small bowel bacterial overgrowth. *Gastroenterology* 1990; **98:** 302–9.

Davies GR, Benson MJ, Gertner DJ et al. Diagnostic and therapeutic push type enteroscopy in clinical use. *Gut* 1995; **37:** 346–52.

Dieterich W, Ehnis T, Bauer M et al. Identification of tissue transglutaminase as the autoantigen of coeliac disease. *Nature Medicine* 1997; **3:** 797–801.

Fine KD, Meyer RL, Lee EC. The prevalence and causes of chronic diarrhea in patients with celiac sprue treated with a gluten-free diet. *Gastroenterology* 1997; **112:** 1830–8.

Holmes GKT, Prior P, Lane MR, Pope D, Allan RN. Malignancy in coeliac disease— effect of a gluten-free diet. *Gut* 1989; **30:** 333–9.

McFarlane XA, Bhalla AK, Reeves DE et al. Osteoporosis in treated adult coeliac disease. *Gut* 1995; **36:** 710–14.

Quigley EMM. Small intestinal transplantation: reflections on an evolving approach to intestinal failure. *Gastroenterology* 1996; **110:** 2009–12.

Ulcerative colitis and Crohn's disease

Allan RN, Rhodes JM, Hanauer S, Keighley M, eds. *Inflammatory Bowel Diseases*. Churchill Livingstone, New York, 1997.

Forbes A. *Clinician's Guide to Inflammatory Bowel Disease*. Chapman & Hall, London, 1997.

Hyde GM, Jewell DP. The management of severe ulcerative colitis. *Alimentary Pharmacology and Therapeutics* 1997; **11:** 419–24.

Jarnerot G. New salicylates as maintenance treatment in ulcerative colitis. *Gut* 1994; **35:** 1155–8.

Johnston D, Williamson MER, Lewis WG, Miller AS, Sagar PM, Holdsworth PJ. Prospective controlled trial of duplicated (J) vs. quadruplicated (W) pelvic ileal reservoirs in restorative proctocolectomy for ulcerative colitis. *Gut* 1996; **38:** 242–7.

Keighley MRB. Review article: the management of pouchitis. *Alimentary Pharmacology and Therapeutics* 1996; **10:** 449–58.

Royall D, Jeejeebhoy KN, Baker JP et al. Comparison of amino acid vs. peptide based enteral diets in active Crohn's disease: clinical and nutritional outcome. *Gut* 1994; **35:** 783–7.

Satsangi J, Grootscholten C, Holt H, Jewell DP. Clinical patterns of familial inflammatory bowel disease. *Gut* 1996; **38:** 738–41.

Satsangi J, Parkes M, Louis E *et al.* Two stage genome-wide search in inflammatory bowel disease provides evidence for susceptibility loci on chromosomes 3, 7 and 12. *Nature Genetics* 1996; **14:** 199–202.

Travis SPL. Insurance risks for ulcerative colitis and Crohn's disease (prognosis and pattern of disease). *Alimentary Pharmacology and Therapeutics* 1997; **11:** 51–60.

Travis SPL, Farrant JM, Ricketts C *et al.* Predicting outcome in severe ulcerative colitis. *Gut* 1996; **38:** 905–10.

Veress B, Lofberg R, Bergman L. Microscopic colitis syndrome. *Gut* 1995; **36:** 880–6.

Large intestine

Eckhauser FE, Knol JA. Surgery for primary and metastatic colorectal cancer. *Gastroenterology Clinics of North America* 1997; **26:** 103–28.

Houlston RS, Murday V, Harcopos C, Williams CB, Slack J. Screening and genetic counselling for relatives of patients with colorectal cancer in a family cancer clinic. *British Medical Journal* 1990; **301:** 366–8.

Lieberman D, Sleisenger MH. Is it time to recommend screening for colorectal cancer? *Lancet* 1996; **348:** 1463.

Lucas CA, Logan ECM, Logan RFA. Audit of the investigation and outcome of iron deficiency anaemia in one health district. *Journal of the Royal College of Physicians of London* 1996; **30:** 33–5.

McFarlane XA, Morris AI. Faecal incontinence and constipation. *Journal of the Royal College of Physicians of London* 1997; **31:** 487–92.

Slevin ML. Adjuvant therapy for colorectal cancer: no more room for nihilism. *British Medical Journal* 1996; **312:** 392–3.

Winawer SJ, Fletcher RH, Miller L *et al.* Colorectal cancer screening: clinical guidelines and rationale. *Gastroenterology* 1997; **112:** 594–642.

Irritable bowel syndrome

Bass C. Somatization. *Medicine International* 1996; **24:** 58–61.

Drossman D. Irritable bowel syndrome: a technical review for practice guideline development. *Gastroenterology* 1997; **112:** 2120–37.

Nanda R, James R, Smith H, Dudley CRK, Jewell DP. Food intolerance and the irritable bowel syndrome. *Gut* 1989; **30:** 1099–104.

Thompson WG. Irritable bowel syndrome: pathogenesis and management. *Lancet* 1993; **341:** 1569–72.

van der Horst HE, van Dulmen AM, Schellevis FG *et al.* Do patients with irritable bowel syndrome in primary care really differ from outpatients with irritable bowel syndrome? *Gut* 1997; **41:** 669–74.

Whorwell PJ. Hypnosis and biofeedback: review in depth. *European Journal of Gastroenterology and Hepatology* 1996; **8:** 513–40.

Gastrointestinal infections

Elliott DE. Schistosomiasis: pathophysiology, diagnosis and treatment. *Gastroenterology Clinics of North America* 1996; **25:** 599–626.

Farthing MJG. Antibiotic-associated diarrhoea: review in depth. *European Journal of Gastroenterology and Hepatology* 1996; **8:** 1033–62.

Wilcox CM, Rabneck L, Friedman S. AGA technical review: malnutrition and cachexia, chronic diarrhea and hepatobiliary disease in patients with human immunodeficiency virus infection. *Gastroenterology* 1996; **111:** 1724–52.

Nutrition

Editorial. Dietary recommendations: how do we move forward? *British Journal of Nutrition* 1990; **64:** 301–5.

Reynolds N, McWhirter JP, Pennington CR. Nutrition support teams: an integral part of developing a gastroenterology service. *Gut* 1995; **37:** 740–2.

Rosenbaum M, Leibel RL, Hirsch J. Medical progress: obesity. *New England Journal of Medicine* 1997; **337:** 396–407.

The gut in systemic disease

Ali GN, Wallace KL, Schwartz R *et al.* Mechanisms of oropharyngeal dysphagia in Parkinson's disease. *Gastroenterology* 1996; **110:** 383–92.

Audibert F, Friedman SA, Frangieh AY, Sibai BM. Clinical utility of strict diagnostic criteria for the HELLP (hemolysis, elevated liver enzymes and low platelets) syndrome. *American Journal of Obstetrics and Gynecology* 1996; **175:** 460–4.

Camilleri M. Gastrointestinal problems in diabetes. *Endocrine and Metabolism Clinics of North America* 1996; **25:** 361–78.

Farthing M, James O. Aging and the alimentary tract (introducing five leading articles on the topic). *Gut* 1997; **41:** 421

Hadjivassilou M, Gibson A, Davies-Jones GAB, Lobo AJ, Stephenson TJ, Milford Ward A. Does cryptic gluten sensitivity play a part in neurological illness? *Lancet* 1996; **347:** 369–71.

Lipscomb G, Loughrey G, Thakker M *et al.* A prospective study of abdominal computerized tomography and colonoscopy in the diagnosis of colonic disease in an elderly population. *European Journal of Gastroenterology and Hepatology* 1996; **8:** 887–92.

Wolf JL. Liver disease in pregnancy. *Medical Clinics of North America* 1996; **80:** 1167–87.

Procedures and investigations

Bateson MC, Bouchier IAD. *Clinical Investigations in Gastroenterology*, 2nd edn. Kluwer Academic Publishers, Dordrecht, 1997.

Cotton PB, Williams CB. *Practical Gastrointestinal Endoscopy*, 4th edn. Blackwell Science, Oxford, 1996.

Douds AC, Joseph AEA, Finlayson C *et al.* Is day case liver biopsy underutilised? *Gut* 1995; **37:** 574–5.

Haggett PJ, Moore NR, Shearman JD, Travis SPL, Jewell DP, Mortensen NJ. Pelvic and perineal complications of Crohn's disease: assessment using magnetic resonance imaging. *Gut* 1995; **36:** 407–10.

Hope RL, Chu G, Hope AH, Newcombe RG, Gillespie PE, Williams SJ. Comparison of three faecal occult blood tests in the detection of colorectal neoplasia. *Gut* 1996; **39:** 722–5.

Rex DK, Rahmani EY, Haseman JH, Lemmel GT, Kaster S, Buckley JS. Relative sensitivity of colonoscopy and barium enema for detection of colorectal cancer in clinical practice. *Gastroenterology* 1997; **112:** 17–23.

Soto JA, Barish MA, Yucel EK *et al.* Magnetic resonance cholangiography: comparison with endoscopic retrograde cholangiopancreatography. *Gastroenterology* 1996; **110:** 598–606.

3 Height and weight charts

- 'Overweight' is defined as 10–19% above the upper limit for either men or women
- 'Obesity' is ≥20% above the upper limit

The desirable weight for height shown in Table A3.1 is based on actuarial data for longevity and good health and should form the basis of advice on body weight

- The body mass index (BMI) (weight(kg)/height^2 (metres), normal range 20–25 kg/m^2) is explained on p. 402. See Fig. 12.1, p. 403

BMI is a more sensitive index of the relationship between body weight and disease and is becoming the accepted standard of reference. Table A3.2 shows values of BMI according to height and weight data.

Table A3.1(a) Height and weight chart for men

Height		Weight					
		Small frame		Medium frame		Large frame	
cm	ft. ins	kg	st. lb	kg	st. lb	kg	st. lb
158	5.2	57.6–60.3	9.2–9.8	59.0–63.5	9.5–10.1	62.1–67.5	9.12–10.10
160	5.3	58.5–61.2	9.4–9.10	59.9–64.4	9.7–10.3	63.0–68.9	10.0–10.13
163	5.4	59.4–62.1	9.6–9.12	60.8–65.3	9.9–10.5	63.9–70.2	10.2–11.2
165	5.5	60.3–63.0	9.8–10.0	61.7–66.6	9.11–10.8	64.8–72.0	10.4–11.6
168	5.6	61.2–63.9	9.10–10.2	62.6–68.0	9.13–10.11	65.7–73.8	10.6–11.10
170	5.7	62.1–65.3	9.12–10.5	63.9–69.3	10.2–11.0	67.1–75.6	10.9–12.0
173	5.8	63.0–66.6	10.0–10.8	65.3–70.7	10.5–11.3	68.4–77.4	10.12–12.4
175	5.9	63.9–68.0	10.2–10.11	66.6–72.0	10.8–11.6	69.8–79.2	11.1–12.8
178	5.10	64.8–69.3	10.4–11.0	68.0–73.4	10.11–11.9	71.1–81.0	11.4–12.12
180	5.11	65.7–70.7	10.6–11.3	69.3–74.7	11.0–11.12	72.5–82.8	11.7–13.2
183	6.0	67.1–72.0	10.9–11.6	70.7–76.5	11.3–12.2	73.8–84.6	11.10–13.6
185	6.1	68.4–73.8	10.12–11.10	72.0–78.3	11.6–12.6	75.6–86.4	12.0–13.10
188	6.2	69.8–75.6	11.1–12.0	73.8–80.1	11.10–12.10	77.4–88.7	12.4–14.1
191	6.3	71.1–77.4	11.4–12.4	75.2–81.9	11.13–13.0	79.2–90.9	12.8–14.6
193	6.4	72.9–79.2	11.8–12.8	77.0–84.2	12.3–13.3	81.5–93.2	12.13–14.11

From 1983 Metropolitan Life Insurance Company height and weight tables, for men aged 25–59 in shoes and wearing indoor clothing.

Table A3.1(b) Height and weight chart for women

Height		Weight					
		Small frame		Medium frame		Large frame	
cm	ft. ins	kg	st. lb	kg	st. lb	kg	st. lb
147	4.10	45.9–50.5	7.4–7.13	49.1–54.5	7.11–8.9	53.1–59.0	8.6–9.5
150	4.11	46.4–50.9	7.5–8.1	50.0–55.4	7.13–8.12	54.0–60.3	8.8–9.8
152	5.0	46.8–51.8	7.6–8.3	50.9–56.7	8.1–9.0	54.9–61.7	8.10–9.11
155	5.1	47.7–53.1	7.8–8.6	51.8–58.1	8.3–9.3	56.3–63.0	8.13–10.0
158	5.2	48.6–54.5	7.10–8.9	53.1–59.4	8.6–9.6	57.6–64.4	9.2–10.3
160	5.3	50.0–55.8	7.13–8.12	54.5–60.8	8.9–9.9	59.0–66.2	9.5–10.7
163	5.4	51.3–57.2	8.2–9.1	55.8–62.1	8.12–9.12	60.3–68.0	9.8–10.11
165	5.5	52.7–58.5	8.5–9.4	57.2–63.5	9.1–10.1	61.7–69.8	9.11–11.1
168	5.6	54.0–59.9	8.8–9.7	58.5–64.8	9.4–10.4	63.0–71.6	10.0–11.5
170	5.7	55.4–61.2	8.11–9.10	59.9–66.2	9.7–10.7	64.4–73.4	10.3–11.9
173	5.8	56.7–62.6	9.0–9.13	61.2–67.5	9.10–10.10	65.7–75.2	10.6–11.13
175	5.9	58.1–63.9	9.3–10.2	62.6–68.9	9.13–10.13	67.1–76.5	10.9–12.2
178	5.10	59.4–65.3	9.5–10.5	63.9–70.2	10.2–11.2	68.4–77.9	10.12–12.5
180	5.11	60.8–66.6	9.8–10.8	65.3–71.6	10.5–11.5	69.8–79.2	11.1–12.8
183	6.0	62.1–68.0	9.11–10.11	66.6–72.9	10.8–11.8	71.1–80.6	11.4–12.11

From 1983 Metropolitan Life Insurance Company height and weight tables, for women aged 25–59 in shoes and wearing indoor clothing.

Table A3.2 Body mass index ready reckoner

	BMI	\multicolumn{10}{c}{Weight (kg) (to the nearest 1 kg)}									
Dangerously overweight	45	101	104	107	110	112	115	118	121	124	127
	44	99	102	104	107	110	113	115	118	121	124
	43	97	99	102	105	107	110	113	116	118	121
	42	95	97	100	102	105	108	110	113	116	119
	41	92	95	97	100	102	105	108	110	113	116
Seriously overweight	40	90	92	95	97	100	102	105	108	110	113
	39	88	90	93	95	97	100	102	105	108	110
	38	86	88	90	93	95	97	100	102	105	107
	37	83	86	88	90	92	95	97	100	102	104
	36	81	83	85	88	90	92	95	97	99	102
	35	79	81	83	85	87	90	92	94	96	99
	34	77	79	81	83	85	87	89	91	94	96
	33	74	76	78	80	82	85	87	89	91	93
	32	72	74	76	78	80	82	84	86	88	90
	31	70	72	74	75	77	79	81	83	85	88
Overweight	30	68	69	71	73	75	77	79	81	83	85
	29	65	67	69	71	72	74	76	78	80	82
	28	63	65	66	68	70	72	74	75	77	79
	27	61	62	64	66	67	69	71	73	74	76
	26	59	60	62	63	65	67	68	70	72	73
Acceptable	25	56	58	59	61	62	64	66	67	69	71
	24	54	55	57	58	60	61	63	65	66	68
	23	52	53	55	56	57	59	60	62	63	65
	22	50	51	52	54	55	56	58	59	61	62
	21	47	49	50	51	52	54	55	57	58	59
	20	45	46	47	49	50	51	53	54	55	56
Underweight	19	43	44	45	46	47	49	50	51	52	54
	18	41	42	43	44	45	46	47	48	50	51
	17	38	39	40	41	42	44	45	46	47	48
Height	m	1.50	1.52	1.54	1.56	1.58	1.60	1.62	1.64	1.66	1.68
	ft ins	4.11	5.0	5.0¾	5.1½	5.2¼	5.3	5.3¾	5.4½	5.5½	5.6

Table A3.2 (continued)

	BMI	Weight (kg) (to the nearest 1 kg)													
Dangerously Overweight	45	130	133	136	139	143	146	149	152	156	159	162	166	169	173
	44	127	130	133	136	139	143	146	149	152	156	159	162	166	169
	43	124	127	130	133	136	139	142	146	149	152	155	159	162	165
	42	121	124	127	130	133	136	139	142	145	148	152	155	158	161
	41	119	121	124	127	130	133	136	139	142	145	148	151	154	158
Seriously Overweight	40	116	118	121	124	127	130	133	135	138	141	144	148	151	154
	39	113	115	118	121	124	126	129	132	135	138	141	144	147	150
	38	110	112	115	118	120	123	126	129	132	134	137	140	143	146
	37	107	110	112	115	117	120	123	125	128	131	134	136	139	142
	36	104	107	109	112	114	117	119	122	125	127	130	133	136	138
	35	101	104	106	108	111	113	116	119	121	124	126	129	132	134
	34	98	101	103	105	108	110	113	115	118	120	123	125	128	131
	33	95	98	100	102	105	107	109	112	114	117	119	122	124	127
	32	93	95	97	99	101	104	106	108	111	113	116	118	120	123
	31	90	92	94	96	98	100	103	105	107	110	112	114	117	119
Overweight	30	87	89	91	93	95	97	99	102	104	106	108	111	113	115
	29	84	86	88	90	92	94	96	98	100	103	105	107	109	111
	28	81	83	85	87	89	91	93	95	97	99	101	103	105	108
	27	78	80	82	84	86	88	89	91	93	95	98	100	102	104
	26	75	77	79	81	82	84	86	88	90	92	94	96	98	100
Acceptable	25	72	74	76	77	79	81	83	85	87	88	90	92	94	96
	24	69	71	73	74	76	78	80	81	83	85	87	89	90	92
	23	67	68	70	71	73	75	76	78	80	81	83	85	87	88
	22	64	65	67	68	70	71	73	75	76	78	79	81	83	85
	21	61	62	64	65	67	68	70	71	73	74	76	77	79	81
	20	58	59	61	62	63	65	66	68	69	71	72	74	75	77
Underweight	19	55	56	58	59	60	62	63	64	66	67	69	70	72	73
	18	52	53	55	56	57	58	60	61	62	64	65	66	68	69
	17	49	50	52	53	54	55	56	58	59	60	61	63	64	65
Height	m	1.70	1.72	1.74	1.76	1.78	1.80	1.82	1.84	1.86	1.88	1.90	1.92	1.94	1.96
	ft ins	5.6¾	5.7¾	5.8½	5.9¼	5.10	5.10¾	5.11¾	6.0½	6.1¼	6.2	6.2¾	6.3¾	6.4½	6.5½

4 Diagnostic dilemmas

When the diagnosis is in doubt, or investigations contribute to rather than resolve the confusion, the following approach is recommended:
- Take a careful history again, paying attention to what the patient says
- Re-examine the patient, paying special attention to lymph nodes, external genitalia and rectal examination, because these areas are often overlooked on the initial examination
- List the investigations and results, in chronological order
- Seek advice if the way ahead remains unclear
- Do not order another test and hope that someone else sees the patient next time!

Index

Page numbers in *italic* refer to figures, those in **bold** refer to tables.